Preventive Cardiology in the Elderly

Guest Editors

MICHAEL W. RICH, MD
GEORGE A. MENSAH, MD

CLINICS IN GERIATRIC MEDICINE

www.geriatric.theclinics.com

November 2009 • Volume 25 • Number 4

SAUNDERS an imprint of ELSEVIER, Inc.

W.B. SAUNDERS COMPANY
A Division of Elsevier Inc.

1600 John F. Kennedy Blvd., Suite 1800. Philadelphia, Pennsylvania 19103-2899

http://www.theclinics.com

CLINICS IN GERIATRIC MEDICINE Volume 25, Number 4
November 2009 ISSN 0749–0690, ISBN-13: 978-1-4377-1386-2, ISBN-10: 1-4377-1386-6

Editor: Yonah Korngold

Clinics in Geriatric Medicine (ISSN 0749-0690) is published quarterly by Elsevier Inc., 360 Park Avenue South, New York, NY 10010-1710. Months of issue are February, May, August, and November. Business and Editorial Offices: 1600 John F. Kennedy Blvd., Suite 1800, Philadelphia, PA 191023-2899. Customer Service Office: 6277 Sea Harbor Drive, Orlando, FL 32887-4800. Periodicals postage paid at New York, NY, and additional mailing offices. Subscription prices is $208.00 per year (US individuals), $353.00 per year (US institutions), $271.00 per year (Canadian individuals), $440.00 per year (Canadian institutions), $288.00 per year (foreign individuals) and $440.00 per year (foreign institutions). Foreign air speed delivery is included in all *Clinics* subscription prices. All prices are subject to change without notice. POSTMASTER: Send address changes to *Clinics in Geriatric Medicine,* Elsevier Health Sciences Division, Subscription Customer Service, 3251 Riverport Lane, Maryland Heights, MO 63043. Telephone: 1-800-654-2452 (U.S. and Canada); 314-447-8871 (outside U.S. and Canada). Fax: 314-447-8029. E-mail: journalscustomerservice-usa@elsevier.com (for print support) or journalsonlinesupport-usa@elsevier.com (for online support).

Reprints. For copies of 100 or more, of articles in this publication, please contact the Commercial Reprints Department, Elsevier Inc., 360 Park Avenue South, New York, New York 10010-1710. Tel.: (212) 633-3812; Fax: (212) 462-1935, email: reprints@elsevier.com.

Clinics in Geriatric Medicine is covered in *MEDLINE/PubMed (Index Medicus), EMBASE/Excerpta Medica, Current Contents/Clinical Medicine (CC/CM),* and the *Cumulative Index to Nursing & Allied Health Literature.*

Printed and bound in the United States of America
Transferred to Digital Print 2011

Contributors

GUEST EDITORS

MICHAEL W. RICH, MD
Cardiovascular Division, Department of Medicine, Washington University School
of Medicine, St Louis, Missouri

GEORGE A. MENSAH, MD
Heart Health and Global Health Policy, Corporate Research and Development, PepsiCo,
Purchase, New York

AUTHORS

STEPHEN D. ANTON, PhD
Assistant Professor, Department of Aging and Geriatric Research, Institute on Aging,
Division of Biology of Aging, University of Florida, Gainesville, Florida

WILBERT S. ARONOW, MD, FACC, FAHA
Department of Medicine, Divisions of Cardiology, Geriatrics, and Pulmonary/Critical Care,
New York Medical College, Valhalla, New York

FARHAN ASLAM, MD
Department of Cardiology, Harvard Medical School, Brigham and Women's/Faulkner
Hospitals, Boston, Massachusetts

ROBERTO BERNABEI, MD
Professor, Department of Gerontology, Geriatrics and Physiatrics, Catholic University
of the Sacred Heart, Rome, Italy

CAROLINE S. BLAUM, MD, MS
Professor and Associate Division Chief, Department of Internal Medicine, Division of
Geriatric Medicine, University of Michigan, Ann Arbor, Michigan; Research Scientist, VA
Ann Arbor Healthcare System Geriatrics Research, Education and Clinical Center
(GRECC), Ann Arbor, Michigan

DAVID M. BUCHNER, MD, MPH
Professor, Department of Kinesiology and Community Health, University of Illinois at
Urbana-Champaign, Illinois

CHRISTY S. CARTER, PhD
Assistant Professor, Department of Aging and Geriatric Research, Institute on Aging,
Division of Biology of Aging, University of Florida, Gainesville, Florida

CHRISTINE T. CIGOLLE, MD, MPH
Lecturer, Department of Family Medicine, University of Michigan, Ann Arbor, Michigan;
Physician Scientist, VA Ann Arbor Healthcare System Geriatrics Research, Education and
Clinical Center (GRECC), Ann Arbor, Michigan

RICKI J. COLMAN, PhD
Associate Scientist, Wisconsin National Primate Research Center, University of Wisconsin, Madison, Wisconsin

CHRISTINA CRUZEN, DVM
Associate Research Animal Veterinarian, Wisconsin National Primate Research Center, University of Wisconsin, Madison, Wisconsin

GREGG C. FONAROW, MD, FACC
Professor of Cardiovascular Medicine, UCLA Division of Cardiology, David Geffen School of Medicine at UCLA, Ahmanson-UCLA Cardiomyopathy Center, Los Angeles, California

JoANNE FOODY, MD, FACC, FAHA
Harvard Medical School, Brigham and Women's/Faulkner Hospitals, Boston, Massachusetts

DANIEL E. FORMAN, MD
Cardiovascular Division, Brigham and Women's Hospital, Boston, Massachusetts; Geriatric Research, Education, and Clinical Center, VA Boston Healthcare System, Boston, Massachusetts

S. MICHAEL GHARACHOLOU, MD
Fellow, Department of Internal Medicine, Division of Cardiology, Duke University Medical Center, Durham, North Carolina; Department of Internal Medicine, Division of Geriatrics, Duke University Medical Center, Durham, North Carolina

JEFFREY B. HALTER, MD
Veterans Administration Health Center, Ann Arbor, Michigan; Associate Professor, Department of Internal Medicine, Associate Chief, Division of Geriatric Medicine, University of Michigan, Ann Arbor, Michigan

ATTIYA HAQUE, MD
Department of Cardiology, Harvard Medical School, Brigham and Women's/Faulkner Hospitals, Boston, Massachusetts

KAMYAR KALANTAR-ZADEH, MD, MPH, PhD
Associate Professor of Medicine, Division of Nephrology and Hypertension, Harbor-UCLA Medical Center, UCLA Schools of Medicine and Public Health, Torrance, California

PETER KRIEKARD, MD
Resident, Department of Internal Medicine, Duke University Medical Center, Durham, North Carolina

L. VERONICA LEE, MD, FACC
Yale University Hospital, New Haven, Connecticut

CHRISTIAAN LEEUWENBURGH, PhD
Professor, Department of Aging and Geriatric Research, Institute on Aging, Division of Biology of Aging, University of Florida, Gainesville, Florida

EMANUELE MARZETTI, MD, PhD
Lecturer, Department of Aging and Geriatric Research, Institute on Aging, Division of Biology of Aging, University of Florida, Gainesville, Florida; Department of Orthopaedics of Traumatology, Catholic University of the Sacred Heart, Rome, Italy

ANNE B. NEWMAN, MD, MPH
Professor of Epidemiology and Medicine, Director, Center for Aging and Population Health, Department of Epidemiology, Graduate School of Public Health, University of Pittsburgh, Pittsburgh, Pennsylvania

ANTIGONE OREOPOULOS, MSc
PhD Candidate, Department of Clinical Epidemiology, School of Public Health, University of Alberta, Edmonton, Alberta, Canada

JEREMY H. PERTMAN, MS
Department of Epidemiology, Harvard School of Public Health, Boston, Massachusetts

ERIC D. PETERSON, MD, MPH
Professor of Medicine, Department of Internal Medicine, Division of Cardiology, Duke Clinical Research Institute, Duke University, Durham, North Carolina

JACOB R. SATTELMAIR, MSc
Department of Epidemiology, Harvard School of Public Health, Boston, Massachusetts

ARYA M. SHARMA, MD, PhD
Professor of Medicine, Division of Endocrinology, Royal Alexandra Hospital, University of Alberta, Edmonton, Alberta, Canada

KERRY J. STEWART, EdD, FAHA, FAACVPR, FACSM, FSGC
Professor, Department of Medicine, Johns Hopkins University School of Medicine, Baltimore, Maryland; Director, Clinical and Research Exercise Physiology, Johns Hopkins Bayview Medical Center, Baltimore, Maryland

MARK A. WILLIAMS, PhD, FACSM, FAACVPR
Professor, Division of Cardiology, Department of Medicine, Creighton University School of Medicine, Omaha, Nebraska; Director, Cardiovascular Disease Prevention and Rehabilitation, Cardiac Center of Creighton University, Omaha, Nebraska

STEPHANIE E. WOHLGEMUTH, PhD
Lecturer, Department of Aging and Geriatric Research, Institute on Aging, University of Florida, Gainesville, Florida

ALI YAZDANYAR, DO
Post-doctoral Scholar, Center for Aging and Population Health, Department of Epidemiology, Graduate School of Public Health, University of Pittsburgh, Pittsburgh, Pennsylvania

Contents

> Cardiovascular disease (CVD) in older Americans imposes a huge burden
> in mortality, morbidity, disability, functional decline, and health care costs.
> In light of the projected growth of the population of older adults over the
> next several decades, the societal burden attributable to CVD will continue
> to rise. There is thus an enormous opportunity to foster successful aging
> and to increase functional life years through expanded efforts aimed at
> CVD prevention. This article provides an overview of the epidemiology of
> CVD in older adults, including an assessment of the impact of CVD on
> mortality, morbidity, and health care costs.

> Many elderly patients have hypertension, although it is more likely to go
> untreated in this population. Treatment goals are the same in elderly pa-
> tients as in younger patients, but elderly patients are more likely to have
> multiple comorbidities, which must be factored into treatment plans.
> This article highlights the unique challenges in treating this population.

> Older adults carry the highest risk for coronary artery disease and the
> highest burden of atherosclerosis. Although most clinical trials of choles-
> terol-lowering therapy have not specifically targeted older persons, growing
> evidence supports treatment of elevated low-density lipoprotein choles-
> terol levels in older patients, especially those at high risk for coronary
> events. The decision to treat a high or high-normal cholesterol level in an el-
> derly individual must be individualized based on chronologic and physio-
> logic age. This article summarizes current data on lipid-lowering therapy
> in older adults and the management of hyperlipidemia in elderly patients.

> Cardiovascular disease is the major cause of death as well as a leading
> cause of disability and impaired quality of life in older adults with diabetes.
> Therefore, preventing cardiovascular events in this population is an impor-
> tant goal of care. Available evidence supports the use of lipid-lowering

agents and treatment of hypertension as effective measures to reduce cardiovascular risk in older adults with diabetes. Glucose control, smoking cessation, weight control, regular physical activity, and a prudent diet are also recommended, although data supporting the efficacy of these interventions are limited. While reducing cardiovascular morbidity and mortality remains a primary objective of preventive cardiology in older adults with diabetes, the impact of these interventions on functional well-being, cognition, and other geriatric syndromes requires further study.

The prevalence of overweight and obesity in the elderly has become a growing concern. Recent evidence indicates that in the elderly, obesity is paradoxically associated with a lower, not higher, mortality risk. Although obesity in the general adult population is associated with higher mortality, this relationship is unclear for persons of advanced age and has lead to great controversy regarding the relationship between obesity and mortality in the elderly, the definition of obesity in the elderly, and the need for its treatment in this population. This article examines the evidence on these controversial issues, explores potential explanations for these findings, discusses the clinical implications, and provides recommendations for further research in this area.

There is strong evidence that regular physical activity reduces risk of cardiovascular disease. Building on the evidence review for the *2008 Physical Activity Guidelines for Americans*, this article summarizes the recommended amounts and types of physical activity for the primary prevention of cardiovascular disease in older adults. Key guidelines are largely based on current understanding of the dose-response relationship between amount of physical activity and risk of chronic disease. In part due to the preventive effects on cardiovascular disease, physical activity has beneficial effects on functional limitations and health-related quality of life in older adults. Gaps in research on physical activity and cardiovascular health are discussed, with an emphasis on the need for research on how sedentary time affects risk of cardiovascular disease and other chronic illnesses.

Aging is associated with a cascade of morphologic and physiologic changes that naturally predispose older adults to progressive weakening, functional decline, morbidity, disability, poor quality of life, and increased mortality. Physical activity moderates such insidious aging patterns and is a vital preventive and therapeutic strategy to optimize health throughout the aging process. Regular exercise provides many physiologic benefits, reduces risk of disease outcomes, and triggers important psychological gains. Advanced age presents distinctive obstacles to maintaining a physically active lifestyle. Individualized exercise strategies and regimens make it possible, however, for every elderly adult to benefit from physical activity.

In older persons with and without cardiovascular disease, muscular strength and endurance contribute to functional independence and quality of life, while reducing disability. Aging skeletal muscle responds to progressive overload through resistance training. In men and women, strength improves through neuromuscular adaptation, muscle fiber hypertrophy, and increased muscle oxidative capacity. The increase in muscle oxidative capacity is due to the combination of strength development and aerobic exercise often used in resistance-type circuit training. Even in the oldest persons, resistance training significantly increases strength and gait velocity, improves balance and coordination, extends walking endurance, and enhances stair-climbing power. This article reviews the physiologic response to resistance training in older adults and discusses the impact of resistance exercise training on cardiovascular risk factors.

Evidence from animal models and preliminary studies in humans indicates that calorie restriction (CR) delays cardiac aging and can prevent cardiovascular disease. These effects are mediated by a wide spectrum of biochemical and cellular adaptations, including redox homeostasis, mitochondrial function, inflammation, apoptosis, and autophagy. Despite the beneficial effects of CR, its large-scale implementation is challenged by applicability issues as well as health concerns. However, preclinical studies indicate that specific compounds, such as resveratrol, may mimic many of the effects of CR, thus potentially obviating the need for drastic food intake reductions. Results from ongoing clinical trials will reveal whether the intriguing alternative of CR mimetics represents a safe and effective strategy to promote cardiovascular health and delay cardiac aging in humans.

Approximately one in three Americans has some form of cardiovascular disease (CVD), accounting for one of every 2.8 deaths in the United States in 2004. Two of the major risk factors for CVD are advancing age and obesity. An intervention able to positively impact both aging and obesity, such as caloric restriction (CR), may prove extremely useful in the fight against CVD. CR is the only environmental or lifestyle intervention that repeatedly has been shown to increase maximum life span and to retard aging in laboratory rodents. This article reviews evidence that CR in nonhuman primates and people has a positive effect on risk factors for CVD.

This article reviews cardiovascular disease (CVD) prevention in older patients, highlighting results from recent clinical studies related to primary and secondary prevention. Many of these studies demonstrated greater absolute reductions in major cardiovascular events among older, higher-risk populations compared with younger patients. Guideline recommendations for CVD risk factor modification are also reviewed with emphasis on issues pertaining to the older adult population.

THE CLINICS ARE NOW AVAILABLE ONLINE!

Access your subscription at:
www.theclinics.com

Preface

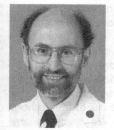 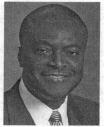

Michael W. Rich, MD   George A. Mensah, MD
Guest Editors

Despite the marked decline in age-adjusted cardiovascular mortality rates over the past 50 years, cardiovascular disease (CVD) remains the leading cause of death in the United States and in other developed countries. Moreover, the burden of CVD is most pronounced in the older adult population. Data from the National Health and Nutrition Examination Survey indicate that the prevalence of CVD exceeds 70% in men and women over 60 years of age, and that it tops 80% among persons 80 years of age or older. In addition, more than 80% of deaths attributable to CVD occur in persons 65 years of age or older and over 50% occur in people age 75 or older. In light of these statistics and the progressive aging of the population, it is evident that the potential benefits of primary and secondary prevention of CVD are perhaps greatest in older adults. The objective of this issue of the *Clinics* is to provide a concise overview of current strategies for CVD prevention in our burgeoning elderly population. Articles in this issue were derived in part from a symposium on preventive cardiology in the elderly held on November 8, 2008, in New Orleans, Louisiana, cosponsored by the Society of Geriatric Cardiology and the Society for Preventive Cardiology, and supported by a grant from the National Institute on Aging.

Drs Yazdanyar and Newman provide an overview of the burden of CVD in older adults, highlighting the imperative to focus on prevention in this population. The next three articles address traditional risk factors for CVD in older individuals, including reviews of hypertension by Dr Aronow, hyperlipidemia by Drs Aslam, Haque, Lee, and Foody, and diabetes mellitus by Drs Cigolle, Blaum, and Halter. Dr Oreopoulos and colleagues then discuss the somewhat controversial issue of obesity and weight management in the elderly. The next three articles address the potential role of exercise in CVD prevention. Drs Sattelmair, Pertman, and Forman provide an overview of currently available evidence in support of regular aerobic exercise as a means for reducing CVD risk in older patients, while Dr Buchner's article provides a concise discussion of guidelines for physical activity in older adults and the impact of exercise in the context of specific cardiovascular conditions. Drs Williams and Stewart then review the evolving role of resistance training and the impact of this exercise modality on cardiovascular risk factors and outcomes. The next two articles examine the

Clin Geriatr Med 25 (2009) xiii–xiv
doi:10.1016/j.cger.2009.08.003
0749-0690/09/$ – see front matter © 2009 Elsevier Inc. All rights reserved.

potential utility of calorie restriction for reducing CVD. Dr Marzetti and colleagues discuss the scientific basis for calorie restriction and the effects of calorie restriction in small laboratory animals. This is followed by a review of currently available data on calorie restriction in nonhuman primates and humans by Drs Cruzen and Colman. Finally, Drs Kriekard, Gharacholou, and Peterson provide a broad overview of current strategies for reducing CVD risk in older adults.

It is hoped that the information provided in this volume will be helpful to clinicians in managing their older patients with cardiovascular risk factors or prevalent CVD. It is also hoped that the issue will serve to stimulate new research initiatives designed to provide novel insights into the potential role of preventive measures for reducing the burden of CVD in older adults. It has been a pleasure working with all of the authors of this issue, as well as with the editorial staff of the *Clinics*. We welcome any comments or feedback that you, the readers, may have.

Michael W. Rich, MD
Cardiovascular Division
Department of Medicine
Washington University School of Medicine
660 South Euclid Avenue, Box 8086
St Louis, MO 63110, USA

George A. Mensah, MD
Heart Health and Global Health Policy
Corporate Research and Development
PepsiCo
700 Anderson Hill Road, Building 6-2
Purchase, NY 10577, USA

E-mail addresses:
mrich@wustl.edu (M.W. Rich)
george.mensah@pepsico.com (G.A. Mensah)

The Burden of Cardiovascular Disease in the Elderly: Morbidity, Mortality, and Costs

Ali Yazdanyar, DO[a], Anne B. Newman, MD, MPH[b],*

KEYWORDS

- Cardiovascular disease • Subclinical disease • Aging
- Morbidity • Mortality • Health care costs • Epidemiology

The age structure of the population in the United States is expected to change dramatically over the next several decades with a nearly two-fold increase in the size of the population aged 65 years or older by 2050.[1] While adults aged 65 to 84 years accounted for 10.9% of the total population in the year 2000, this proportion is estimated to increase to approximately 16% by 2050. Moreover, it is anticipated that individuals aged 85 years or older will account for 4.3% of the population in the 2050, representing a more than two-fold increase from 2010.[1] In absolute terms, and considering the projected growth of the overall population, the number of adults aged 85 years or older is estimated to increase from approximately 5.8 million in 2010 to 19 million by 2050, a 228% increase.[1] These projected changes in the United States' age distribution translate into a significant burden in morbidity, mortality, and costs related to cardiovascular diseases (CVD).

The age-related increase in CVD morbidity and mortality can be appreciated by consideration of the population-based, disease-specific incidence and prevalence rates of CVD, including coronary heart disease (CHD), peripheral arterial disease (PAD), heart failure (HF), valvular heart disease, and stroke. Similarly insightful is a review of the associations between age and several measures of subclinical CVD, such as coronary artery calcification and the ankle brachial index (ABI). The impact of CVD on successful aging versus frailty, hospitalization rates, and cost will provide an important additional perspective.

[a] Center for Aging and Population Health, Department of Epidemiology, Graduate School of Public Health, University of Pittsburgh, Room 518, 130 North Bellefield Avenue, Pittsburgh, PA 15213, USA
[b] Center for Aging and Population Health, Department of Epidemiology, Graduate School of Public Health, University of Pittsburgh, Room 532, 130 North Bellefield Avenue, Pittsburgh, PA 15213, USA
* Corresponding author.
E-mail address: newmana@edc.pitt.edu (A.B. Newman).

Clin Geriatr Med 25 (2009) 563–577
doi:10.1016/j.cger.2009.07.007   geriatric.theclinics.com

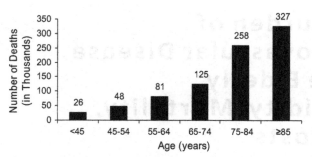

Fig. 1. Number of Deaths (in thousands) caused by Cardiovascular Diseases by Age in 2005. (*Data from* American Heart Association. Heart Disease and Stroke Statistics-2009 Update. Dallas, Texas: American Heart Association; 2009.)

Data presented in this article are derived primarily from population-based epidemiologic studies of community-dwelling adults in the United States, including those focusing on older adults, such as the Cardiovascular Health Study (CHS).[2]

MORBIDITY AND MORTALITY
Cardiovascular Disease

In 2005 CVD was the underlying cause of death in 864,480 of the approximately 2.5 million total deaths in the United States, and adults aged 65 years or older accounted for 82% of all deaths attributable to CVD (**Fig. 1**). In morbidity, an estimated 80 million Americans have at least one form of CVD, and nearly one half of these are aged 60 years or older,[3] reflecting a marked increase in the incidence and prevalence of CVD with advancing age. The prevalence of CVD, including hypertension, CHD, HF, and stroke increases from approximately 40% in men and women aged 40 to 59 years, to 70% to 75% in persons aged 60 to 79 years, and to 79% to 86% among those aged

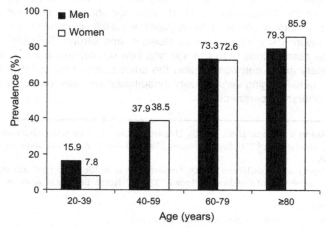

Fig. 2. Prevalence of cardiovascular disease in adults aged 20 years and older by age and sex. Cardiovascular disease includes coronary heart disease, heart failure, stroke, and hypertension.

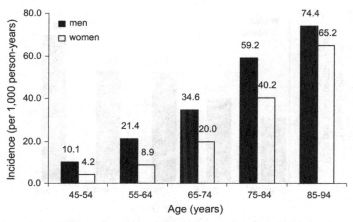

Fig. 3. Incidence of Cardiovascular disease in adults aged 45 years and older by age and sex. Cardiovascular disease includes coronary heart disease, heart failure, and stroke or intracerebral hemorrhage. (*Data from* American Heart Association. Heart Disease and Stroke Statistics-2009 Update. Dallas, Texas: American Heart Association; 2009.)

80 years or older (**Fig. 2**).[3] Similarly, the incidence of CVD, including CHD, HF, and stroke or intracerebral hemorrhage increases from 4 to 10 per 1000 person-years in adults aged 45 to 54 years to 65 to 75 per 1000 person-years in adults aged 85 to 94 years (**Fig. 3**).[3,4]

Coronary Heart Disease

CHD accounts for more than half of all CVD-related deaths. In 2005, CHD was the primary cause of 445,687 deaths, of which nearly 82% were in individuals aged 65 years or older.[3] The prevalence of CHD increases markedly with age in men and women (**Fig. 4**).[3] Similarly, the incidence of CHD increases with age among older adults, irrespective of race or gender (**Figs. 5** and **6**).[5] Even at the age of 70 years, the lifetime risk of a first CHD event is 34.9% in men and 24.2% in women.[6]

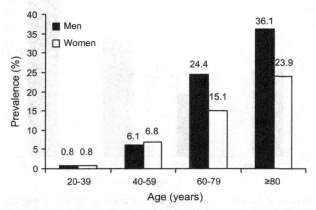

Fig. 4. Prevalence of coronary heart disease in adults aged 20 years and older by age and sex. (*Data from* American Heart Association. Heart Disease and Stroke Statistics-2009 Update. Dallas, Texas: American Heart Association; 2009.)

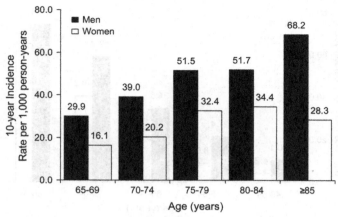

Fig. 5. 10-Year Incidence Rate for Coronary Heart Disease in Caucasians by Age and Gender in the Cardiovascular Health Study. (*Data from* Arnold AM, Psaty BM, Kuller LH, et al. Incidence of cardiovascular disease in older Americans: the cardiovascular health study. J Am Geriatr Soc 2005;53(2):211–8; with permission.)

Myocardial Infarction

Prevalence

The prevalence of myocardial infarction (MI) increases with age, and there is nearly a sevenfold higher prevalence among individuals aged 65 to74 years relative to those aged 35 to 44 years.[7] The pattern of age-related increase in MI prevalence extends into the oldest age groups, and the magnitude is greater in women. In the CHS, MI prevalence increased from 9.7% in women aged 65 to 69 years to nearly 18% in those aged 85 years or older, representing an increase of nearly twofold.[8]

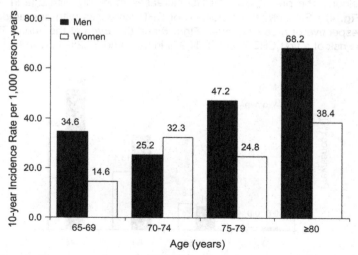

Fig. 6. 10-Year Incidence Rate for Coronary Heart Disease in African Americans by Age and Gender in the Cardiovascular Health Study. (*Data from* Arnold AM, Psaty BM, Kuller LH, et al. Incidence of cardiovascular disease in older Americans: the cardiovascular health study. J Am Geriatr Soc 2005;53(2):211–8; with permission.)

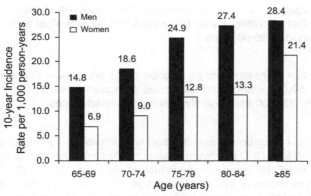

Fig. 7. 10-Year Incidence Rate for Myocardial Infarction in Caucasians by Age and Gender in the Cardiovascular Health Study. (*Data from* Arnold AM, Psaty BM, Kuller LH, et al. Incidence of cardiovascular disease in older Americans: the cardiovascular health study. J Am Geriatr Soc 2005;53(2):211–8; with permission.)

Incidence

Nearly 0.5 million persons aged 75 years or older are diagnosed with an MI each year, accounting for more than one third of all MI in the United States. Relative to individuals aged 35 to 44 years, men and women aged 65 to 74 years have an approximately tenfold greater MI incidence rate. This represents an increase from approximately 1.0 to nearly 10 per 1000 person-years in men and from 0.3 to 0.7 to 5.1 to 7.2 per 1000 person-years in women.[3] Data from the CHS indicate that the age-related increase in MI incidence continues into the oldest age groups, with twofold to threefold increases in persons aged 80 years or older compared with those aged 65 to 69 years. (**Figs. 7** and **8**).[5]

Prognosis

MI in the elderly is associated with poor short- and long-term prognosis in morbidity and mortality.[3,9] The proportion of patients aged 70 years or older with recurrent MI, stroke, or HF within 5 years following a first MI is one and a half to three times greater

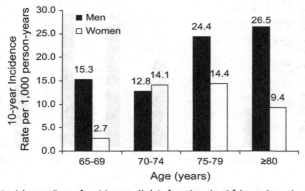

Fig. 8. 10-Year Incidence Rate for Myocardial Infarction in African Americans by Age and Gender in the Cardiovascular Health Study. (*Data from* Arnold AM, Psaty BM, Kuller LH, et al. Incidence of cardiovascular disease in older Americans: the cardiovascular health study. J Am Geriatr Soc 2005;53(2):211–8; with permission.)

than in those aged 40 to 69 years. Likewise, the proportion of individuals aged 70 years or older that die within 1 year following a first MI is twofold to threefold higher than in those aged 40 to 69 years.[3]

Heart failure
In 2005, HF, which is predominantly a disorder of the elderly, was the primary cause of approximately 59,000 deaths and was listed as a primary or contributory cause of death on nearly 300,000 death certificates in the United States.[3,10]

Prevalence
The aging of the population in combination with improved survival in patients who have CVD, particularly CHD and hypertension, has led to an increase in the prevalence and incidence of HF. HF is uncommon in individuals aged 20 to 39 (0.1%–0.2%), but the prevalence increases progressively with age: 5% to 10% in persons aged 60 to 79 years and 12% to 14% in those aged 80 years or older.[3] In the CHS, the prevalence of HF increased from 12% in men and 6% in women aged 65 to 69 years to 18% in men and 14% in women aged 85 years or older.[8]

Incidence
Older adults without HF have an approximately one in five lifetime risk for developing HF.[11] At 80 years of age, men without HF have a 20.2% risk for developing HF, which is close to the 21.0% lifetime risk for 40-year-old men. However, relative to younger adults, the short-term risk of HF is much greater in the elderly. For example, the 5-year risk of incident HF for an 80-year-old person is approximately 8%, whereas the risk for a 40 year old is only 0.2% (ie, a 40-fold difference).

In the CHS, the 10-year incidence of HF increased by up to sixfold across age strata,[5] with similar increases in men and women and in Caucasians and African Americans (**Figs. 9** and **10**). In Caucasians and African Americans, men had a higher 10-year incidence of HF than women. While the overall incidence rate of HF was higher in Caucasian men than in African American men, the reverse was true in women.

Stroke
Stroke is the third leading cause of death and a leading cause of long-term disability in the United States. While the prevalence of stroke is below 3% in adults aged 20 to 59

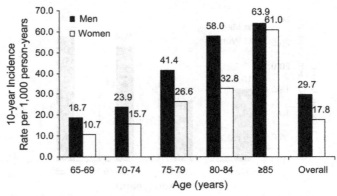

Fig. 9. 10-Year Incidence Rate for Congestive Heart Failure in Caucasians by Age and Gender in the Cardiovascular Health Study. (*Data from* Arnold AM, Psaty BM, Kuller LH, et al. Incidence of cardiovascular disease in older Americans: the cardiovascular health study. J Am Geriatr Soc 2005;53(2):211–8; with permission.)

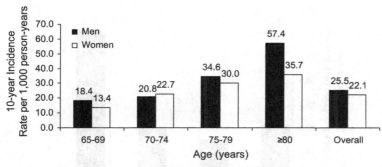

Fig. 10. 10-Year Incidence Rate for Congestive Heart Failure in African Americans by Age and Gender in the Cardiovascular Health Study. (*Data from* Arnold AM, Psaty BM, Kuller LH, et al. Incidence of cardiovascular disease in older Americans: the cardiovascular health study. J Am Geriatr Soc 2005;53(2):211–8; with permission.)

years, it increases to approximately 8% by 60 to 79 years, and reaches 13% to 17% among persons aged 80 years or older.[3]

The overall 10-year incidence of stroke in the CHS ranged from 13.7 to 14.7 per 1000 person-years.[5] Notably, after 75 years of age, the 10-year incidence of stroke tended to be higher in women than in men. Stroke incidence rates also increased twofold to fivefold across age groups (**Figs. 11 and 12**).[5]

Peripheral arterial disease
PAD is a significant predictor of cardiovascular and overall mortality. In addition, PAD is associated with limitations in physical function and with reduced health-related quality of life.[12,13] PAD, diagnosed by an ABI less than 0.9, was present in 12.4% of 5084 CHS participants.[14] In the CHS, the prevalence of an ABI less than 0.9 among

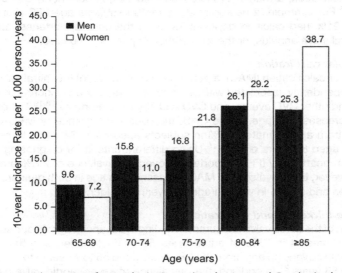

Fig. 11. 10-Year Incidence Rate for Stroke in Caucasians by Age and Gender in the Cardiovascular Health Study. (*Data from* Arnold AM, Psaty BM, Kuller LH, et al. Incidence of cardiovascular disease in older Americans: the cardiovascular health study. J Am Geriatr Soc 2005;53(2):211–8; with permission.)

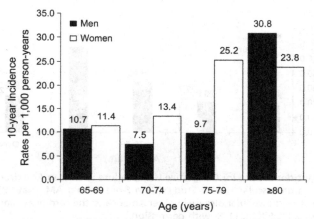

Fig. 12. 10-Year Incidence Rate for Stroke in African Americans by Age and Gender in the Cardiovascular Health Study. (*Data from* Arnold AM, Psaty BM, Kuller LH, et al. Incidence of cardiovascular disease in older Americans: the cardiovascular health study. J Am Geriatr Soc 2005;53(2):211–8; with permission.)

men without clinical CVD increased almost threefold from 65 to 69 years old to 85 years or older, reaching approximately 30% in the latter age group. In women, the increase in prevalence of PAD with age was even more striking, with nearly 40% of women aged 85 or older having an abnormal ABI, representing an eightfold increase relative to the 65- to 69-year age group.

Valvular Heart Disease

Cardiac calcification
Cardiac calcification, a marker of increased CVD risk, is commonly detected in the elderly.[15,16] For example, a necropsy study of 490 subjects aged 80 years or older found that 91% had calcified deposits involving the coronary arteries, aortic valve cusps, mitral valve annulus, or the left ventricular papillary muscles.[17]

Mitral annular calcification
Mitral annular calcification (MAC), a degenerative condition of the mitral valve support ring, is independently associated with one and one half to twofold increases in the risk of stroke and other CVD events, and CVD and all-cause mortality.[18,19] The prevalence of MAC increases with age. In the CHS, the overall prevalence of MAC was 42%, increasing from approximately 35% in subjects aged 65 to 74 years to nearly 60% in subjects aged 85 years or over.[15] Using different criteria for diagnosing MAC, the Framingham heart study (FHS) reported an overall prevalence of 2.8% among 5694 adults. However, the prevalence of MAC increased with age in both genders, reaching 6.0% in men and 22.4% in women aged 80 years or older.[20]

Aortic valve thickening and calcification
Calcification of the aortic valve is a common finding in advanced age. In one study, calcification was present in 53% of adults aged 55 years or older, and the proportion increased with advancing age, from 28% in adults aged 55 to 71 years to 75% in adults aged 85 to 86 years.[21] In addition, the prevalence of severe aortic valve calcification increased from 7% in persons aged 55 to 71 years to 19% in persons aged 85 to 86 years.

Aortic valve sclerosis, defined as increased echogenicity and leaflet thickness without restriction of leaflet motion, is associated with an approximately 50% increase in the risk of CVD death and incident MI.[22] Aortic valve sclerosis was present in 26% of CHS participants, increasing from 20% in subjects aged 65 to 74 years, to 35% in subjects aged 75 to 84 years, and to 48% in those aged 85 years or older.[23]

Aortic stenosis

In 2005, diseases of the heart valves accounted for 93,000 hospital discharges and nearly 21,000 deaths, of which approximately 13,000 were caused by aortic valve disease.[3] In the CHS, the prevalence of aortic stenosis (AS), defined as an increased systolic velocity across the aortic valve ($\geq$2.5 m/s by Doppler echocardiography), increased from 1.3% in participants aged 65 to 74 years, to 2.4% in those aged 75 to 84, and to 4% among those aged 85 years or older.[23]

The Helsinki Ageing Study reported the prevalence of moderate or severe AS among 197 participants aged 75 to 76 years, 155 participants aged 80 to 81 years, and 124 participants aged 85 to 86 years.[21] Moderate and severe AS were defined as calculated aortic valve areas less than or equal to 1.2 cm^2 and less than or equal to 0.8 cm^2, respectively. The overall prevalence rates of moderate and severe AS were 4.8% and 2.9%. The prevalence of at least moderate AS increased from 2.5% in subjects aged 75 to 76 years, to 3.9% in subjects aged 80 to 81 years, and to 8.1% in subjects aged 85 to 86 years. Prevalence rates for severe AS for these age categories were 0.5%, 2.6%, and 5.6%, respectively.

Valvular regurgitation

In the FHS, the prevalence of valvular regurgitation involving the mitral, tricuspid, and aortic valves was determined in participants aged 26 to 83 years using Doppler echocardiography.[24] In men, the prevalence of at least mild severity mitral regurgitation increased more than fourfold from 8.9% in subjects aged 26 to 39 years to 39.3% in those aged 70 to 83 years. The prevalence of at least mild tricuspid regurgitation increased from 13.0% in participants aged 26 to 39 years to 27.3% in those aged 70 to 83 years. Similarly, the prevalence of aortic valve regurgitation increased from 0% in subjects aged 26 to 39 years to 14.4% in subjects aged 70 to 83 years. In women, the prevalence of at least mild mitral, tricuspid, and aortic valve regurgitation in those aged 26 to 39 years was 9.7%, 14.4%, and 0%, respectively. By 70 to 83 years of age, prevalence rates increased to 23.6%, 29.5%, and 16.9%, respectively. The age-related increase in prevalence of valvular heart disease has also been confirmed by a pooled analysis of echocardiographic data from 11,911 participants in three epidemiologic studies representing various age groups, including the Coronary Artery Risk Development in Young Adults study, Atherosclerosis Risk in Communities study, and the CHS.[25]

In contrast to most other forms of valvular heart disease, the prevalence of mitral valve prolapse (MVP) has not been observed to vary significantly with age.[26] Among 3491 FHS participants with a mean age of 54.7 years (range: 26–84 years), the overall prevalence of MVP was 2.4%. MVP prevalence rates were similar across age decades from 30 to 80 years.

Electrocardiographic Abnormalities and Arrhythmias

Resting electrocardiogram

Abnormalities on the resting electrocardiogram (ECG) are quite common in older adults. Evaluation of ECG from 5150 CHS participants revealed that the overall prevalence of any ECG abnormality was 28.7%.[27] Prevalence rates of specific ECG abnormalities were 8.7% for ventricular conduction defects, 5.3% for first-degree atrioventricular block, 3.2% for atrial fibrillation (AF), 6.3% for isolated major ST-T wave abnormalities, 4.2% for left ventricular hypertrophy, and 5.2% for major Q/QS waves.

The prevalence of ECG abnormalities in men and women with known coronary artery disease (CAD) and hypertension (HTN) was 44.5% and 31.3%, respectively. In comparison, the prevalence of ECG abnormalities in men and women free of CAD and HTN was lower at 25.0% and 14.3%. In men free of CAD and HTN, the prevalence of ECG abnormalities increased from 16.0% in those aged 65 to 69 years, to 27.5% in those aged 75 to 79 years, and 45.9% in those aged 85 years or older. Likewise, in women free of CAD and HTN, prevalence of ECG abnormalities increased from 10.5% in those aged 65 to 69 years, to 20.2% in those aged 75 to 79 years, and 31.6% in those aged 85 years or older.

Ambulatory Electrocardiogram

Twenty-four hour ambulatory electrocardiography was performed in 1372 CHS participants and revealed that supraventricular ectopic beats and minor supraventricular arrhythmias were extremely common, occurring in approximately 97% of older adults.[28] Similarly, ventricular ectopic activity was present in 82% of the CHS population. Frequent ectopic beats, defined as greater than or equal to 15 beats per hour, were recorded in nearly half of men and women and were more commonly of supraventricular origin. Supraventricular arrhythmias were observed in 57.1% and 55.5% of men and women, respectively. There was an age-related increase in the prevalence of supraventricular arrhythmias, such that by 80 years old or older more than three quarters of subjects manifested supraventricular arrhythmias. Supraventricular tachycardia (SVT) of at least three beats was seen in 47.7% of men and 49.9% women. Ventricular arrhythmias were observed in 28.5% of men and 15.6% of women. Prevalence rates for ventricular tachycardia, defined as greater than or equal to three consecutive complexes, were 13% and 4.3% in men and women, respectively. Conversely, serious arrhythmias, such as sustained ventricular tachycardia ($\geq$15 complexes) and complete atrioventricular block, were rarely detected ($\leq$0.5%) in CHS participants.

Atrial Fibrillation

Prevalence

In 2005, AF was estimated to affect 2.2 million Americans, but it is projected that by 2050 the number of individuals with AF will exceed 10 million, primarily because of population aging.[3,29] In the CHS, the overall prevalence rates of AF in men and women were 6.2% and 4.8%, respectively.[30] The prevalence of AF varied by CVD status such that the prevalence in women with clinical CVD was 8.7%, compared with 4.5% in those with subclinical CVD, and 1.1% in women without evidence for CVD. The prevalence of AF in men was 9.4% in those with clinical CVD, 4.7% in those with subclinical CVD, and 2.7% in those without CVD. Regardless of CVD status, the overall prevalence of AF increased with age, from 5.9% in men and 2.8% in women aged 65 to 69 years, to 8.0% in men and 6.7% in women aged 80 years or older.

Incidence

The lifetime risk for AF in persons without HF or MI is approximately 15% at 40 years of age and also at 80 years of age.[31] Overall incidence rates of AF in the CHS men and women were 26.4 and 14.1 per 1000 person-years, respectively.[32] There is an age-associated increase in the incidence of AF in both genders, such that the incidence increases from 12.3 per 1000 person-years in men aged 65 to 69 years to 58.7 per 1000 person-years by 80 years old or older. Similarly, the incidence in women increases from 10.9 per 1000 person-years in the 65- to 69-year age group to 25.1 per 1000 person-years in women aged 80 years or older.

FRAILTY AND SUCCESSFUL AGING

CVD is the second leading cause of disability among older adults (after arthritis), and it is an important cause of a decline in self-reported health. Certain features of aging are in part a reflection of not only clinical but also subclinical atherosclerotic burden. As with clinical CVD, the burden of subclinical CVD, evidenced by low ABI or high coronary artery calcium score, increases progressively with age in men and women.[33–36]

Data from the CHS also implicate CVD, clinical and subclinical, as contributing to dementia and functional decline, manifested by loss of independence and the ability to perform routine activities of daily living. Further, there is a growing body of evidence linking CVD with frailty, a clinical syndrome associated with marked loss of physiologic reserve and an increased risk for disability, institutionalization, and death.[37] In CHS, for example, compared to people 65 years old or older with a normal ABI (ie, ≥ 0.9), those with an ABI less than 0.8 had more than a threefold increased risk of frailty.[37] Viewed another way, the presence of subclinical CVD among participants in CHS was associated with a loss of approximately 6.5 years of successful life (ie, with good health and function) in women and 5.6 years in men.[38]

MORTALITY

In the United States, CVD accounts for more deaths than any other major cause, and CHD and stroke account for approximately two thirds of CVD deaths.[3] The remaining CVD deaths are caused by HF (7%), high blood pressure (7%), diseases of the arteries (4%), and miscellaneous causes (14%).[3] As noted earlier, in 2005 approximately 80% of the 864,000 CVD deaths occurred in individuals aged 65 years or older and nearly 40% occurred in persons aged 85 years or older.[3] Furthermore, mortality rates from CHD, HF, and stroke are nearly twofold higher in the 75- to 84-year age group compared to the 65- to 74-year age group.[7]

In 2004, 48% of all deaths in Americans aged 85 years or older were ascribed to CVD, compared with only 20% in those aged 35 to 44 years.[7] Among women, more than 200,000 of the 454,613 total CVD deaths occurred in those aged 85 years and older age. In men, approximately 100,000 of the 409,867 total CVD deaths were in those aged 85 years and older.[3] Thus, CVD exacts an exceptionally high toll in the very elderly, particularly among women.

HOSPITALIZATIONS

CVD accounted for 6.2 million hospital discharges in 2006, more than any other disease category.[3] Approximately 75% of admissions for HF occur in people aged 65 years or older, with more than half occurring in people aged 75 years or older. Persons over 65 years old also account for more than 60% of admissions for acute MI and 75% of admissions for heart rhythm disorders. Likewise, in 2006, persons aged 65 years or older accounted for more than half of hospital discharges listing a major cardiac-related procedure as the principal procedure for the hospitalization. More specifically, persons aged 65 years or older accounted for 85% of pacemaker insertions, 61% of implantable defibrillators, 53% of coronary bypass operations, 51% of percutaneous coronary interventions, 60% of cardiac valve procedures, and 75% of endarterectomies.[39]

COSTS

In 2009, the cost of CVD and stroke, including direct and indirect costs, is expected to exceed $475 billion (**Fig. 13**), making CVD the most expensive disease category in the

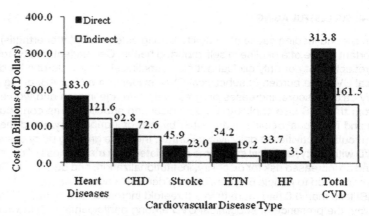

Fig. 13. Estimated Direct and Indirect Costs in Billions of Dollars of Cardiovascular Disease and Stroke. Heart Disease category includes coronary heart disease, heart failure, stroke, and part of hypertensive disease, cardiac dysrhythmias, rheumatic heart disease, cardiomyopathy, pulmonary heart disease, and other or ill-defined heart disease. (*Data from* American Heart Association. Heart Disease and Stroke Statistics-2009 Update. Dallas, Texas: American Heart Association; 2009.)

United States.[3] Direct costs, including hospital, nursing home, professional fees, drugs, and other costs, will total more than $313 billion. Indirect costs, including costs arising from disability and loss of productivity, will approach $161.5 billion. CHD accounts for the largest proportion of the total cost burden at approximately $165.4 billion, followed by hypertensive disease at $73.4 billion, stroke at $68.9 billion, and HF at $37.2 billion.

In light of the high prevalence rates and substantial morbidity associated with CVD among older adults, it is not surprising that the costs attributable to CVD in the elderly are extremely high. Most of the total expenditures for circulatory diseases, nearly three quarters, are for persons aged 65 years or older.[40] In addition, approximately one quarter of all personal health care expenditures are for diseases of the circulatory system, and this proportion increases with age such that by 85 years old circulatory diseases account for about one third of all personal health care expenses.[40] Moreover, with the growth in size of the older adult population in the United States, it has been projected that expenditures for the treatment of heart disease will increase 46% by 2025 relative to 1999.[41]

SUMMARY

CVD in older Americans imposes a huge burden in mortality, morbidity, disability, functional decline, and health care costs. Thus, there is an enormous opportunity to foster successful aging and to increase functional life years through expanded efforts aimed at CVD prevention. It follows that active life expectancy, rather than survival alone, should be included as a pivotal outcome in clinical trials involving older adults.

REFERENCES

1. U.S. Census Bureau. U.S. population projections: 2010 to 2050. Washington, DC: U.S. Department of Commerce; 2008. Available at: http://www.census.gov/population/www/projections/summarytables.html. Accessed April 15, 2009.

2. Fried LP, Borhani NO, Enright P, et al. The Cardiovascular Health Study: design and rationale. Ann Epidemiol 1991;1(3):263–76.
3. Lloyd-Jones D, Adams R, Carnethon M, et al. Heart disease and stroke statistics–2009 update: a report from the American Heart Association Statistics Committee and Stroke Statistics Subcommittee. Circulation 2009;119(3):e21–181.
4. National Institute of Health, National Heart, Lung, and Blood Institute. Incidence and prevalence: 2006 chart book on cardiovascular and lung diseases. Bethesda (MD): National Heart, Lung, and Blood Institute; 2006. Available at: http://www.nhlbi.nih.gov/rsources/docs/06a_ip_chtbk.pdf. Accessed March 9, 2009.
5. Arnold AM, Psaty BM, Kuller LH, et al. Incidence of cardiovascular disease in older Americans: the cardiovascular health study. J Am Geriatr Soc 2005;53(2):211–8.
6. Lloyd-Jones DM, Larson MG, Beiser A, et al. Lifetime risk of developing coronary heart disease. Lancet 1999;353:89–92.
7. National Heart, Lung, and Blood Institute. Morbidity and mortality: 2007 chart book on cardiovascular, lung, and blood diseases. Bethesda (MD): National Institutes of Health; 2007.
8. Mittelmark MB, Psaty BM, Rautaharju PM, et al. Prevalence of cardiovascular diseases among older adults. The Cardiovascular Health Study. Am J Epidemiol 1993;137(3):311–7.
9. Rich MW, Bosner MS, Chung MK, et al. Is age an independent predictor of early and late mortality in patients with acute myocardial infarction? Am J Med 1992;92(1):7–13.
10. National Center for Health Statistics. Centers for Disease Control and Prevention. Compressed mortality file: underlying cause of death. Available at: http://wonder.cdc.gov/mortSQL.html. Accessed March 9, 2009.
11. Lloyd-Jones DM, Larson MG, Leip EP, et al. Lifetime risk for developing congestive heart failure: the Framingham Heart Study. Circulation 2002;106(24):3068–72.
12. Breek JC, Hamming JF, De Vries J, et al. Quality of life in patients with intermittent claudication using the World Health Organisation (WHO) questionnaire. Eur J Vasc Endovasc Surg 2001;21(2):118–22.
13. Izquierdo-Porrera AM, Gardner AW, Bradham DD, et al. Relationship between objective measures of peripheral arterial disease severity to self-reported quality of life in older adults with intermittent claudication. J Vasc Surg 2005;41(4):625–30.
14. Newman AB, Siscovick DS, Manolio TA, et al. Ankle-arm index as a marker of atherosclerosis in the Cardiovascular Health Study. Cardiovascular Heart Study (CHS) Collaborative Research Group. Circulation 1993;88(3):837–45.
15. Barasch E, Gottdiener JS, Larsen EK, et al. Clinical significance of calcification of the fibrous skeleton of the heart and aortosclerosis in community dwelling elderly. The Cardiovascular Health Study (CHS). Am Heart J 2006;151(1):39–47.
16. Roberts WC. The senile cardiac calcification syndrome. Am J Cardiol 1986;58(6):572–4.
17. Roberts WC, Shirani J. Comparison of cardiac findings at necropsy in octogenarians, nonagenarians, and centenarians. Am J Cardiol 1998;82(5):627–31.
18. Fox CS, Vasan RS, Parise H, et al. Mitral annular calcification predicts cardiovascular morbidity and mortality. Circulation 2003;107:1492–6.
19. Benjamin EJ, Plehn JF, D'Agostino RB, et al. Mitral annular calcification and the risk of stroke in an elderly cohort. N Engl J Med 1992;327:374–9.
20. Savage DD, Garrison RJ, Castelli WP, et al. Prevalence of submitral (anular) calcium and its correlates in a general population-based sample (the Framingham Study). Am J Cardiol 1983;51(8):1375–8.

21. Lindroos M, Kupari M, Heikkila J, et al. Prevalence of aortic valve abnormalities in the elderly: an echocardiographic study of a random population sample. J Am Coll Cardiol 1993;21(5):1220–5.
22. Otto CM, Lind BK, Kitzman DW, et al. Association of aortic-valve sclerosis with cardiovascular mortality and morbidity in the elderly. N Engl J Med 1999;341:142–7.
23. Stewart BF, Siscovick D, Lind BK, et al. Clinical factors associated with calcific aortic valve disease. Cardiovascular Health Study. J Am Coll Cardiol 1997; 29(3):630–4.
24. Singh JP, Evans JC, Levy D, et al. Prevalence and clinical determinants of mitral, tricuspid, and aortic regurgitation (the Framingham Heart Study). Am J Cardiol 1999;83(6):897–902.
25. Nkomo VT, Gardin JM, Skelton TN, et al. Burden of valvular heart diseases: a population-based study. Lancet 2006;368(9540):1005–11.
26. Freed LA, Levy D, Levine RA, et al. Prevalence and clinical outcome of mitral-valve prolapse. N Engl J Med 1999;341(1):1–7.
27. Furberg CD, Manolio TA, Psaty BM, et al. Major electrocardiographic abnormalities in persons aged 65 years and older (the Cardiovascular Health Study). Cardiovascular Health Study Collaborative Research Group. Am J Cardiol 1992;69(16):1329–35.
28. Manolio TA, Furberg CD, Rautaharju PM, et al. Cardiac arrhythmias on 24-h ambulatory electrocardiography in older women and men: the Cardiovascular Health Study. J Am Coll Cardiol 1994;23(4):916–25.
29. Miyasaka Y, Barnes ME, Gersh BJ, et al. Secular trends in incidence of atrial fibrillation in Olmstead County, Minnesota, 1980 to 2000, and implications on the projections for future prevalence. Circulation 2006;114:119–25.
30. Furberg CD, Psaty BM, Manolio TA, et al. Prevalence of atrial fibrillation in elderly subjects (the Cardiovascular Health Study). Am J Cardiol 1994;74(3):236–41.
31. Lloyd-Jones DM, Wang TJ, Leip AP, et al. Lifetime risk for development of atrial fibrillation. Circulation 2004;110:1042–6.
32. Psaty BM, Manolio TA, Kuller LH, et al. Incidence of and risk factors for atrial fibrillation in older adults. Circulation 1997;96(7):2455–61.
33. Kuller L, Borhani N, Furberg C, et al. Prevalence of subclinical atherosclerosis and cardiovascular disease and association with risk factors in the Cardiovascular Health Study. Am J Epidemiol 1994;139(12):1164–79.
34. Newman AB, Naydeck BL, Sutton-Tyrrell K, et al. Coronary artery calcification in older adults to age 99: prevalence and risk factors. Circulation 2001;104(22): 2679–84.
35. Yue NC, Arnold AM, Longstreth WT Jr, et al. Sulcal, ventricular, and white matter changes at MR imaging in the aging brain: data from the cardiovascular health study. Radiology 1997;202(1):33–9.
36. Bryan RN, Wells SW, Miller TJ, et al. Infarct-like lesions in the brain: prevalence and anatomic characteristics at MR imaging of the elderly–data from the Cardiovascular Health Study. Radiology 1997;202(1):47–54.
37. Newman AB, Gottdiener JS, McBurnie MA, et al. Associations of subclinical cardiovascular disease with frailty. J Gerontol A Biol Sci Med Sci 2001;56(3): M158–66.
38. Newman AB, Arnold AM, Naydeck BL, et al. "Successful aging": effect of subclinical cardiovascular disease. Arch Intern Med 2003;163(19):2315–22.
39. Agency for Healthcare Research and Quality. Healthcare Cost and Utilization Project. HCUPnet. Available at: http://www.hcup.ahrq.gov/HCUPnet.jsp. Accessed March 15, 2009.

40. Hodgson TA, Cohen AJ. Medical care expenditures for selected circulatory diseases: opportunities for reducing national health expenditures. Med Care 1999;37(10):994–1012.
41. Steinwachs DM, Collins-Nakai RL, Cohn LH, et al. The future of cardiology: utilization and costs of care. J Am Coll Cardiol 2000;35(5 Suppl B):91B–8B.

Hypertension in the Elderly

Wilbert S. Aronow, MD, FACC, FAHA

KEYWORDS

- Hypertension • Antihypertensive drugs • Diuretics
- Beta blockers • Angiotensin-converting enzyme inhibitors
- Angiotensin receptor blockers

As in younger people, hypertension in the elderly is defined as a systolic blood pressure of greater than or equal to 140 mm Hg or a diastolic blood pressure of greater than or equal to 90 mm Hg based on the mean of two or more properly measured seated blood pressure readings on each of two or more office visits.[1] Stage 1 hypertension is a systolic blood pressure of 140 to 159 mm Hg or a diastolic blood pressure of 90 to 99 mm Hg.[1] Stage 2 hypertension is a systolic blood pressure of greater than or equal to 160 mm Hg or a diastolic blood pressure of greater than or equal to 100 mm Hg.[1] Prehypertension is a systolic blood pressure of 120 to 139 mm Hg or a diastolic blood pressure of 80 to 89 mm Hg.[1]

Pseudohypertension in the elderly refers to a falsely high systolic blood pressure that results from markedly sclerotic arteries that do not collapse during inflation of the blood pressure cuff. Pseudohypertension can be confirmed by measuring intra-arterial pressure. The Osler maneuver is neither sensitive nor specific in diagnosing pseudohypertension. White coat hypertension is diagnosed when the office blood pressure is elevated persistently, but daytime ambulatory blood pressure readings are normal. Ambulatory blood pressure monitoring is recommended to confirm white coat hypertension in persons with office hypertension but no target organ damage. The main indications for ambulatory blood pressure monitoring in the elderly are to confirm the diagnosis of hypertension and to assist with management. Home recordings of blood pressure also should be obtained to ensure that blood pressure is controlled adequately while avoiding excessive blood pressure reduction in the elderly.

PATHOPHYSIOLOGY

An increase in systolic blood pressure in elderly persons is related in part to an age-associated increase in central arterial stiffness caused by structural alterations within the arterial media (including changes in the amount and nature of collagen, increased

Department of Medicine, Divisions of Cardiology, Geriatrics, and Pulmonary/Critical Care, New York Medical College, Macy Pavilion, Room 138, Valhalla, NY 10595, USA
E-mail address: wsaronow@aol.com

Clin Geriatr Med 25 (2009) 579–590
doi:10.1016/j.cger.2009.07.006
0749-0690/09/$ – see front matter © 2009 Elsevier Inc. All rights reserved.

interstitial fibrosis and calcification, and degradation of elastin fibers).[2] The increased wall stiffness and tortuosity of the aorta and large arteries with aging often are reflected by an increased systolic blood pressure and widened pulse pressure. Elderly persons with hypertension are more likely than those without hypertension to have increased left ventricular mass, increased peripheral resistance, decreased baroreceptor sensitivity, increased characteristic aortic impedance at rest, decreased left ventricular early diastolic filling rate and volume, increased left atrial dimension, and reduced cardiovascular response to catecholamines.[2]

Decreased baroreflex sensitivity with age and with hypertension leads to an impaired baroreflex-mediated increase in heart rate and total systemic vascular resistance in response to decreased blood pressure.[3] Therefore, elderly persons are more likely than younger persons to develop orthostatic and postprandial hypotension when treated with antihypertensive medications.[4]

Hypertension in the elderly also accelerates the age-dependent decline in renal function. Of 143 older persons, mean age 73 years, with hypertension in an academic nursing home, 60 (42%) had moderate (33%) or severe (9%) renal insufficiency with an estimated glomerular filtration rate of less than 60 mL/min/1.73 m^2 or less than 30 mL/min/1.73 m^2, respectively.[5] Renal artery stenosis is also an important cause of secondary hypertension in the elderly.[6]

PREVALENCE

The prevalence of hypertension increases with age, affecting 64% of men and 76% of women aged 75 years and older in the United States.[7] In the Framingham Heart Study, 90% of persons with a normal blood pressure at 55 years of age eventually developed hypertension.[8] In a study of 1819 older persons, mean age 80 years, living in the community and seen in an academic geriatrics practice, 58% had hypertension, including 37% with isolated systolic hypertension.[9] Target organ damage, clinical cardiovascular disease, or diabetes mellitus was present in 70% of those with hypertension.[9] In an academic nursing home, the prevalence of hypertension was 60% in one study[10] and 71% in another study[11]; in persons with diabetes mellitus, the prevalence was 76%.[12]

HYPERTENSION AND RISK OF CARDIOVASCULAR DISEASE

As systolic or diastolic blood pressure increases in elderly persons, so too does the risk for cardiovascular morbidity and mortality.[13] Increased systolic blood pressure and pulse pressure are stronger risk factors for cardiovascular morbidity and mortality in elderly persons than is increased diastolic blood pressure.[14,15] An increased pulse pressure found in older persons with isolated systolic hypertension indicates reduced vascular compliance in the large arteries and is a better marker of risk than systolic or diastolic blood pressure.[14,15] The Cardiovascular Health Study found in 5202 older men and women that a brachial systolic blood pressure higher than 169 mm Hg was associated with a risk-adjusted 1.6-fold higher mortality rate compared with a blood pressure of less than 129 mm Hg.[16] In contrast, observational data from one study showed that a lower systolic blood pressure was associated with greater mortality in persons aged 85 years and older.[17] The optimal blood pressure in very elderly persons requires further investigation.

Hypertension in elderly persons is a major risk factor for coronary events,[1,18–22] stroke,[1,18,22–25] heart failure (HF),[1,18,26,27] and peripheral arterial disease.[28–32] Compared with younger patients who have hypertension, the prevalence of target organ damage and clinical cardiovascular disease is higher in elderly patients, as is the incidence of new cardiovascular events. Despite the increased risk, however, elderly persons have the lowest rate of blood pressure control.[1,33]

Barriers to treatment of hypertension include physicians not recognizing that most elderly persons should be treated according to recommended guidelines to reduce cardiovascular morbidity and mortality. Prevalent comorbidities, polypharmacy, and the high cost of medications also contribute to lower blood pressure control rates in the elderly.[34]

EFFECT OF ANTIHYPERTENSIVE THERAPY IN REDUCING CARDIOVASCULAR EVENTS

Numerous prospective, double-blind, randomized, placebo-controlled studies have demonstrated that antihypertensive drug therapy decreases the development of new coronary events, stroke, and HF in elderly persons.[1,35–46] Treatment of hypertension in older persons is associated with a greater absolute decrease in cardiovascular events, including coronary events, stroke, HF, and renal insufficiency, and a greater reduction in dementia,[47] than are seen in younger persons.

Therapy with antihypertensive drugs reduces the incidence of all strokes by 36% in older persons, with similar effects in men and women and in persons older than 80 years.[24] The data also suggest that reduction of stroke in older persons with hypertension is related more to lowering the blood pressure than to the type of antihypertensive drugs used.[24]

In the Perindopril Protection Against Recurrent Stroke Study,[48] perindopril plus indapamide reduced stroke-related dementia by 34% and cognitive decline by 45%. In the Systolic Hypertension in Europe trial,[49] nitrendipine decreased dementia by 55% at 3.9-year follow-up. In 1900 older African Americans, antihypertensive drug treatment decreased cognitive impairment by 38%.[50] In the Rotterdam Study,[51] antihypertensive drugs decreased vascular dementia by 70%. The Study on Cognition and Prognosis in the Elderly, however, showed no difference in cognitive function in patients treated with candesartan versus placebo.[52] In addition, a substudy of the Hypertension in the Very Elderly Trial (HYVET) showed that antihypertensive drug therapy reduced dementia by 14%, but the effect was not significant.[53]

Despite multiple large randomized trials, treatment of hypertension in patients age 80 or older remained controversial[54,55] until the publication of HYVET.[46] In HYVET, 3845 individuals aged 80 years and older (mean age 83.6 years) with a sustained systolic blood pressure of 160 mm Hg or higher were randomized to indapamide (sustained-release 1.5 mg) or matching placebo.[46] Perindopril 2 mg or 4 mg, or matching placebo, was added if needed to achieve the target blood pressure of 150/80 mm Hg. The study was terminated early after a median follow-up of 1.8 years. Antihypertensive drug treatment reduced the incidence of the primary end point (fatal or nonfatal stroke) by 30% ($P = .06$). Antihypertensive drug treatment reduced fatal stroke by 39% ($P = .05$), all-cause mortality by 21% ($P = .02$), death from cardiovascular causes by 23% ($P = .06$), and heart failure by 64% ($P<.001$). The significant 21% reduction in all-cause mortality by antihypertensive drug treatment was unexpected. The benefits of antihypertensive drug treatment appeared during the first year of follow-up.

The prevalence of cardiovascular disease was only 12% at baseline in HYVET patients (ie, much lower than generally reported in community-based samples of octogenarians). For example, in a cohort of patients with hypertension, mean age 80 years, in a university geriatrics practice, 70% had cardiovascular disease, target organ damage, or diabetes mellitus.[9] The absolute reduction in cardiovascular events resulting from antihypertensive drug therapy in an elderly population with a high prevalence of cardiovascular disease could be much greater than observed in HYVET.

Although the results of HYVET clearly indicate that hypertensive patients aged 80 years and older should be treated with antihypertensive drug therapy, the study does not provide data on target blood pressure. Should the target blood pressure be 150/80 mm Hg (as in HYVET), less than 140/90 mm Hg (as recommended by Joint National Committee on Detection, Evaluation, and Treatment of Hypertension 7th Report [JNC 7]), or an even lower value?[56] Further research is needed to answer this question.

USE OF ANTIHYPERTENSIVE DRUG THERAPY IN THE ELDERLY

According to JNC 7,[1] the goal of treatment of hypertension in elderly persons is to reduce the blood pressure to less than 140/90 mm Hg and to less than 130/80 mm Hg in those with diabetes mellitus or chronic renal insufficiency.

Lifestyle modification in the elderly should be used to prevent mild hypertension and to reduce the dose levels of drugs needed to control hypertension. Weight reduction, consuming a diet rich in fruits, vegetables, and low-fat dairy products with a decreased content of saturated fat and total fat, dietary sodium reduction, regular aerobic physical activity, and limiting consumption of alcohol are recommended.[1]

Most elderly persons with hypertension will need two or more antihypertensive drugs to control their blood pressure.[1,11] It is important to measure blood pressure in both arms and to use the arm with the higher blood pressure during follow-up.[57] It is also important to measure blood pressure in the upright position and in the sitting position to check for orthostatic hypotension.

JNC 7 recommends that diuretics be used as initial drugs for treating elderly persons with hypertension and no associated medical conditions, because these drugs have been shown to reduce cardiovascular events and mortality in controlled clinical trials.[1] Elderly persons with hypertension, however, have a high prevalence of associated medical conditions, and these conditions should be considered in the selection of antihypertensive drug therapy.[1] If the blood pressure is more than 20/10 mm Hg above the goal blood pressure, drug therapy should be initiated with two antihypertensive agents, one of which should be a thiazide-type diuretic.[1]

The initial antihypertensive drug should be given at the lowest dose and gradually increased to the maximum dose. If the antihypertensive response to the initial drug is inadequate after reaching the full dose of drug, a second drug from another class should be given if the person is tolerating the initial drug. If there is no therapeutic response or if there are significant adverse effects, a drug from another class should be substituted. If a diuretic is not the initial drug, it usually is indicated as the second drug. If the antihypertensive response is inadequate after reaching the full dose of two classes of drugs, a third drug from another class should be added.

Before adding new antihypertensive drugs, the physician should consider possible reasons for inadequate response to antihypertensive drug therapy, including nonadherence to therapy, volume overload, drug interactions (use of nonsteroidal anti-inflammatory drugs, caffeine, antidepressants, nasal decongestants, sympathomimetics,), and associated conditions such as increasing obesity, smoking, excessive ethanol intake, and insulin resistance.[1] Causes of secondary hypertension should be identified and treated in accordance with current guidelines.[1,6]

ADVERSE EFFECTS OF ANTIHYPERTENSIVE DRUG THERAPY

In general, first-line anti-hypertensive agents, including diuretics, angiotensin-converting enzyme inhibitors (ACEIs), angiotensin receptor blockers (ARBs), calcium channel blockers (CCBs), and beta blockers, are tolerated well in most elderly patients. Compared with younger patients, however, older patients are at increased risk for serious adverse effects, including drug interactions related to the use of multiple medications.

Falls or syncope in elderly persons may be caused by orthostatic or postprandial hypotension, and frail elderly persons are at increased risk for these adverse consequences of antihypertensive therapy.[4] Blood pressure should be measured in the upright position, especially after eating. Marked orthostasis or postprandial hypotension should prompt a reduction in drug dosage or substitution of another antihypertensive agent.

Age-related alterations in renal function predispose elderly patients to electrolyte abnormalities, including hypokalemia, hyponatremia, and hypomagnesemia with both thiazide-like and loop diuretics. Similarly, older patients are at increased risk for hyperkalemia with potassium-sparing diuretics, and these agents should be used very cautiously or not at all in patients receiving ACEIs or ARBs.

Diuretics, ACEIs, and ARBs also can lead to worsening renal function in elderly patients, especially those with pre-existing renal insufficiency. Additional risk factors for worsening renal function include renal artery stenosis (usually bilateral), polycystic kidney disease, decreased absolute or effective arterial blood volume, sepsis, and use of nonsteroidal anti-inflammatory drugs, cyclosporine, or tacrolimus.[58–60] The risk of worsening renal function, and the risk of hyperkalemia, is similar with ACEIs and ARBs. Approximately 5% to 10% of patients develop a dry cough during long-term therapy with ACEIs; this adverse effect is uncommon with ARBs.

Beta blockers depress the sinus node and the atrioventricular node and are contraindicated in patients with severe sinus bradycardia, sinoatrial disease, or marked first-degree, second-degree, or third-degree atrioventricular block.[61] Beta blockers also should not be given to patients with bronchial asthma or to patients with lung disease with severe bronchospasm.[61] In addition, beta blockers may cause fatigue, exercise intolerance, or confusion in the elderly.

Short-acting dihydropyridine CCBs have the potential to increase cardiovascular events and should be avoided.[62] In the absence of compelling indications for their use (eg, refractory angina), CCBs additionally should be avoided in patients with decreased left ventricular systolic function (ejection fraction less 40%)[63–67] Like beta blockers, verapamil and diltiazem depress the sinus and atrioventricular nodes and are contraindicated in patients with significant bradyarrhythmias.[63] Verapamil may cause constipation in older patients. The venodilatory effects of dihydropyridine CCBs may cause dependent edema that, in some cases, may be difficult to distinguish from HF.

In the Antihypertensive and Lipid-Lowering Treatment to Prevent Heart Attack Trial (ALLHAT), the doxazosin arm involving 9067 patients was stopped prematurely at a median of 3.3 years.[68] Compared with the diuretic chlorthalidone, the alpha blocker doxazosin was associated with significant increases in HF (204%), stroke (19%), combined cardiovascular disease events (including coronary heart disease death, nonfatal myocardial infarction, stroke, angina pectoris, coronary revascularization, HF, or peripheral arterial disease; 25%), angina pectoris (16%), and coronary revascularization (15%). Based on these findings, alpha blockers should not be used as first-line agents to treat hypertension in the elderly. They may play an adjunctive role in older men with concomitant prostatic hypertrophy, however.

Centrally acting agents, such as clonidine, reserpine, and guanethidine, should not be used as monotherapy in elderly patients, because they have been associated with a high incidence of significant adverse effects, including sedation, depression, and constipation.[69] Direct vasodilators, including hydralazine and minoxidil, may cause headache, fluid retention, tachycardia, and angina pectoris. Hydralazine may cause a lupus-like syndrome in 5% to 10% of patients during long-term use.[70] Minoxidil may cause hirsutism and pericardial effusion.[71]

USE OF ANTIHYPERTENSIVE DRUGS IN PERSONS WITH ASSOCIATED MEDICAL CONDITIONS

Elderly persons with prior myocardial infarction should be treated with beta blockers and ACEIs.[1,66,72–76] In a prospective observational study of 1212 elderly men and women with prior myocardial infarction and hypertension treated with beta blockers, ACEIs, diuretics, CCBs, or alpha blockers, at 40-month follow-up, the incidence of new coronary events in elderly persons treated with a single antihypertensive drug was lowest in those treated with beta blockers or ACEIs.[66] In elderly persons treated with two antihypertensive drugs, the incidence of new coronary events was lowest in those treated with beta blockers plus ACE inhibitors.[66]

Beta blockers should be used to treat elderly persons with HF or complex ventricular arrhythmias with either normal or reduced LVEF.[77–81] Beta-blockers also are

---

Box 1
Some key points for treating hypertension in elderly persons

1. Hypertension in elderly persons is a major risk factor for coronary events, stroke, heart failure, peripheral arterial disease, and dementia.

2. Increased systolic blood pressure and pulse pressure are stronger risk factors for cardiovascular morbidity and mortality in elderly persons than is increased diastolic blood pressure.

3. White coat hypertension is common in elderly persons and is diagnosed when office blood pressures are persistently elevated, but daytime ambulatory blood pressures are normal.

4. Home blood pressure recordings are useful for ensuring that blood pressure is controlled adequately while avoiding excessive blood pressure reduction.

5. Elderly persons with hypertension, including those older than age 80 years, should be treated with antihypertensive drug therapy to reduce cardiovascular morbidity and mortality.

6. JNC 7 recommends that the goal of treatment of hypertension in elderly persons is to lower the blood pressure to less than 140/90 mm Hg and to less than 130/80 mm Hg in those with diabetes mellitus or chronic renal insufficiency.

7. Most elderly persons with hypertension will need two or more antihypertensive drugs to control their blood pressure.

8. JNC 7 recommends that diuretics should be used as initial drugs for treating elderly persons with hypertension and no associated medical conditions, because these drugs have been demonstrated to reduce cardiovascular events and mortality in controlled clinical trials.

9. Elderly persons with hypertension have a high prevalence of associated medical conditions, and these conditions should be considered in the selection of antihypertensive drug therapy.

10. If the blood pressure is more than 20/10 mm Hg above the blood pressure goal, drug therapy should be initiated with two antihypertensive agents, one of which should be a thiazide diuretic.

11. Measure blood pressure in the upright and sitting positions in both arms, and use the arm with the higher blood pressure during follow-up.

12. Treat other modifiable cardiovascular risk factors to reduce cardiovascular events and mortality.

indicated in elderly persons with hypertension who have angina pectoris,[82] myocardial ischemia,[83] supraventricular tachyarrhythmias such as atrial fibrillation with a rapid ventricular rate,[84,85] hyperthyroidism,[86] preoperative hypertension,[1] migraine,[1] or essential tremor.[1]

In addition to beta blockers, elderly persons with HF should be treated with diuretics and either an ACEI or ARB.[87] ACEIs or ARBs should be administered to elderly persons with diabetes mellitus, chronic renal insufficiency, or proteinuria.[1,75,88,89] Diuretics and ACEIs are recommended by JNC 7 to prevent recurrent stroke in elderly persons with hypertension.[1,48] Thiazide diuretics should be used in elderly persons with hypertension and osteoporosis.[1]

In addition to controlling blood pressure, it is essential to treat other cardiovascular risk factors in elderly persons, including dyslipidemia,[90,91] diabetes mellitus,[12,92-95] and tobacco use.[90]

SUMMARY

Numerous double-blind, randomized, placebo-controlled studies have documented that antihypertensive drug therapy reduces cardiovascular events in elderly persons, including octogenarians. Currently recommended treatment goals in elderly persons with hypertension are identical to those in younger patients, and include lowering the blood pressure to less than 140/90 mm Hg in most patients and to less than 130/80 mm Hg in those with diabetes or chronic renal insufficiency. All antihypertensive drugs may predispose the elderly person to develop symptomatic orthostatic hypotension and postprandial hypotension, thereby increasing the risk for falls and syncope. Although most commonly used antihypertensive drugs are tolerated well by elderly patients, adverse effects are common, and depend upon the specific drugs and drug dosages used, prevalent comorbidities, and the potential for drug–drug interactions. **Box 1** summarizes 12 key points for treating hypertension in elderly persons.

REFERENCES

1. Chobanian AV, Bakris GL, Black HR, et al. The seventh report of the Joint National Committee on Prevention, Detection, Evaluation, and Treatment of High Blood Pressure. The JNC 7 Report. JAMA 2003;289:2560–72.
2. Lakatta EG. Mechanisms of hypertension in the elderly. J Am Geriatr Soc 1989;37:780–90.
3. Gribbin B, Pickering GT, Sleight P, et al. Effect of age and high blood pressure on baroreflex sensitivity in man. Circ Res 1971;29:424–31.
4. Aronow WS. Dizziness and syncope. In: Hazzard WR, Blass JP, Ettinger WH Jr, et al, editors. Principles of geriatric medicine and gerontology. 4th edition. New York: McGraw-Hill, Incorporated; 1998. p. 1519–34.
5. Joseph J, Koka M, Aronow WS. Prevalence of moderate and severe renal insufficiency in older persons with hypertension, diabetes mellitus, coronary artery disease, peripheral arterial disease, ischemic stroke, or congestive heart failure in an academic nursing home. J Am Med Dir Assoc 2008;9:257–9.
6. Chiong JR, Aronow WS, Khan IA, et al. Secondary hypertension: current diagnosis and treatment. Int J Cardiol 2008;124:6–21.
7. Lloyd-Jones D, Adams R, Carnethon M, et al. Heart disease and stroke statistics—2009 update: a report from the American Heart Association Statistics Committee and Stroke Statistics Subcommittee. Circulation 2009;119:e21–181.

8. Vasan RS, Larson MG, Leip EP, et al. Impact of high–normal blood pressure on the risk of cardiovascular disease. N Engl J Med 2001;345:1291–7.

9. Mendelson G, Ness J, Aronow WS. Drug treatment of hypertension in older persons in an academic hospital-based geriatrics practice. J Am Geriatr Soc 1999;47:597–9.

10. Aronow WS, Ahn C, Gutstein H. Prevalence and incidence of cardiovascular disease in 1160 older men and 2464 older women in a long-term health care facility. J Gerontol A Biol Sci Med Sci 2002;57A:M45–6.

11. Koka M, Joseph J, Aronow WS. Adequacy of control of hypertension in an academic nursing home. J Am Med Dir Assoc 2007;8:538–40.

12. Joseph J, Koka M, Aronow WS. Prevalence of a hemoglobin A_{1c} <7.0%, of a blood pressure <130/80 mm Hg, and of a serum low-density lipoprotein cholesterol <100 mg/dL in older patients with diabetes mellitus in an academic nursing home. J Am Med Dir Assoc 2008;9:51–4.

13. National High Blood Pressure Education Program Working Group. National High Blood Pressure Education Program working group report on hypertension in the elderly. Hypertens 1994;23:275–85.

14. Madhavan S, Ooi WL, Cohen H, et al. Relation of pulse pressure and blood pressure reduction to the incidence of myocardial infarction. Hypertens 1994;23:395–401.

15. Rigaud AS, Forette B. Hypertension in older adults. J Gerontol A Biol Sci Med Sci 2001;56:M217–25.

16. Fried LP, Kronmal RA, Newman AB, et al. Risk factors for 5-year mortality in older adults. The Cardiovascular Health Study. JAMA 1998;279:585–92.

17. Molander L, Lovheim H, Norman T, et al. Lower systolic blood pressure is associated with greater mortality in people aged 85 and older. J Am Geriatr Soc 2008;56:1853–9.

18. Aronow WS, Ahn C, Kronzon I, et al. Congestive heart failure, coronary events, and atherothrombotic brain infarction in elderly blacks and whites with systemic hypertension and with and without echocardiographic and electrocardiographic evidence of left ventricular hypertrophy. Am J Cardiol 1991;67:295–9.

19. Aronow WS, Ahn C. Risk factors for new coronary events in a large cohort of very elderly patients with and without coronary artery disease. Am J Cardiol 1996;77:864–6.

20. Vokonas PS, Kannel WB. Epidemiology of coronary heart disease in the elderly. In: Aronow WS, Fleg JL, Rich MW, editors. Cardiovascular disease in the elderly. 4th edition. New York: Informa Healthcare; 2008. p. 215–41.

21. Franklin SS, Larson MG, Khan SA, et al. Does the relation of blood pressure to coronary heart disease risk change with aging? The Framingham Heart Study. Circulation 2001;103:1245–9.

22. Psaty BM, Furberg CD, Kuller LH, et al. Association between blood pressure level and the risk of myocardial infarction, stroke, and total mortality: the Cardiovascular Health Study. Arch Intern Med 2001;161:1183–92.

23. Aronow WS, Ahn C, Gutstein H. Risk factors for new atherothrombotic brain infarction in 664 older men and 1488 older women. Am J Cardiol 1996;77:1381–3.

24. Aronow WS, Frishman WH. Treatment of hypertension and prevention of ischemic stroke. Curr Cardiol Rep 2004;6:124–9.

25. Wolf PA. Cerebrovascular disease in the elderly. In: Tresch DD, Aronow WS, editors. Cardiovascular disease in the elderly patient. New York: Marcel Dekker, Incorporated; 1994. p. 125–47.

26. Aronow WS, Ahn C, Kronzon I. Comparison of incidences of congestive heart failure in older African Americans, Hispanics, and whites. Am J Cardiol 1999;84:611–2.

27. Levy D, Larson MG, Vasan RS, et al. The progression from hypertension to congestive heart failure. JAMA 1996;275:1557–62.
28. Stokes J III, Kannel WB, Wolf PA, et al. The relative importance of selected risk factors for various manifestations of cardiovascular disease among men and women from 35 to 64 years old: 30 years of follow-up in the Framingham Study. Circulation 1987;75(Suppl V):V65–73.
29. Aronow WS, Sales FF, Etienne F, et al. Prevalence of peripheral arterial disease and its correlation with risk factors for peripheral arterial disease in elderly patients in a long-term health care facility. Am J Cardiol 1988;62:644–6.
30. Ness J, Aronow WS, Ahn C. Risk factors for peripheral arterial disease in an academic hospital-based geriatrics practice. J Am Geriatr Soc 2000;48:312–4.
31. Ness J, Aronow WS, Newkirk E, et al. Prevalence of symptomatic peripheral arterial disease, modifiable risk factors, and appropriate use of drugs in the treatment of peripheral arterial disease in older persons seen in a university general medicine clinic. J Gerontol A Biol Sci Med Sci 2005;60:M255–7.
32. Aronow WS, Ahmed MI, Ekundayo OJ, et al. A propensity-matched study of the association of peripheral arterial disease with cardiovascular outcomes in community-dwelling older adults. Am J Cardiol 2009;103:130–5.
33. Hyman DJ, Pavlik VN. Characteristics of patients with uncontrolled hypertension in the United States. N Engl J Med 2001;345:479–86.
34. Gandelman G, Aronow WS, Varma R. Prevalence of adequate blood pressure control in self-pay or Medicare patients versus Medicaid or private insurance patients with systemic hypertension followed in a university cardiology or general medicine clinic. Am J Cardiol 2004;94:815–6.
35. Report by the Management Committee. The Australian therapeutic trial in mild hypertension. Lancet 1980;1:1261–7.
36. Medical Research Council Working Party. MRC trial of mild hypertension: principal results. Br Med J 1985;291:97–104.
37. MRC Working Party. Medical Research Council Trial of treatment of hypertension in older adults: principal results. Br Med J 1992;304:405–12.
38. Amery A, Birkenhager W, Brixko P, et al. Morbidity and mortality results from the European Working Party on High Blood Pressure in the Elderly Trial. Lancet 1985; 1:1349–54.
39. Coope J, Warrender TS. Randomised trial of the treatment of hypertension in elderly patients in primary care. Br Med J 1986;293:1145–51.
40. Dahlof B, Lindholm LH, Hansson L, et al. Morbidity and mortality in the Swedish Trial in Old Patients With Hypertension (STOP Hypertension). Lancet 1991;338:1281–5.
41. SHEP Cooperative Research Group. Prevention of stroke by antihypertensive drug treatment in older persons with isolated systolic hypertension. Final results of the Systolic Hypertension in the Elderly Program (SHEP). JAMA 1991;265:3255–64.
42. Kostis JB, Davis BR, Cutler J, et al. Prevention of heart failure by antihypertensive drug treatment in older persons with isolated systolic hypertension. JAMA 1997; 278:212–6.
43. Perry HM Jr, Davis BR, Price TR, et al. Effect of treating isolated systolic hypertension on the risk of developing various types and subtypes of stroke. The Systolic Hypertension in the Elderly Program (SHEP). JAMA 2000;284:465–71.
44. Staessen JA, Fagard R, Thijs L, et al. Randomised double-blind comparison of placebo and active treatment for older patients with isolated systolic hypertension. Lancet 1997;350:757–64.
45. Wang J-G, Staessen JA, Gong L, et al. Chinese trial on isolated systolic hypertension in the elderly. Arch Intern Med 2000;160:211–20.

46. Beckett NS, Peters R, Fletcher AE, et al. Treatment of hypertension in patients 80 years of age or older. N Engl J Med 2008;358:1887–98.
47. Aronow WS, Frishman WH. Effect of antihypertensive drug treatment on cognitive function. Clin Geriatr 2006;14(11):25–8.
48. Progress Collaborative Group. Randomised trial of a perindopril-based blood pressure-lowering regimen among 6105 individuals with previous stroke or transient ischaemic attack. Lancet 2001;358:1033–41.
49. Forette F, Seux ML, Staessen JA, et al. The prevention of dementia with antihypertensive treatment. New evidence from the Systolic Hypertension in Europe (Syst-Eur) study. Arch Intern Med 2002;162:2046–52.
50. Murray MD, Lane KA, Gao S, et al. Preservation of cognitive function with antihypertensive medications. A longitudinal analysis of a community-based sample of African Americans. Arch Intern Med 2002;162:2090–6.
51. Veld BA, Ruitenberg A, Holman A, et al. Antihypertensive drugs and incidence of dementia: the Rotterdam Study. Neurobiol Aging 2001;22:407–12.
52. Saxby BK, Harrington F, Wesnes KA, et al. Candesartan and cognitive decline in older patients with hypertension: a substudy of the SCOPE trial. Neurology 2008; 70:1858–66.
53. Peters R, Beckett N, Forette F, et al. Incident dementia and blood pressure lowering in the Hypertension in the Very elderly Trial cognitive function assessment (HYVET-COG): a double-blind, placebo-controlled trial. Lancet Neurol 2008;7:683–9.
54. Aronow WS. What is the appropriate treatment of hypertension in elders? [editorial]. J Gerontol A Biol Sci Med Sci 2002;57:M483–6.
55. Goodwin JS. Embracing complexity: a consideration of hypertension in the very old. J Gerontol A Biol Sci Med Sci 2003;58:M653–8.
56. Aronow WS. Older age should not be a barrier to the treatment of hypertension. Nat Clin Pract Cardiovasc Med 2008;5:514–5.
57. Mendelson G, Nassimiha D, Aronow WS. Simultaneous measurements of blood pressures in right and left brachial arteries. Cardiol Rev 2004;12:276–8.
58. Palmer BF. Renal dysfunction complicating the treatment of hypertension. N Engl J Med 2002;347:1256–61.
59. Hricick DE, Browning PJ, Kopelman R, et al. Captopril-induced functional renal insufficiency in patients with bilateral renal artery stenosis or renal artery stenosis in a solitary kidney. N Engl J Med 1983;308:373–6.
60. Toto RD, Mitchell HC, Lee HC, et al. Reversible renal insufficiency due to angiotensin-converting enzyme inhibitors in hypertensive nephrosclerosis. Ann Intern Med 1991;115:513–9.
61. Rosendorff C, Black HR, Cannon CP, et al. Treatment of hypertension in the prevention and management of ischemic heart disease. A scientific statement from the American Heart Association Council for High Blood Pressure Research and the Councils on Clinical Cardiology and Epidemiology and Prevention. Circulation 2007;115:2761–88.
62. Pahor M, Guralnik JM, Corti C, et al. Long-term survival and use of antihypertensive medications in older persons. J Am Geriatr Soc 1995;43:1191–7.
63. Aronow WS. Verapamil as an antiarrhythmic agent. In: Gould LA, editor. Drug treatment of cardiac arrhythmias. Mount Kisco (NY): Futura Publishing Company, Incorporated; 1983. p. 325–41.
64. The Multicenter Diltiazem Postinfarction Trial Research Group. The effect of diltiazem on mortality and reinfarction after myocardial infarction. N Engl J Med 1988; 319:385–92.

65. Goldstein RE, Boccuzzi SJ, Cruess D, et al. Diltiazem increases late-onset congestive heart failure in postinfarction patients with early reduction in ejection fraction. Circulation 1991;83:52–60.
66. Aronow WS, Ahn C. Incidence of new coronary events in older persons with prior myocardial infarction and systemic hypertension treated with beta blockers, angiotensin-converting enzyme inhibitors, diuretics, calcium antagonists, and alpha blockers. Am J Cardiol 2002;89:1207–9.
67. Elkayam U, Amin J, Mehra A, et al. A prospective, randomized, double-blind, crossover study to compare the efficacy and safety of chronic nifedipine therapy with that of isosorbide dinitrate and their combination in the treatment of chronic congestive heart failure. Circulation 1990;82:1954–61.
68. ALLHAT Officers and Coordinators for the ALLHAT Collaborative Research Group. Major cardiovascular events in hypertensive patients randomized to doxazosin vs chlorthalidone. The Antihypertensive and Lipid-Lowering Treatment to Prevent Heart Attack Trial (ALLHAT). JAMA 2000;283:1967–75.
69. Frishman WH, Aronow WS, Cheng-Lai A. Cardiovascular drug therapy in the elderly. In: Aronow WS, Fleg JL, Rich MW, editors. Cardiovascular disease in the elderly. fourth edition. New York: Informa Healthcare; 2008. p. 99–135.
70. Cameron HA, Ramsay LE. The lupus syndrome induced by hydralazine: a common complication with low-dose treatment. Br Med J (Clin Res Ed) 1984; 289:410–2.
71. Krehlik JM, Hindson DA, Crowley JJ Jr, et al. Minoxidil-associated pericarditis and fatal cardiac tamponade. West J Med 1986;143:527–9.
72. Ryan TJ, Antman EM, Brooks NH, et al. 1999 update: ACC/AHA guidelines for the management of patients with acute myocardial infarction: executive summary and recommendations. A report of the American College of Cardiology/American Heart Association Task Force on Practice Guidelines (Committee on Management of Acute Myocardial Infarction). Circulation 1999;100:1016–30.
73. Aronow WS, Ahn C. Effect of beta blockers on incidence of new coronary events in older persons with prior myocardial infarction and diabetes mellitus. Am J Cardiol 2001;87:780–1.
74. Aronow WS, Ahn C. Effect of beta blockers on incidence of new coronary events in older persons with prior myocardial infarction and symptomatic peripheral arterial disease. Am J Cardiol 2001;87:1284–6.
75. The Heart Outcomes Prevention Evaluation Study Investigators. Effects of an angiotensin-converting enzyme inhibitor, ramipril on cardiovascular events in high-risk patients. N Engl J Med 2000;342:145–53.
76. Aronow WS, Ahn C, Kronzon I. Effect of beta blockers alone, of angiotensin-converting enzyme inhibitors alone, and of beta blockers plus angiotensin-converting enzyme inhibitors on new coronary events and on congestive heart failure in older persons with healed myocardial infarcts and asymptomatic left ventricular systolic dysfunction. Am J Cardiol 2001;88:1298–300.
77. Kennedy HL, Brooks MM, Barker AH, et al. Beta-blocker therapy in the Cardiac Arrhythmia Suppression Trial. Am J Cardiol 1994;74:674–80.
78. Aronow WS, Ahn C, Mercando AD, et al. Effect of propranolol versus no antiarrhythmic drug on sudden cardiac death, total cardiac death, and total death in patients ≥62 years of age with heart disease, complex ventricular arrhythmias, and left ventricular ejection fraction ≥40%. Am J Cardiol 1994;74:267–70.
79. MERIT-HF Study Group. Effect of metoprolol CR/XL in chronic heart failure: Metoprolol CR/XL Randomised Intervention Trial in Congestive Heart Failure (MERIT-HF) Lancet 1999;353:2001–7

80. Flather MD, Shibata MC, Coats AJS, et al. Randomized trial to determine the effect of nebivolol on mortality and cardiovascular hospital admission in elderly patients with heart failure (SENIORS). Eur Heart J 2005;26:215–25.
81. Aronow WS, Ahn C, Kronzon I. Effect of propranolol versus no propranolol on total mortality plus nonfatal myocardial infarction in older patients with prior myocardial infarction, congestive heart failure, and left ventricular ejection fraction ≥40% treated with diuretics plus angiotensin-converting-enzyme inhibitors. Am J Cardiol 1997;80:207–9.
82. Aronow WS, Frishman WH. Angina in the elderly. In: Aronow WS, Fleg JL, Rich MW, editors. Cardiovascular disease in the elderly. fourth edition. New York: Informa Healthcare; 2008. p. 269–92.
83. Aronow WS, Ahn C, Mercando AD, et al. Decrease of mortality by propranolol in patients with heart disease and complex ventricular arrhythmias is more an anti-ischemic than an antiarrhythmic effect. Am J Cardiol 1994;74:613–5.
84. Aronow WS. Treatment of atrial fibrillation. Part 1. Cardiol Rev 2008;16:181–8.
85. Aronow WS. Treatment of atrial fibrillation and atrial flutter. Part 2. Cardiol Rev 2008;16:230–9.
86. Aronow WS. The heart and thyroid disease. Clin Geriatr Med 1995;11:219–29.
87. Hunt SA, Baker DW, Chin MH, et al. ACC/AHA guidelines for the evaluation and management of chronic heart failure in the adult: executive summary. A report of the American College of Cardiology/American Heart Association Task Force on Practice Guidelines (Committee to Revise the 1995 Guidelines for the Evaluation and Management of Heart Failure). Developed in collaboration with the International Society for Heart and Lung Transplantation. Endorsed by the Heart Failure Society of America. J Am Coll Cardiol 2001;38:2101–13.
88. Agodoa LY, Appel L, Bakris GL, et al. Effect of ramipril versus amlodipine on renal outcomes in hypertensive nephrosclerosis. A randomized controlled trial. JAMA 2001;285:2719–28.
89. Brenner BM, Cooper ME, de Zeeuw D, et al. Effects of losartan on renal and cardiovascular outcomes in patients with type 2 diabetes and nephropathy. N Engl J Med 2001;345:861–9.
90. Smith SC Jr, Allen J, Blair SN, et al. ACC/AHA guidelines for secondary prevention for patients with coronary and other atherosclerotic vascular disease: 2006 update: endorsed by the National Heart, Lung, and Blood Institute. Circulation 2006;113:2363–72.
91. Grundy SM, Cleeman JI, Merz CNB, et al. Implications of recent clinical trials for the National Cholesterol Education Program Adult Treatment Panel III guidelines. Circulation 2004;110:227–39.
92. American Diabetes Association. Standards of medical care for patients with diabetes mellitus. Diabetes Care 2003;26(Suppl 1):S33–50.
93. Stratton IM, Adler AI, Neil HA, et al. Association of glycaemia with macrovascular and microvascular complications of type 2 diabetes (UKPDS 35): prospective observational study. Br Med J 2000;321:405–12.
94. Ravipati G, Aronow WS, Ahn C, et al. Association of hemoglobin A_{1c} level with the severity of coronary artery disease in patients with diabetes mellitus. Am J Cardiol 2006;97:968–9.
95. Aronow WS, Ahn C, Weiss MB, et al. Relation of hemoglobin A_{1c} levels to severity of peripheral arterial disease in patients with diabetes mellitus. Am J Cardiol 2007;99:1468–9.

Hyperlipidemia in Older Adults

Farhan Aslam, MD[a], Attiya Haque, MD[a], L. Veronica Lee, MD, FACC[b],
JoAnne Foody, MD, FACC, FAHA[a],*

KEYWORDS

- Cholesterol • Coronary artery disease • Blood pressure
- Control • Procedure

Coronary artery disease (CAD) is the leading cause of morbidity and mortality in older individuals.[1] The highest incidence and prevalence is found in adults older than 65 years, with approximately 80% of deaths caused by CAD occurring in this age group. This statistic is concerning because older adults constitute the fastest growing segment of the United States population, increasing by approximately 3% per year.

Elevations in serum lipids are a significant risk factor for CAD and are present in approximately 25% of men and 42% of women older than 65 years.[2] Although clinical trials of cholesterol-lowering therapies have shown consistent benefits for patients who have established CAD and those who do not, these trials have typically excluded patients older than 65 years. This apparent age bias stems from concerns regarding life expectancy, comorbidity, safety of lipid-lowering agents, and cost-effectiveness of preventive care in the elderly. In fact, the absolute risk for CAD increases dramatically with age in men and women. Thus, the absolute number of persons who might benefit from cholesterol lowering is potentially greater in the elderly.[3]

AGE-RELATED CHANGES IN LIPOPROTEIN METABOLISM

Lipoprotein metabolism undergoes several hepatic and hormone-mediated changes with aging. Longitudinal studies have shown that total cholesterol levels increase in men after the onset of puberty until approximately 50 years of age, followed by a plateau until 70 years of age, when the serum cholesterol concentration falls slightly. Although the latter change is suspected to be an artifact resulting from CAD deaths in hypercholesterolemic men,[4] the most important factor influencing cholesterol is believed to be weight change.[5] Reductions in total and low-density lipoprotein (LDL) cholesterol levels and increases in high-density lipoprotein (HDL) cholesterol concentrations in older men occur primarily in those who have lost weight, and are independent of age.

---

[a] Department of Cardiology, Harvard Medical School, Brigham and Women's/Faulkner Hospitals, 1153 Centre Street, Suite 4930, Boston, MA 02130, USA
[b] Yale University Hospital, 20 York Street, New Haven, CT 06510, USA
* Corresponding author.
E-mail address: jfoody@partners.org (J. Foody).

Clin Geriatr Med 25 (2009) 591–606
doi:10.1016/j.cger.2009.08.001
0749-0690/09/$ – see front matter © 2009 Elsevier Inc. All rights reserved.
geriatric.theclinics.com

In women, the serum total cholesterol concentration is slightly higher than in men before 20 to 25 years of age. From age 25 to 55 years, serum cholesterol levels rise, although at a slower rate than in men. Total cholesterol levels are similar in women and men 55 to 60 years of age and higher in women than in men after 60 years of age.

Age-related changes in the total serum cholesterol concentration primarily result from an increase in LDL cholesterol levels. HDL cholesterol levels do not vary much with age, being approximately 10 mg/dL higher in women than men throughout life. The mechanisms responsible for the progressive age-related elevation in LDL cholesterol have not been fully explained; however, data support a primary role for a decrease in the fractional catabolic rate of LDL cholesterol. This reduction in LDL cholesterol catabolism is believed to result from diminished activity of hepatic LDL cholesterol receptors.[6]

HYPERLIPIDEMIA IN OLDER ADULTS AND ASSOCIATION WITH CORONARY ARTERY DISEASE

The association between hyperlipidemia and CAD in older men and women has been shown in several large epidemiologic studies. In the Framingham Heart Study, among patients aged 65 years and older who had prior myocardial infarction, serum total cholesterol was strongly related to death from CAD and all-cause mortality.[7] The relative risk for developing symptomatic CAD was 1.5 in men and 2.3 in women, with a total cholesterol level in the 90th percentile compared with those who had a plasma total cholesterol concentration lower than 200 mg/dL. In another study involving 1793 older men and women (mean age, 81 years), each 10 mg/dL increment in LDL cholesterol was associated with a 1.28-fold greater probability of having CAD.[8]

Low HDL cholesterol is also an independent risk factor for CAD in older adults. This finding was illustrated in a prospective cohort study of 2527 women and 1377 men older than 70 years that examined the effect of total and HDL cholesterol on the death rate from CAD.[9] In this study, an elevated total cholesterol concentration (>240 mg/dL) correlated significantly with CAD mortality in women (relative risk, 1.8), but not in men (relative risk, 1.1) after a mean follow-up of 4.4 years. The relative risk for coronary mortality for those who had low HDL-cholesterol levels (<35 mg/dL) was 4.9 in men and 2.0 in women. Hypertriglyceridemia was also shown to be an independent risk factor for new coronary events in older adults, especially women.[10]

Some reports have observed a U- or J-shaped curve in the elderly, in which lower total cholesterol levels are paradoxically associated with an increase in cardiovascular risk. In a longitudinal study of 4066 older men and women, for example, death from CAD increased at total serum cholesterol levels lower than 160 mg/dL.[11] However, after adjusting for CAD risk factors and serum iron and albumin (to account for comorbid diseases and frailty), the apparent increased risk at lower total cholesterol concentrations disappeared.

MANAGEMENT OF HYPERLIPIDEMIA IN OLDER ADULTS

Older people vary markedly in their functional age. At one extreme are vigorous, independent, physiologically robust persons in their 80s or even 90s who are as fit and resilient as individuals who are much younger. At the other extreme, many older patients have multisystem disease and limited reserve. Clinical judgment must therefore dominate treatment decisions in elderly patients. If a patient has other serious illnesses that impart a poor prognosis for quality or duration of life, withholding aggressive cholesterol management may be prudent. Conversely, if a patient older than 75 years is in otherwise relatively good health, cholesterol-lowering therapy can be considered.

Treatment of hyperlipidemia involves lifestyle modification and pharmacotherapy when indicated. Lifestyle modification in elderly individuals should include healthy eating habits, regular exercise, and maintenance of a healthy body weight. The updated National Cholesterol Education Program III (NCEP III) guidelines[12] are summarized in **Table 1**.

Table 1
Adult Treatment Panel III low-density lipoprotein cholesterol goals and cut-points for therapeutic lifestyle changes and drug therapy in different risk categories and proposed modifications based on recent clinical trial evidence

Risk Category	LDL-C Goal	Initiate TLC	Consider Drug Therapy[h]
High risk: CHD[a] or CHD risk equivalents[b] (10-year risk >20%)	<100 mg/dL (optional goal: <70 mg/dL)[f]	>100 mg/dL[g]	>100 mg/dL[i] (<100 mg/dL: consider drug options)[h]
Moderately high risk: 2+ risk factors[c] (10-year risk 10% to 20%)[d]	<130 mg/dL	<130 mg/dL[g]	>130 mg/dL (100–129 mg/dL; consider drug options)[j]
Moderate risk: 2+ risk factors[c] (10-year risk <10%)[d]	<130 mg/dL	<130 mg/dL	>160 mg/dL
Lower risk: 0–1 risk factor[e]	<160 mg/dL	<160 mg/dL	>190 mg/dL (160–189 mg/dL: LDL-lowering drug optional)

Abbreviations: CHD, coronary heart disease; HDL-C, high-density lipoprotein cholesterol; LDL-C, low-density lipoprotein cholesterol.

[a] CHD includes history of myocardial infarction, unstable angina, stable angina, coronary artery procedures (angioplasty or bypass surgery), or evidence of clinically significant myocardial ischemia.

[b] CHD risk equivalents include clinical manifestations of noncoronary forms of atherosclerotic disease (peripheral arterial disease, abdominal aortic aneurysm, and carotid artery disease [transient ischemic attacks or stroke of carotid origin or >50% obstruction of a carotid artery]), diabetes, and 2+ risk factors with 10-year risk for hard CHD >20%.

[c] Risk factors include cigarette smoking, hypertension (BP >140/90 mm Hg or on antihypertensive medication), low HDL cholesterol (<40 mg/dL), family history of premature CHD (CHD in male first-degree relative <55 years of age; CHD in female first-degree relative <65 years of age), and age (men <45 years; women <55 years).

[d] Electronic 10-year risk calculators are available at www.nhlbi.nih.gov/guidelines/cholesterol.

[e] Almost all people who have 0 or 1 risk factor have a 10-year risk <10%, and 10-year risk assessment in people who have 0 or 1 risk factor is therefore not necessary.

[f] Very high-risk favors the optional LDL cholesterol goal of <70 mg/dL, and in patients who have high triglycerides, non-HDL cholesterol <100 mg/dL. Optional LDL cholesterol goal <100 mg/dL.

[g] Any person at high risk or moderately high risk who has lifestyle-related risk factors (eg, obesity, physical inactivity, elevated triglyceride, low HDL cholesterol, metabolic syndrome) is a candidate for therapeutic lifestyle changes to modify these risk factors, regardless of LDL cholesterol level.

[h] When LDL-lowering drug therapy is used, it is advised that intensity of therapy be sufficient to achieve at least a 30% to 40% reduction in LDL cholesterol levels.

[i] If baseline LDL cholesterol is <100 mg/dL, institution of an LDL-lowering drug is a therapeutic option on the basis of available clinical trial results. If a high-risk person has high triglycerides or low HDL cholesterol, combining a fibrate or nicotinic acid with an LDL-lowering drug can be considered.

[j] For moderately high-risk persons, when LDL cholesterol level is 100 to 129 mg/dL, at baseline or on lifestyle therapy, initiation of an LDL-lowering drug to achieve an LDL cholesterol level <100 mg/dL is a therapeutic option based on available clinical trial results.

Adapted from Grundy SM, Cleeman JI, Merz CNB et al. Implications of recent clinical trials for the National Cholesterol Education Program Adult Treatment Panel III guidelines. Circulation. 2004;110:227–39; with permission.

DIETARY THERAPY FOR HYPERLIPIDEMIA

No data show that diet alone reduces cardiovascular events in older persons.[13] Nonetheless, dietary modification is considered an integral component of an overall strategy to reduce cardiovascular risk. Dietary treatment of hyperlipidemia involves initiating the NCEP therapeutic lifestyle change (TLC) diet. Cholesterol intake should be less than 200 mg daily. Less than 30% of total caloric intake should be from fatty acids. Saturated fatty acids should constitute less than 7% of total calories, polyunsaturated fatty acids up to 10% of total calories, and monounsaturated fatty acids 10% to 20% of total calories. Protein intake should account for 10% to 20% of total calories. The diet should be balanced and rich in fruits, vegetables, and whole grains, and malnutrition should be avoided.[14]

EXERCISE TRAINING AND REHABILITATION

Compared with younger patients, older patients who have CAD typically have markedly reduced exercise capacity and overall physical function.[15] Conversely, exercise training programs significantly improve exercise capacity and overall fitness in elderly patients.[16,17] In addition, cardiac rehabilitation and exercise training programs improve plasma lipids levels and reduce the prevalence of metabolic syndrome.[18] In older patients who have CAD, these programs generally produce modest but statistically significant reductions in total cholesterol (−5%), triglycerides (−15%), LDL cholesterol (−3%), and the LDL/HDL cholesterol ratio (−8%), and increases in HDL cholesterol (+6%).[19,20] These changes, although modest, seem to be additive to those obtained with pharmacologic therapy. In addition, exercise training is associated with reductions in subsequent hospitalization costs, cardiovascular morbidity and mortality, obesity indices (body mass index, −1.5% and percent body fat, −5%), and improvements in exercise capacity (+35%), behavioral characteristics (depression, anxiety, somatization, and hostility), and overall quality of life.[21,22]

PLANT STANOLS AND STEROLS

Plant sterols and stanols, which are derived from wood, vegetable oils, corn, rice, squash, and other plants, resemble cholesterol structurally. They are minimally absorbed and reduce intestinal cholesterol absorption.[23] In a 1995 study involving 153 patients who had mild hypercholesterolemia,[24] subjects replaced 24 g of daily fat with an 8-g serving of margarine containing 1 g of plant stanols during each of their three daily meals. At the end of 1 year, total cholesterol and LDL cholesterol levels were reduced by 10% and 14%, respectively.

Other studies have indicated that plant stanol esters are highly effective adjuncts to statin therapy, typically producing 10% to 15% additional reductions in LDL cholesterol.[25] Based on these findings, clinicians should consider using plant stanols/sterols in conjunction with standard dietary therapy, particularly for treating mildly elevated LDL -cholesterol levels in older patients.

SOLUBLE FIBER

Epidemiologic evidence strongly supports an inverse association between dietary fiber intake and the incidence of cardiovascular diseases.[26] Dietary fiber is plant material that is resistant to gastrointestinal enzymatic digestion and can be divided into two general categories: insoluble fibers (cellulose and lignan), commonly found in foods such as wheat and bran, which have laxative effects but do not substantially lower lipid levels; and water-soluble fibers (pectins, gums, and mucilages), found in legumes, beans, peas, oatmeal, cereal grain (especially oats and barley), and certain fruits, which have bulk-forming laxative effects and substantial lipid-lowering effects.

In clinical studies, soluble fibers were shown to reduce total cholesterol by 10% to 15%.[27,28] Increased consumption of soluble fibers may provide sufficient treatment for some older patients who have mildly elevated levels of LDL cholesterol, and may also be considered for patients who require additional lowering of LDL cholesterol despite appropriate medical therapy.

LIPID-LOWERING MEDICATIONS

Although lipid-lowering drugs have proven benefit, they are markedly underused in older patients. For example, in a prospective study of 500 patients who had a mean age of 81 years and a history of Q-wave myocardial infarction,[29] 67% had a serum LDL cholesterol concentration greater than 125 mg/dL, but only 5% were treated with a lipid-lowering drug. A retrospective cohort study of 396,077 high-risk older patients (ie, those who had history of cardiovascular disease or diabetes mellitus) showed that prescription of statins decreased with increasing age and as cardiovascular risk increased. Thus, older patients likely to derive the greatest benefit from lipid-lowering medications were least likely to receive them.[30]

STATINS

Statins suppress cholesterol biosynthesis by competitively inhibiting 3-hydroxy-3-methyl-glutaryl-coenzyme A (HMG-CoA) reductase, the enzyme that catalyzes the conversion of HMG-CoA to mevalonate, a precursor of sterols, including cholesterol. This action induces up-regulation of LDL cholesterol receptors in the liver, resulting in increased clearance of LDL cholesterol from the plasma, thereby decreasing total plasma cholesterol and LDL cholesterol levels. Through reducing high serum LDL cholesterol levels and increasing HDL cholesterol levels, statins can slow the rate of progression and promote regression of coronary atherosclerosis and also stabilize atherosclerotic plaque that is prone to rupture.[31–33] Statins reduce endothelial dysfunction,[34–36] decrease platelet aggregation and deposition, and help maintain a favorable balance between prothrombotic and fibrinolytic activity.[37] Irrespective of age, statins are first-line treatment for hyperlipidemia.

Statins are a cost-effective therapy for preventing recurrent CAD-related events in older patients.[38] For a patient 70 years of age, the cost of statin therapy per year of life gained ranges from $3800 to $13,300, which is within the range of acceptable therapeutic cost in the United States. Although primary and secondary prevention trials of LDL cholesterol–lowering therapies have shown a reduction in cardiac events and all-cause mortality, most studies included only small numbers of older subjects, or none at all. Nevertheless, subgroup analysis of trials that included older individuals suggests that the benefits from lipid-lowering therapy are similar in older and younger patients (**Tables 2** and **3**).

PRIMARY PREVENTION TRIALS
The Prospective Study of Pravastatin in the Elderly at Risk Trial

The Prospective Study of Pravastatin in the Elderly at Risk (PROSPER) trial was designed to determine whether pravastatin 40 mg/d reduces coronary and cerebral events in older patients who have preexisting vascular disease or who are at high risk for vascular disease and stroke.[39] This double-blind trial randomized 5804 patients to either placebo (n = 2913) or 40 mg of pravastatin (n = 2891). The primary

Table 2
Prospective, randomized, double-blinded, placebo-controlled primary prevention trials of statins for reducing cardiovascular events

Study	Patients	Drug Dose	Major Results
The prospective Study of Pravastatin in the Elderly at Risk (PROSPER) Trial	5408 patients aged >70 y who have or are at high risk for cardiovascular disease	Pravastatin, 40 mg/d	Pravastatin achieved a 15% relative risk reduction in the primary end point at 3.2 y follow-up. Treated patients had coronary events significantly reduced by 19% and coronary mortality by 24%
West of Scotland Coronary Prevention Study	6595 men aged up to 64 y with no heart disease	Pravastatin, 40 mg/d	Pravastatin reduced all-cause mortality ($P = .051$) and significantly reduced nonfatal MI, death from all cardiovascular causes, and death from CAD
Air Force/Texas Coronary Atherosclerosis Prevention Study	5608 men and 997 women who had no heart disease, 22% aged 65–73 y	Lovastatin, 20–40 mg/d	Lovastatin significantly reduced fatal or nonfatal MI, unstable angina, or sudden cardiac death (primary composite end point), and coronary revascularization, unstable angina, fatal and nonfatal MI, fatal and nonfatal cardiovascular events, and fatal and nonfatal coronary events (secondary end points)

Abbreviations: CABG, coronary artery bypass graft surgery; CAD, coronary artery disease; MI, myocardial infarction.

composite end point was definite or suspected death from coronary heart disease (CHD), nonfatal myocardial infarction, or fatal or nonfatal stroke.

Pravastatin therapy lowered LDL cholesterol levels by 34%, total cholesterol by 23%, and triglycerides by 13%, and increased HDL cholesterol by 5% at 3 months follow-up. Pravastatin was well tolerated and achieved a 15% relative risk reduction in the primary end point at 3.2 years follow-up. Coronary events were significantly reduced by 19%, and coronary mortality was reduced by 24%; however, this therapy had no effect on stroke or cognitive function. The PROSPER study clearly showed that the benefits of statin therapy observed among middle-aged adults also extend to older patients (>70 years) (see **Table 2**).

West of Scotland Coronary Prevention Study

The West of Scotland Coronary Prevention Study randomized 6595 middle-aged men 45 to 64 years of age who had hypercholesterolemia but no heart disease to pravastatin 40 mg/d or placebo.[40] Mean follow-up was 4.9 years (up to 6.2 years). Pravastatin significantly decreased serum total cholesterol by 20%, LDL cholesterol by 26%, and triglycerides by 12%, while increasing HDL cholesterol by 5%. Compared with placebo, pravastatin reduced all-cause mortality by 22% (P = .051), significantly reduced death from all cardiovascular causes by 32% and death from CAD or nonfatal myocardial infarction by 31%, and insignificantly decreased stroke by 10%.

Air Force/Texas Coronary Atherosclerosis Prevention Study

The Air Force/Texas Coronary Atherosclerosis Prevention Study randomized 6605 men and women (22% aged 65–73 years) who had no cardiovascular disease (mean serum total cholesterol level, 221 mg/dL; mean LDL cholesterol level, 150 mg/dL; and mean HDL cholesterol level, 36 mg/dL in men and 40 mg/dL in women) to lovastatin 20 to 40 mg/d or placebo.[41] Mean follow-up was 5.2 years (up to 7.2 years). Lovastatin significantly decreased serum total cholesterol by 18%, LDL cholesterol by 25%, and triglycerides by 15%, and increased HDL cholesterol by 6%. Compared with placebo, lovastatin significantly reduced major coronary events, defined as fatal or nonfatal MI, unstable angina, or sudden cardiac death, by 37% in patients aged 65 years or older.

SECONDARY PREVENTION TRIALS
Scandinavian Simvastatin Survival Study

The Scandinavian Simvastatin Survival Study included 1021 patients (total study population 4,444) aged 65 to 70 years who had angina or a previous myocardial infarction and hypercholesterolemia (baseline plasma total cholesterol levels between 212 and 309 mg/dL).[42] In this subgroup, treatment with simvastatin reduced all-cause mortality by 34%, CAD mortality by 43%, major coronary events by 34%, and the number of revascularization procedures by 41% (see **Table 3**).

Cholesterol and Recurrent Events Trial

The Cholesterol and Recurrent Events trial randomized 4159 men and women (51% aged 60–75 years) who had prior myocardial infarction, serum total cholesterol levels more than 240 mg/dL, and serum LDL cholesterol levels of 115 mg/dL or higher to pravastatin 40 mg/d or placebo.[43–45] Median follow-up was 5 years (up to 6.2 years). Pravastatin significantly reduced total cholesterol by 20% (from 209 to 167 mg/dL), LDL cholesterol by 32% (from 139 to 98 mg/dL), and triglycerides by 14% (from 155 to 135 mg/dL), and significantly increased HDL cholesterol by 5% (from 39 to 41 mg/dL).

Subgroup analysis of the 1283 patients aged 65 to 75 years at study entry showed that compared with placebo, pravastatin significantly reduced CAD mortality by 45%, CAD death or nonfatal myocardial infarction by 39%, major coronary events by 32%, coronary revascularization by 32%, and stroke by 40%.[44] Effects on unstable angina and heart failure did not reach statistical significance. In a subset of 576 postmenopausal women, pravastatin significantly reduced coronary death or nonfatal

Table 3
Prospective, randomized, double-blinded, placebo-controlled secondary prevention trials of statins for reducing cardiovascular events

Study	Patients	Drug Dose	Major Results
Scandinavian Simvastatin Survival Study	4444 (18.6% women) who had CAD, 1021 aged 65–70 y	Simvastatin, 20–40 mg/d	Simvastatin significantly reduced all-cause mortality, CAD mortality, major coronary events, nonfatal MI, any acute CAD-related event, any atherosclerosis-related end point, coronary revascularization, and stroke
Cholesterol and Recurrent Events	4159 (13.8% women) who had MI,1283 aged 65–75 y	Pravastatin, 40 mg/d	Pravastatin significantly reduced CAD mortality, CAD death or nonfatal MI, major coronary events, coronary revascularization, and stroke
Collaborative Atorvastatin Diabetes Study (CARDS)	2838 patients who had type II diabetes	Atorvastatin, 10 mg/d	Atorvastatin reduced incident major cardiovascular events by 37% in patients younger than 65 y and by 38% in patients aged 65 and older
Long-Term Intervention With Pravastatin in Ischemic Disease	9014 (16.8% women) who had MI or unstable angina, 3514 aged 65–75 y	Pravastatin, 40 mg/d	Pravastatin significantly reduced all-cause mortality, CAD death, death from cardiovascular disease, fatal and nonfatal MI, coronary revascularization, hospitalization for unstable angina, and stroke

(continued on next page)

Study	Patients	Drug Dose	Major Results
Table 3 _(continued)_			
Post Coronary Artery Bypass Graft trial	1351 (8% women) aged up to 74 y post-CABG	Lovastatin, 40–80 mg/d versus 2.5–5.0 mg/d	Aggressive lipid-lowering treatment significantly reduced the percentage of grafts with progression of atherosclerosis and the composite end point of death from cardiovascular or unknown causes or nonfatal MI, stroke, or coronary revascularization compared with moderate lipid-lowering treatment
Simvastatin/ Enalapril Coronary Atherosclerosis trial	394 (10.9% women) with angiographic CAD, 57% aged 60–75 y	Simvastatin, 10–40 mg/d	Simvastatin caused a significant slowing in progression of coronary atherosclerosis

Abbreviations: CABG, coronary artery bypass graft surgery; CAD, coronary artery disease; MI, myocardial infarction.

myocardial infarction by 41%, all coronary events by 46%, coronary angioplasty by 48%, coronary artery bypass graft surgery by 40%, and stroke by 56%.[45]

Collaborative Atorvastatin Diabetes Study

The Collaborative Atorvastatin Diabetes Study randomized patients who had type 2 diabetes but no known CAD to atorvastatin 10 mg/d or placebo. Compared with placebo, atorvastatin reduced the incidence of major cardiovascular events by 37% in patients younger than 65 years and by 38% in patients aged 65 years and older.[46]

The Long-term Intervention with Pravastatin in Ischemic Disease Trial

The double-blind, randomized Long-term Intervention with Pravastatin in Ischemic Disease trial compared the effects of pravastatin (40 mg/d) with those of placebo over a mean follow-up period of 6.1 years in 9014 patients 31 to 75 years of age.[47] The incidence of all cardiovascular outcomes was consistently lower among patients assigned to receive pravastatin, including myocardial infarction (reduction in risk, 29%; $P<.001$), death from CAD or nonfatal myocardial infarction (24% reduction; $P<.001$), stroke (19% reduction; $P = .048$), and coronary revascularization (20% reduction; $P<.001$).

The benefits of pravastatin in patients aged 65 years and older were equal to or exceeded those in younger patients. For every 1000 patients aged 65 to 75 years at baseline, 6 years of pravastatin therapy prevented 43 deaths, 33 myocardial infarctions, 32 hospitalizations for unstable angina, 34 myocardial revascularization procedures, and 13 strokes. Pravastatin prevented a total of 133 major cardiovascular events in this age group,[48] compared with 23 deaths and 107 major cardiovascular events prevented per 1000 patients aged 31 to 64 years.

In a subsequent economic analysis, pravastatin was more cost-effective in older patients because of the greater number of cardiovascular events avoided.[49]

The Post Coronary Artery Bypass Graft Trial

The Post Coronary Artery Bypass Graft trial studied 1351 patients who had undergone bypass surgery 1 to 11 years before baseline and who had LDL cholesterol level between 130 and 175 mg/dL and at least one patent vein graft as seen on angiography.[50] Patients were assigned to aggressive or moderate treatment to lower LDL cholesterol levels (with lovastatin and, if needed, cholestyramine). Angiography was repeated an average of 4.3 years after baseline. The primary angiographic outcome was the mean percentage per patient of grafts with a decrease of 0.6 mm or more in lumen diameter.

Results showed that the mean LDL cholesterol level of patients who underwent aggressive treatment ranged from 93 to 97 mg/dL; with moderate treatment, this level ranged from 132 to 136 mg/dL ($P<.001$). The mean percentage of grafts with progression of atherosclerosis was 27% for patients whose LDL cholesterol level was lowered with aggressive treatment and 39% for those who underwent moderate treatment ($P<.001$). The rate of revascularization over 4 years was 29% lower in the group whose LDL cholesterol level was lowered aggressively than in the group undergoing moderate treatment (6.5% vs 9.2%; $P = .03$).

Simvastatin/Enalapril Coronary Atherosclerosis Trial

The randomized, placebo-controlled clinical trial, Simvastatin/Enalapril Coronary Atherosclerosis, compared the effect of simvastatin on coronary atherosclerosis with that of placebo in 394 patients who had paired coronary angiograms taken an average of 4 years apart.[51] The effects of treatment were examined on the following prespecified subgroups: sex, age (<65 years vs ≥65 years), smoking status (current or previous vs never), history of diabetes mellitus or hypertension, and severity of coronary artery lesions (diameter ≥50% vs <50%). All subgroups treated with simvastatin had significantly smaller decreases in the average minimum diameters, between closeout and baseline angiograms, compared with those treated with placebo.

ADVERSE EFFECTS OF STATINS

Common side effects of statins include headache, upset stomach, fatigue, flu-like symptoms, and myalgias (without increases in creatine kinase [CK]).One or both liver transaminases may be elevated to more than three times the upper limit of normal on two consecutive occasions in 0.5% of patients taking low doses to as high as 2.5% in patients taking high doses of statins.[52] Whether statin-induced elevations in liver enzymes constitute true hepatotoxicity has not been determined.

Serious liver dysfunction or failure is rare and not clearly related to statin therapy. Enzyme levels frequently return to normal after dose reduction or even with continuation of therapy. If transaminase elevation persists, discontinuation of therapy for a short period is advised until levels return to normal, after which statin therapy may be reinitiated. Baseline liver function tests should be obtained before starting statin therapy, at 12 weeks after initiating therapy, after any dosage increase, and at 12-month intervals thereafter. Because of a higher risk for adverse effects, statins should be used cautiously in persons who have a history of liver disease or excessive alcohol intake.[53]

Myopathy, defined as muscle symptoms (weakness, aching, or soreness) in conjunction with CK elevations greater than 10 times the upper limit of normal, occurs in fewer than 0.2% of persons taking statins. Rare cases of rhabdomyolysis, myoglobinuria, acute renal necrosis, and death have been reported. Myopathy is more likely to occur at higher dosages in patients who have renal impairment when a statin is combined with a fibrate, when drugs affecting statin metabolism are given concurrently (eg, macrolide antibiotics, antifungal medications), and in elderly women.[54] All patients started on statins should be instructed to promptly report muscle symptoms or brown urine. CK should be measured and, if myopathy is present or strongly suspected, the statin should be discontinued immediately.

In some patients who have statin-induced myopathy, supplementation with coenzyme Q10 and vitamin D has shown promising results. In a randomized double-blinded study of patients treated with statins and reporting myopathic pain, coenzyme Q10 supplementation (100 mg/d for 30 days) decreased muscle pain by 40% and improved the interference of pain with daily life activities by 38%.[55]

Ezetimibe

Ezetimibe reduces intestinal cholesterol absorption by approximately 50%, and ezetimibe, 10 mg daily, lowers LDL cholesterol by 15% to 20% when used as monotherapy and by an additional 20% to 25% when added to statin therapy.[56] Ezetimibe also slightly raises HDL cholesterol and reduces triglyceride levels by approximately 10%. Ezetimibe also lowers C-reactive protein (CRP), an important inflammatory risk factor for cardiovascular disease.[57] Ezetimibe can be safely added to statin therapy without significant drug interactions. However, the effect of ezetimibe on the progression of atherosclerosis and on clinical outcomes remains unknown. In patients who had familial hypercholesterolemia, combined therapy with ezetimibe and simvastatin did not result in greater changes in carotid intima-media thickness compared with simvastatin alone, despite significantly greater reductions in LDL cholesterol and CRP.[58]

Niacin

Nicotinic acid, or niacin, is perhaps the most underused agent to treat patients who have hyperlipidemia. Niacin significantly improves all components of the lipid profile, including lowering total and LDL cholesterol by 15% and triglycerides by 25% to 30%, and increasing HDL cholesterol by 25% to 30%. Niacin also lowers CRP by 15% to 25%.[59]

However, side effects with are frequent, although not life-threatening. In particular, cutaneous flushing occurs in up to 50% of patients. This effect can be minimized by premedication with low-dose aspirin, using lower doses of niacin sustained-release formulations, and by slowly increasing the dose over weeks to months. Ingestion of wheat-containing snacks before taking niacin and avoidance of alcohol have also been found to decrease the occurrence of flushing. Short-acting niacin preparations at therapeutic doses have also been associated with an increased risk for hepatic toxicity. When niacin is used in combination with statins, the risk for myopathy may be mildly increased, which can be minimized by using a statin that is more hydrophilic and less metabolized by the cytochrome P450 3A4 system, such as rosuvastatin and pravastatin.

Fibrates

Fibric acid derivatives (fibrates), are the preferred drugs for treating severe hypertrigly-ceridemia, because triglyceride levels may be lowered by more than 50%, with concomitant increases in HDL cholesterol of up to 10%.[60] However, fibrate therapy has not been shown to reduce total mortality in either primary or secondary prevention studies. In the United States, gemfibrozil and fenofibrate are currently approved for the treatment of dyslipidemia. Gemfibrozil has been shown to improve outcomes in patients who have CAD[61,62] and costs less than fenofibrate. However, gemfibrozil has minimal to no effect on LDL cholesterol and is associated with a higher risk of drug interactions with statins in older patients (including increased risk for myopathy and rhabdomyolysis), especially with agents that are more lipophilic, undergo metabolism through the cytochrome P450 system, or require glucuronidation (eg, atorvastatin, simvastatin).

Fenofibrate is administered once daily and has slightly greater effects on triglycerides and HDL cholesterol than gemfibrozil. Fenofibrate is also considerably less likely to cause drug interactions when prescribed with statins. Conversely, fenofibrate has not been shown to reduce cardiovascular event rates.

Bile Acid Sequestrants

Bile acid sequestrants include cholestyramine and colestipol. This class of drugs act through binding bile acids in the intestine, thereby interrupting enterohepatic circulation of bile acids and increasing the conversion of cholesterol into bile acids in the liver.

The Lipid Research Clinics Coronary Primary Prevention trial randomized 3806 asymptomatic men aged 35 to 59 years who had a serum total cholesterol level of 265 mg/dL or higher to cholestyramine 24 g/d or placebo.[63] Reductions in total and in LDL cholesterol were 8.5% and 12.6% greater, respectively, in patients treated with cholestyramine than in those treated with placebo. During 7.4 years of follow-up, cholestyramine was associated with a significant 19% reduction in CAD death or nonfatal myocardial infarction.

Drug Interactions and Side Effects

Older patients are frequently treated with multiple medications and are therefore at increased risk for drug interactions. For example, macrolide antibiotics can increase statin blood levels and thus the risk for muscle toxicity. Additionally, older patients may have greater susceptibility to medication side effects, such as bloating and constipation associated with bile acid sequestrants, and hyperglycemia and gout with niacin.

Older patients may be at increased risk for myopathy and rhabdomyolysis with the combined use of a statin and a fibrate, particularly gemfibrozil. This risk is enhanced at high statin doses, in the presence of renal insufficiency, and when using drugs that interfere with statin metabolism.[64] The risk for toxicity can be minimized through using the lowest effective doses of the statin and fibrate to achieve treatment goals, dosing the fibrate in the morning and the statin in the evening (based on theoretical considerations but without clinical evidence for reduced muscle toxicity), and avoiding statins in patients who have impaired renal or hepatic function (including alcoholics).

SUMMARY

The NCEP III guidelines emphasize the importance of including older patients in the management of lipid disorders. Older patients have the highest risk for CAD and the highest burden of atherosclerotic disease. Although clinical trials of cholesterol-lowering therapy have not specifically targeted older persons, growing evidence supports treatment of elevated LDL cholesterol levels in older patients, especially those at high risk for coronary events. The decision to treat a high or high-normal cholesterol level in an elderly individual must be individualized, based on chronologic and physiologic age. For primary prevention, the first line of therapy is dietary modification, regular physical activity, and weight control. In patients at higher risk, drug therapy should be considered. As in younger patients, statins are first-line agents for treating most older patients who have elevated total or LDL cholesterol. Other medications can be added as needed to achieve target levels of LDL cholesterol, HDL cholesterol, and triglycerides.

REFERENCES

1. Castelli WP, Wilson PW, Levy D, et al. Cardiovascular risk factors in the elderly. Am J Cardiol 1989;63:12–6.
2. Katzel LI, Goldberg AP, Hazzard WR, et al. Principals of geriatric medicine and gerontology. 5th edition. New York: McGraw-Hill Inc; 2003. p. 875–91.
3. Grundy SM, Cleeman JI, Rifkind BM, et al. Cholesterol lowering in the elderly population. Coordinating Committee of the National Cholesterol Education Program. Arch Intern Med 1999;159:1670.
4. Kreisberg RA, Kasim S. Cholesterol metabolism and aging. Am J Med 1987;82:54.
5. Ferrara A, Elizabeth BC, Shan J. Total, LDL, and HDL cholesterol decrease with age in older men and women. The Rancho Bernardo Study 1984–1994. Circulation 1997;96:37.
6. Ericsson S, Eriksson M, Vitols S, et al. Influence of age on the metabolism of plasma low density lipoproteins in healthy males. J Clin Invest 1991;87:591.
7. Wong ND, Wilson PW, Kannel WB. Serum cholesterol as a prognostic factor after myocardial infarction; the Framingham Study. Ann Intern Med 1991;115:687–93.
8. Aronow WS, Ahn C. Correlation of serum lipids with the presence and absence of coronary artery disease in 1,793 men and women aged >62 years. Am J Cardiol 1994;73:702–3.
9. Corti MC, Guralnik JM, Salive ME, et al. HDL cholesterol predicts coronary heart disease mortality in older persons. JAMA 1995;274:539.
10. Aronow WS, Ahn C. Risk factors for new coronary events in large cohort of very elderly patients with and without coronary artery disease. Am J Cardiol 1996;77:866.
11. Corti MC, Guralnik JM, Salive ME, et al. Clarifying the direct relation between total cholesterol levels and death from coronary heart disease in older persons. Ann Intern Med 1997;126:753.
12. Grundy SM, Cleeman JI, Merz CNB, et al. Implications of recent clinical trials for the National Cholesterol Education Program Adult Treatment Panel III guidelines. Circulation 2004;110:227–39.
13. Buckley DA, Kelber ST, Goodwin JS. The use of dietary restrictions in malnourished nursing home patients. J Am Geriatr Soc 1994;42:1100–2.
14. Wilson MM, Vaswani S, Morley JE, et al. Prevalence and causes of undernutrition in medical outpatients. Am J Med 1998;104:56–63.
15. Lavie CJ. Treatment of hyperlipidemia in elderly persons with exercise training, non pharmacologic therapy and drug combinations. Am J Geriatr Cardiol 2004;13(3 Suppl 1):29–33.

16. Lavie CJ, Milani RV, Cassidy MM, et al. Benefits of cardiac rehabilitation and exercise training in older persons. Am J Geriatr Cardiol 1995;4:42–8.
17. Lavic CJ, Milani RV. Effects of cardiac rehabilitation programs on exercise capacity, coronary risk factors, behavioral characteristics, and quality of life in a large elderly cohort. Am J Cardiol 1995;76:177–9.
18. Milani RV, Lavie CJ. Prevalence and profile of metabolic syndrome in patients following acute coronary events and effects of therapeutic lifestyle change with cardiac rehabilitation. Am J Cardiol 2003;92:50–4.
19. Milani RV, Lavie CJ. Prevalence and effects or nonpharmacologic treatment of "isolated" low-HDL cholesterol in patients with coronary artery disease. J Cardiopulm Rehabil 1995;15:439–44.
20. Lavie CJ, Milani RV. Effects of nonpharmacologic therapy with cardiac rehabilitation and exercise training in patients with low levels of high-density lipoprotein cholesterol. Am J Cardiol 1997;78:1286–8.
21. Ades P, Huang D, Weaver SO. Cardiac rehabilitation participation predicts lower rehospitalization costs. Am Heart J 1992;123:916–21.
22. O'Connor GT, Buring JE, Yusuf S, et al. An overview of randomized trials of rehabilitation with exercise after myocardial infarction. Circulation 1989;80:234–44.
23. Cater NB, Grundyh SM. Lowering serum cholesterol with plant sterols and stanols historical perspectives. Postgrad Med 1998;6–14.
24. Miettinen TA, Puska P, Gylling H, et al. Reduction of serum cholesterol with sitostanol-ester margarine in a mildly hypercholesterolemic population. N Engl J Med 1995;333(20):1306–12.
25. Gylling H, Radhakrishnan R, Miettinen TA. Reduction of serum cholesterol in postmenopausal women with previous myocardial infarction and cholesterol malabsorption induced by dietary sitostanol ester margarine. Women and dietary sitostanol. Circulation 1997;96(12):4226–31.
26. O'Keefe J, Lavie CJ. Dietary prevention of coronary artery disease. How to help patients modify eating habits and reduce cholesterol. Postgrad Med 1989;85:243–61.
27. Anderson JW, Story L, Sieling B, et al. Hypercholesterolemic effects of oat-bran or bean intake for hypercholesterolemic men. Am J Clin Nutr 1984;40(6):1146–55.
28. Anderson JW, Zettwoch N, Feldman T, et al. Cholesterol lowering effects of psyllium hydrophilic mucilloid for hypercholesterolemic men. Arch Intern Med 1988;148(2):292–6.
29. Aronow WS. Underutilization of lipid-lowering drugs in older persons with prior myocardial infarction and a serum low-density lipoprotein cholesterol >125 mg/dL. Am J Cardiol 1998;82:668–74.
30. Ko DT, Mamdani M, Alter DA. Lipid-lowering therapy with statins in high-risk elderly patients: the treatment-risk paradox. JAMA 2004;291:1864.
31. Pitt B, Mancini GB, Ellis SG, et al. Pravastatin limitation of atherosclerosis in the coronary arteries (PLAC 1): reduction in atherosclerosis progression and clinical events. J Am Coll Cardiol 1995;26:1133–9.
32. Tamura A, Mikuriya Y, Nasu M, et al. Effect of Pravastatin (10 mg/d) on progression of coronary atherosclerosis in patients with serum total cholesterol levels from 160 to 220 mg/dl and angiographically documented coronary artery disease. Am J Cardiol 1997;79:893–6.
33. Walter DH, Schachinger V, Elsner M, et al. Effect of statin therapy on restenosis after coronary stent implantation. Am J Cardiol 2000;85:962–8.
34. Vaughan CJ, Gotto AM, Basson CT. The evolving role of statins in the management of atherosclerosis. J Am Coll Cardiol 2000;35:1–10.

35. Anderson TJ, Meredith IT, Yeung AC, et al. The effect of cholesterol lowering and anti-oxidant therapy on endothelium dependant coronary vasomotion. N Engl J Med 1995;332:488–93.

36. Dupuis J, Tardif JC, Cernacek P, et al. Cholesterol reduction rapidly improves endothelial function after acute coronary syndromes. The RECIFE (Reduction of Cholesterol in Ischemia and Function of Endothelium) trial. Circulation 1999;99: 3227–33.

37. Rosenson RS, Tangney CC. Antiatherothrombotic properties of statins. Implications of cardiovascular event reduction. JAMA 1998;279:1643–50.

38. Johannesson M, Jönsson B, Kjekshus J, et al. Cost effectiveness of simvastatin treatment to lower cholesterol levels in patients with coronary heart disease. Scandinavian Simvastatin Survival Study Group. N Engl J Med 1997;336(5): 332–6.

39. Shepherd J, Blauw GJ, Murphy MB, et al. Pravastatin in elderly individuals at risk of vascular disease (PROSPER): a randomized controlled trial. Lancet 2002;360: 1623–30.

40. Shepherd J, Cobbe SM, Ford I, et al. Prevention of coronary heart disease with pravastatin in men with hypercholesterolemia. N Engl J Med 1995;333:1301–7.

41. Downs JR, Clearfield M, Weis S, et al. Primary prevention of acute coronary events with lovastatin in men and with average cholesterol levels. Results of AFCAPS/TexCAPS. JAMA 1998;279:1615–22.

42. SSSS Group. Randomised trial of cholesterol lowering in 4444 patients with coronary heart disease: the Scandinavian Simvastatin Survival Study (4S). Lancet 1994;344:1383.

43. Sacks FM, Pfeffer MA, Moye LA, et al. The effect of pravastatin on coronary events after myocardial infarction in patients with average cholesterol levels. N Engl J Med 1996;335:1001–9.

44. Lewis SJ, Moye LA, Sacks FM, et al. Effect of pravastatin on cardiovascular events in older patients with myocardial infarction and cholesterol levels in the average range. Results of the Cholesterol and Recurrent Events (CARE) trial. Ann Intern Med 1998;129:681–9.

45. Lewis SJ, Sacks FM, Mitchell JS, et al. Effect of pravastatin on cardiovascular events in women after myocardial infarction: the Cholesterol and Recurrent Events (CARE) trial. J Am Coll Cardiol 1998;32:140–6.

46. Neil HA, DeMicco DA, Luo D, et al. Analysis of efficacy and safety in patients aged 65–75 years at randomization: Collaborative Atorvastatin Diabetes Study (CARDS). Diabetes Care 2006;29:2378.

47. The Long-Term Intervention with Pravastatin in Ischemic Disease (LIPID) Study Group. Prevention of cardiovascular events and death with pravastatin in patients with coronary heart disease and a broad range of initial cholesterol levels. N Engl J Med 1998;339:1349–57.

48. Hunt D, Young P, Simes J, et al. For the LIPID Investigators. Benefits of pravastatin on cardiovascular events and mortality in older patients with coronary heart disease are equal to or exceed those seen in younger patients: results from the LIPID trial. Ann Intern Med 2001;134:931–40.

49. Tonkin AM, Eckermann S, White H, et al. Cost-effectiveness of cholesterol-lowering therapy with pravastatin in patients with previous acute coronary syndromes aged 65 to 74 years compared with younger patients: results from the LIPID study. Am Heart J 2006;151:1305–12.

50. The Post Coronary Artery Bypass Graft Trial Investigators. The effect of aggressive lowering of low-density lipoprotein cholesterol levels and low-dose

anticoagulation on obstructive changes in saphenous-vein coronary-artery bypass grafts. N Engl J Med 1997;336:153–63.

51. Burton JR, Teo KK, Buller CE, et al. Effects of long term cholesterol lowering on coronary atherosclerosis in patient risk factor subgroups: the Simvastatin/enalapril Coronary Atherosclerosis Trial (SCAT). Can J Cardiol 2003;19(5):487–91.

52. Alexander K, Iddo Z, Frida G, et al. Declining frequency of liver enzyme abnormalities with statins: experience from general practice in Jerusalem. Eur J Gastroenterol Hepatol 2008;20:1002–5.

53. Ballantyne CM, Corsini A, Davidson MH, et al. Risk for myopathy with statin therapy in high-risk patients. Arch Intern Med 2003;163:553–64.

54. Lemaitre RN, Psaty BM, Heckbert SR, et al. Therapy with hydroxymethylglutaryl coenzyme a reductase inhibitors (statins) and associated risk of incident cardiovascular events in older adults: evidence from the cardiovascular health study. Arch Intern Med 2002;162:1395.

55. Caso G, Kelly P, McNurlan MA, et al. Effect of coenzyme q10 on myopathic symptoms in patients treated with statins. Am J Cardiol 2007;99:1409–12.

56. Ballantyne CM, Houri J, Notarbartolo A, et al. Effect of ezetimibe co-administered with atonastatin in 628 patients with primary hypercholesterolemia: a prospective, randomized double-blind trial. Circulation 2003;107(19):2409–15.

57. Sager PT, Melani L, Lipka L, et al. Effect of co-administration of ezetimibe and simvastatin on high-sensitivity C-reactive protein. Am J Cardiol 2003;92:1414–8.

58. Kastelein JP, Akdim F, Stroes ES, et al. Simvastatin with or without ezetimibe in familial hypercholesterolemia. N Engl J Med 2008;358:1431–43.

59. Lavie CJ, Milani RV. Lipid lowering drugs: nicotinic acid. Cardiovascular Drug Therapy. 2nd edition. Philadelphia: W.B. Saunders Company; 1996. p. 1061–7.

60. Mannimen V, Elo MO, Frick MH, et al. Lipid alterations and decline in the incidence of coronary heart disease in the Helsinki Heart Study. JAMA 1988; 260:641–51.

61. Milani RV, Lavie CJ. Lipid lowering drugs: gemfibrozil. Cardiovascular Drug Therapy. 2nd edition. Philadelphia: WB Saunders Company; 1996. p. 1098–101.

62. Bloomfield H, Robins SJ, Collins D, et al. Gemfibrozil for the secondary prevention of coronary heart disease in men with low levels of high-density lipoprotein cholesterol. N Engl J Med 1999;341(6):410–8.

63. Lipids Research Clinics Program. The Lipid Research Clinics Coronary Primary Prevention Trial Results. Reduction in incidence of coronary heart disease. JAMA 1984;251:351–64.

64. Bays HE, Stein EA. Pharmacotherapy for dyslipidemia: current therapies and future agents. Expert Opin Pharmacother 2003;4:1901–38.

Diabetes and Cardiovascular Disease Prevention in Older Adults

Christine T. Cigolle, MD, MPH[a,b,*], Caroline S. Blaum, MD, MS[b,c], Jeffrey B. Halter, MD[d]

KEYWORDS

- Diabetes mellitus • Cardiovascular disease
- Prevention • Aging

Diabetes mellitus is a major risk factor for cardiovascular disease and mortality. Type 2 diabetes, the focus of this article, has its greatest prevalence and incidence in the older adult population, in whom it is frequently accompanied by dyslipidemia and hypertension, comorbid conditions with their own risk for cardiovascular events. Preventing cardiovascular disease due to diabetes in the older adult population may be achieved, first, by preventing or delaying the onset of diabetes, and second, by preventing cardiovascular events in those who have already developed diabetes.

Preventing the incidence and progression of cardiovascular disease in older adults with type 2 diabetes faces 3 challenges. First, prevention may require a comprehensive strategy, involving multiple ongoing interventions. Second, much of the evidence underlying the current management guidelines for older adults with diabetes has been extrapolated from data from other groups (eg, middle-age adults with diabetes, older-age adults without diabetes). Most of the major prospective trials have not included large numbers of older adults (eg, 70 years and older) or have excluded those with a substantial burden of comorbid diseases. Third, older adults with diabetes are a heterogeneous population.[1] Older adults with diabetes vary in age (young-old

[a] Department of Family Medicine, University of Michigan, 300 North Ingalls Building, Room 919, Ann Arbor, MI 48109-2007, USA
[b] VA Ann Arbor Healthcare System Geriatrics Research, Education and Clinical Center (GRECC), 2215 Fuller Road, Ann Arbor, Michigan 48105, USA
[c] Department of Internal Medicine, Division of Geriatric Medicine, University of Michigan, 300 North Ingalls Building, Room 914, Ann Arbor, MI 48109-2007, USA
[d] Department of Internal Medicine, Division of Geriatric Medicine, University of Michigan, 300 North Ingalls Building, Room 913, Ann Arbor, MI, USA
* Corresponding author. Department of Family Medicine, University of Michigan, 300 North Ingalls Building, Room 919, Ann Arbor, MI 48109-2007.
E-mail address: ccigolle@umich.edu (C.T. Cigolle).

Clin Geriatr Med 25 (2009) 607–641
doi:10.1016/j.cger.2009.09.001
0749-0690/09/$ – see front matter © 2009 Published by Elsevier Inc.

geriatric.theclinics.com

[65–70 years old] vs old-old [80 years and older]), age of onset and duration of diabetes, comorbid disease burden, and life expectancy. Older adults also vary in their burden of geriatric conditions such as cognitive impairment, falling, and functional impairment (basic activities of daily living [ADLs] and instrumental activities of daily living [IADLs]) and in their reliance on and access to caregiver support. The same characteristics that may limit participation by older adults in clinical trials also make it difficult for some older adults to implement a multi-intervention diabetes management plan.

The evidence base demonstrating the effectiveness of specific interventions in preventing cardiovascular disease in older adults with diabetes is limited. This article examines the evidence for interventions addressing the key modifiable risk factors. The article concludes with a discussion on individualizing and prioritizing the interventions in the overall health management plans of older adult patients with diabetes.

DIABETES: PATHOPHYSIOLOGY, DIAGNOSIS, AND EPIDEMIOLOGY

Type 2 diabetes is a metabolic disease defined by the presence of hyperglycemia. Type 2 diabetes is characterized by impaired insulin secretion and varying degrees of insulin resistance; it is also characterized by its long-term complications that are microvascular (nephropathy, retinopathy) and macrovascular (cardiac, cerebral, peripheral). Type 2 diabetes is frequently accompanied by other cardiovascular disease risk factors such as dyslipidemia, elevated blood pressure, and obesity. The disease is also frequently accompanied by lifestyle factors such as physical inactivity and use of cigarettes.

The continuum from normal glucose regulation to diabetes has an intermediate prediabetes phase (impaired fasting glucose [IFG], impaired glucose tolerance [IGT]). IFG is defined as fasting plasma glucose of 100 to 125 mg/dL.[2] IGT is defined as 2-hour plasma glucose of 140 to 199 mg/dL during an oral glucose tolerance test (OGTT).[2] These prediabetes conditions are themselves associated with an increased risk for cardiovascular disease. Diabetes is diagnosed by meeting 1 of 3 criteria: (1) fasting plasma glucose ≥126 mg/dL, (2) hyperglycemia symptoms and random fasting glucose ≥200 mg/dL, or (3) 2-hour plasma glucose ≥200 mg/dL during an OGTT.[2] There is no present consensus on the use of glycated hemoglobin levels (eg, hemoglobin A1c) to diagnose diabetes.

Diabetes has its greatest prevalence and incidence in the older adult population. Approximately 18% of adults 65 to 74 years old and 17% of those 75 years and older had diagnosed diabetes in 2006.[3] Drawing on the National Health and Nutrition Examination Survey (NHANES), the National Health Interview Survey (NHIS), and other data sources, the Centers for Disease Control and Prevention (CDC) estimated that 12 million, or 23%, of all adults age 60 years and older had diagnosed or undiagnosed diabetes in 2007.[4] Of these, approximately 95% had type 2 diabetes.[4] In 2007, the incidence rate for the development of diabetes in adults 65 to 79 years old was 12.5 per 1000, compared with 4.4 in those 18 to 44 years old and 11.7 in those 45 to 64 years old.[5] Diabetes incidence data are not available from the CDC for adults 80 years and older, the most rapidly growing segment of the population.

DIABETES AND CARDIOVASCULAR DISEASE: EPIDEMIOLOGY

Diabetes is a significant risk factor for cardiovascular disease. However, the precise role of diabetes in causing cardiovascular disease in older adults is less clear. In part, this uncertainty is due to the heterogeneity of diabetes in older adults (eg, diabetes onset in middle-age vs old age, presence of comorbid dyslipidemia and hypertension). This uncertainty is also due to cohort effects and the changing demography of the aging population.[6] Competing risks of mortality in the older adult population (eg, malignancy) are now more successfully treated, and older adults with chronic diseases have increasing life expectancy.

The Cardiovascular Health Study followed 5888 adults age 65 years and older (mean age 73 years).[7] Based on clinical history and measurement of fasting plasma glucose, 15% of male participants had IFG, 9% newly diagnosed diabetes, and 10% known diabetes. Among female participants 13% had IFG, 7% newly diagnosed diabetes, and 7% known diabetes. At baseline, the prevalence of clinical cardiac disease among participants with glucose disorders was: for men, IFG 28%, newly diagnosed diabetes 36%, and known diabetes 44% (compared with 29% for those without diabetes or IFG); and for women, IFG 25%, newly diagnosed diabetes 25%, and known diabetes 42% (compared with 19%). The prevalence of subclinical cardiac disease was: for men, IFG 30%, newly diagnosed diabetes 35%, and known diabetes 29% (compared with 24% for those without diabetes or IFG); and for women, IFG 22%, newly diagnosed diabetes 26%, and known diabetes 29% (compared with 19%). After adjusting for age and race, odds ratios for the prevalence of clinical and subclinical cardiac disease among men and women with glucose disorders, compared with those without diabetes or IFG, ranged from 0.95 to 3.01, generally increasing with the severity of the glucose disorder. (Note that a sizeable proportion of the older adults in the comparison group—the group not having diabetes or IFG by fasting plasma glucose testing—would have diabetes or IGT by OGTT and would therefore not be considered normoglycemic.) Ten-year follow-up study of participants with diabetes revealed that those with subclinical cardiac disease had a very high incidence of coronary heart disease, compared with moderate or no increased incidence among those not meeting criteria for subclinical disease.[8]

These findings have implications for interventions targeting modifiable risk factors for cardiovascular disease in older adults with glucose disorders. First, subclinical cardiac disease and risk for progression of cardiac disease can occur before the development of glucose elevations in the diabetes range. Thus, there may be benefit in targeting modifiable risk factors in those having IFG/IGT.[8]

Second, the prevalence of cardiac disease (whether diagnosed or undiagnosed/subclinical) in older adults with diabetes is sufficiently high that preventative interventions could generally be regarded as secondary prevention. The traditional understanding of the terms primary prevention and secondary prevention is that the former applies to actions taken to prevent a disease in individuals not having the disease, and the latter to actions taken to slow progression and prevent complications in individuals having the disease. Use of this terminology can be confusing with respect to diabetes and cardiac disease. The prevalence of subclinical cardiac disease is high among older adults with diabetes. Primary prevention studies of older adults with diabetes are likely to include a sizeable subset with unknown cardiac disease. Thus, interventions that target modifiable risk factors for cardiac disease in this group could be viewed as secondary, that is, preventing the progression of undiagnosed disease.

PREVENTING OR DELAYING THE ONSET OF DIABETES TO DECREASE THE RISK FOR CARDIOVASCULAR DISEASE

IFG and IGT represent part of the long asymptomatic phase that adults pass through before formal diagnosis with diabetes. This intermediate phase is critical, as IFG and IGT are risk factors for progression to diabetes and for cardiovascular disease. Interventions at this stage can have clinical impact by delaying or preventing progression to diabetes and by addressing comorbid risk factors (dyslipidemia, elevated blood pressure, obesity). Several diabetes prevention trials have investigated the efficacy of intensive lifestyle interventions or medications.[9-16] For example, the Diabetes Prevention Program (DPP) examined a lifestyle intervention including both weight loss (5%–10%) and exercise (30 minutes of moderate physical activity daily).[11] Compared with controls, the relative risk of converting to diabetes was 0.42 for those in the lifestyle intervention arm. In post hoc analysis, the lifestyle intervention appeared to be especially effective in adults older than 60 years, with a relative risk of converting to diabetes of only 0.29.[17]

All of the diabetes prevention trials, both lifestyle and medication, have been performed in predominantly middle-age populations (range of mean ages, 43–55 years old) with no studies or substudies in older adults.[9-16] An American Diabetes Association (ADA) Consensus Development Panel has recommended lifestyle interventions for those with IFG/IGT to prevent or delay diabetes, but did not specifically address older adults.[18] The only medication that was considered safe and effective in preventing diabetes, metformin, was recommended only for adults younger than 60 years, as metformin was relatively ineffective among older adults in the DPP.

The diabetes prevention trials have focused primarily on the reduction in the conversion to diabetes. No large prospective trials on diabetes prevention have conclusively demonstrated a reduction in the incidence of cardiovascular disease among participants of any age.[18] Long-term follow-up of the DPP population is in progress.

MODIFIABLE RISK FACTORS FOR CARDIOVASCULAR DISEASE IN OLDER ADULTS WITH DIABETES: EXAMINING THE EVIDENCE

Over the past 2 decades, multiple large prospective clinical trials have investigated modifiable risk factors for cardiovascular disease in adults with diabetes. Findings from these trials may be limited in their applicability to older adults with diabetes because many of the trials

- did not include substantial numbers of older adults (especially those 70 years and older) and are therefore underpowered to yield reliable findings for this age group
- did not include adults with complex health status (comorbid diseases and conditions, cognitive impairment, functional impairment, and so forth)
- did not perform analyses of the older adult subgroup (eg, those 65 years and older)
- employed varying primary and secondary outcomes (eg, composite outcomes, outcomes including other vascular disease such as stroke and peripheral arterial disease, and so forth), making comparison of the trials and generalizability of the findings difficult

In general, as the age of the diabetes patient increases, the evidence base for targeting modifiable risk factors decreases. Thus, for the oldest-old (80 years and older), the fasting growing segment of the population and among whom the prevalence of diabetes is high, very little evidence exists about the efficacy of interventions targeting cardiovascular risk factors. Clinicians caring for older adults with diabetes are faced with a challenge. There is frequently a lack of evidence supporting the efficacy of interventions in the older adult population. Yet, many older adults with diabetes who are at high risk for cardiac events are functional and active, and have substantial remaining life expectancy, making it reasonable to extrapolate to this group findings about prevention from younger age groups.

The present review article makes extensive use of tables (**Tables 1–6**) to summarize key clinical trials, highlighting characteristics of the trials most relevant to older adults with diabetes. The tables organize data from the trials as follows:

- The trial name, acronym, and sample size
- Dates of trial enrollment and ending (noting when and why trials were prematurely terminated)
- Relevant inclusion criteria, focusing on the age of the subjects and their comorbid conditions (except where noted, all the trials listed were limited to adults with type 2 diabetes)
- The intervention, indicating whether the focus was risk factor modification, the use of a specific medication, or both
- Pertinent cardiovascular outcomes (although stroke was often specified as a cardiovascular outcome for many of the trials, stroke is not listed in the tables as it is not a cardiac outcome)
- Key findings, including the degree of risk factor modification where relevant, the effect on cardiovascular risk, and the findings from any subgroup analysis of older adults.

Multiple Risk Factor Control

The Steno-2 trial studied the effects of an intensive, individualized, long-term multifactorial intervention targeting multiple modifiable cardiovascular risk factors in adults with diabetes (see **Table 1**).[19] The lifestyle intervention included dietary (low fat, low saturated fat), physical activity (regular light to moderate exercise), and smoking cessation components. Participants were placed on aspirin and on angiotensin-converting enzyme inhibitors or angiotensin-II receptor antagonists. Further stepwise pharmacologic interventions addressed elevated blood sugar, dyslipidemia, and elevated blood pressure. Participants were 40 to 65 years old at baseline, with a mean age of 55 years. Follow-up at 8 years found an absolute reduction of 20% in cardiovascular events; 5 patients would need to be treated for this time length to prevent one event.[20] Follow-up at 10 years found an absolute reduction of 13% in cardiovascular mortality.[21] Odds ratios from proportional hazards models were adjusted for age. There are no similar trials that have targeted multiple risk factors and that have in addition enrolled substantial numbers of older adults.

Glycemic Control

Elevated blood glucose is the cardiovascular risk factor for which the findings from clinical trials are most difficult to interpret (see **Table 2**). Data from large, epidemiologic studies of adults with diabetes indicate that higher glucose levels are associated with higher rates of cardiovascular disease.

In 2008, the United Kingdom Prospective Diabetes Study (UKPDS) released 10-year follow-up findings.[27] Subjects undergoing intensive glucose management had reduced mortality from any cause and reduced incidence of myocardial infarction; this was true for participants in the sulfonylurea and/or insulin group and in the metformin group. Of note, the baseline glycated hemoglobin levels for both intensive treatment groups (sulfonylurea-insulin group 7.9%, metformin group 8.4%) and for their respective standard treatment groups (8.5% and 8.9%) converged early during follow-up, so that reductions in mortality and myocardial infarctions may represent a "legacy effect"

Table 1
Trials of multiple risk factor control in adults with type 2 diabetes mellitus: participation of older adults

Study	Year	Participants	Intervention	Cardiovascular Outcomes	Findings
Steno-2 Study[19-21] N = 160	1992–1993; trial ended in 2001	40–65 y old, mean age 55 ± 7 y Microalbuminuria	Comprehensive intensive therapy, GHb <6.5%, total cholesterol <175 mg/dL, triglycerides <150 mg/dL, BP <130/80, renin-angiotensin system blocker, aspirin, low fat diet, exercise, smoking cessation	Death from any cause, CV death, composite of CVD events	Reduction in death from any cause (20% absolute risk reduction, 46% adjusted relative risk reduction) Reduction in CV death (13% absolute risk reduction, 57% relative risk reduction) Reduction in CVD events (29% absolute risk reduction, 59% relative risk reduction) Proportional-hazards model adjusted for age

Abbreviations: BP, blood pressure; CV, cardiovascular; CVD, cardiovascular disease; GHb, glycated hemoglobin.

from previous differences in degree of glycemic control. The generalizability of the UKPDS findings to older adults is limited by the young age and relatively good overall health of UKPDS participants. The maximum age at initial enrollment was 65 years, with a mean age of 63 years at the beginning of the post-trial monitoring phase in 1997. The 10-year follow-up study did not include an older adult subgroup analysis.

Two later studies were designed to examine the role of glycemic control in preventing cardiovascular disease in older adults with diabetes, many of whom had comorbidities: the action to control cardiovascular risk in diabetes (ACCORD) trial[22,23] and the action in diabetes and vascular disease (ADVANCE) trial.[24] Subjects in both studies either had or were at high risk for cardiovascular disease. In both studies, subjects in the intensive glucose control arms achieved a glycated hemoglobin level of 6.4%. However, neither study was able to detect a reduction in major cardiovascular events or macrovascular events. Further, mortality was increased in the intensive glucose control arm of the ACCORD trial, resulting in premature termination of this phase of the study. No simple explanation for the increased mortality was evident. Both ACCORD and ADVANCE enrolled older adults, with a mean age of 62 years for ACCORD and 66 years for ADVANCE.[22,24] The ACCORD trial did not include an older adult subgroup analysis. The ADVANCE trial reported that the effects of intensive glucose control on major vascular events across participant subgroups, including age, were consistent with the trial's overall findings.[24] Both studies were somewhat underpowered as overall event rates were lower than predicted. Thus, sample sizes may not have been adequate to detect an effect. Also, additional follow-up time may be required for glycemic control to show benefit.

A third trial, the veterans affairs diabetes trial (VADT), also recently concluded.[25,26] The intervention, to reduce the glycated hemoglobin by 1.5 percentage points (to 6.9%), was achieved. Consistent with the findings from ACCORD and ADVANCE, there was no significant reduction in any cardiovascular outcome, nor was there reduction in death from any cause. The trial did not include an older adult subgroup analysis.

The PROspective pioglitAzone clinical trial In macroVascular Events (PROactive) study demonstrated reduction in secondary cardiovascular disease outcomes for adults with diabetes who already had macrovascular disease.[28,29] However, participants in the pioglitazone arm had a substantial increase in heart failure, and the medication had no effect on the study's primary cardiovascular outcomes. (The primary end point of the study was time from randomization to all-cause mortality, nonfatal myocardial infarction [including silent infarction], nonfatal stroke, acute coronary syndrome, coronary/peripheral arterial interventions, or amputation above the ankle. Secondary end points included time to the first event or death from any cause, nonfatal myocardial infarction [excluding silent infarction], and nonfatal stroke; time to cardiovascular death; and time to individual components of the primary composite end point.[28,29])

The ADA and the American College of Cardiology released a statement on the ACCORD, ADVANCE, and VADT, drawing some tentative conclusions that may be particularly relevant to older adults with diabetes.[2,22,24,26,112,113] First, controlling blood glucose seems to confer more modest benefit in preventing cardiovascular disease than other modifiable risk factors. Second, the more recent studies have targeted the flatter portion of the curve relating blood glucose level with risk for cardiovascular disease (ie, decrease in glycated hemoglobin level from 7% to 6% compared with a decrease from 9% to 7%). Third, "subset analyses of ACCORD, ADVANCE, and VADT suggest the hypothesis that patients with shorter duration of type 2 diabetes and without established atherosclerosis might reap cardiovascular

Table 2
Trials of glucose control in adults with type 2 diabetes mellitus: participation of older adults

Study	Year	Participants	Intervention	Cardiovascular Outcomes	Findings
Action to Control Cardiovascular Risk in Diabetes (ACCORD)[22,23] N = 10251	2001–2005; glucose control study terminated prematurely in 2008	40–79 y old with CVD, OR 55–79 y old with atherosclerosis, LVH, albuminuria, or ≥2 other CV risk factors Mean age 62 ± 7 y GHb ≥7.5%	Intensive therapy, GHb target of <6.0% (vs standard therapy, GHb target of 7.0%–7.9%)	CV death, nonfatal MI	Increase in mortality (resulting in premature termination of glucose control study) No reduction in major CV events Achieved GHb level of 6.4% No older adult subgroup analysis
Action in Diabetes and Vascular disease (ADVANCE)[24] N = 11140	2001–2003; trial ended in 2008	55 years or older, mean age 66 ± 6 y Age at diabetes diagnosis ≥30 y old History of major CVD or ≥1 other CVD risk factors	Intensive therapy, GHb target of ≤6.5% (vs standard therapy)	CV death, nonfatal MI	No reduction in death from any cause, CV death, or major macrovascular events Achieved GHb level of 6.4% Increase in hypoglycemic events and hospitalizations Findings were consistent across participant subgroups, including age

Study	Dates	Population	Intervention	Outcome	Results
Veterans Affairs Diabetes Trial (VADT)[25,26] N = 1791	2000–2003; trial ended in 2008	≥41 y old, mean age 60 ± 9 y. Inadequate response to maximal doses of oral agent ± insulin GHb ≥7.5%	Intensive therapy, reduction of 1.5 in % GHb (vs standard therapy, GHb target of <9%)	CV death, MI, new/worsening HF, CV surgery, inoperable CAD	No reduction in any CV outcome. No reduction in death from any cause. Achieved target of reduction of 1.5 in % GHb (to 6.9%). Increase in hypoglycemic events. No older adult subgroup analysis
United Kingdom Prospective Diabetes Study (UKPDS), 10-y follow-up study[27] N = 4209 (N = 3277 for post-trial follow-up)	1977–1991; trial ended in 1997; 10-y follow-up study in 2007	25–65 y old, mean age 62 ± 8, at beginning of 10-y follow-up. Newly diagnosed diabetes	Intensive therapy, via: Sulfonylurea/Insulin, or Metformin (vs standard therapy)	Death from any cause, MI	Reduction in death from any cause and reduction in MI for intensive treatment by sulfonylurea/insulin group (15%, 13%) and for intensive treatment by metformin group (33%, 27%). Reductions were sustained from the post-trial phase. GHb differences rapidly converged during follow-up, so reductions were a "legacy effect." No older adult subgroup analysis

(continued on next page)

Table 2
(*continued*)

Study	Year	Participants	Intervention	Cardiovascular Outcomes	Findings
PROspective pioglitAzone Clinical Trial In macroVascular Events (PROactive)[28] N = 5238	2001–2002; followed up into 2005	35–75 y old, mean age 62 ± 8 HbA1c >6.5% Evidence of extensive macrovascular disease	Stepwise Pioglitazone to maximum doses (vs placebo)	Death from any cause, nonfatal MI, ACS, CABG or PCI	Reduction in the composite of death from any cause, nonfatal MI, and stroke (16%) (secondary outcome) Reduction of 0.8 in % HbA1c Findings consistent in subgroup analyses, including age
PROspective pioglitAzone Clinical Trial In macroVascular Events (PROactive), subanalysis of participants with previous MI[29] N = 2445	Same	35–75 y old, mean age 62 ± 8 HbA1c >6.5% Previous MI	Same	Death from any cause, nonfatal MI, ACS, CABG or PCI	Reduction in fatal and nonfatal MI (28%) and in ACS (37%) Reduction of 0.8 in % GHb Adjustment for advanced age made no difference to estimate of treatment effect/hazard ratio

Abbreviations: ACS, acute coronary syndrome; CABG, coronary artery bypass graft; CAD, coronary artery disease; CV, cardiovascular; CVD, cardiovascular disease; GHb, glycated hemoglobin; HbA1c, hemoglobin A1c; HF, heart failure; LVH, left ventricular hypertrophy; MI, myocardial infarction; PCI, percutaneous coronary intervention.

benefit from intensive glycemic control. It is conversely possible that potential risks of intensive glycemic control may outweigh its benefits in other patients, such as those with a very long duration of diabetes, known history of severe hypoglycemia, advanced atherosclerosis, and advanced age/frailty."[113] However, this hypothesis regarding differential effectiveness and risk of glucose lowering requires definitive testing.

Lipid Control

Multiple trials have investigated dyslipidemia as a modifiable risk factor in the primary and secondary prevention of cardiovascular disease.[30–67,114–117] However, there are no large trials of lipid-lowering interventions specifically in older adults with diabetes.

Benefit for older adults with diabetes has been extrapolated from trials of older adults at risk for cardiovascular disease that include but are not limited to those with diabetes. For example, the prospective study of pravastatin in the elderly at risk (PROSPER), a primary and secondary prevention trial whose participants were 70 to 82 years old, found a 15% reduction in coronary artery disease events among those receiving pravastatin.[117]

Findings from trials (or trial substudies) of adults with diabetes have also been extrapolated to older adults. **Table 3** summarizes lipid-lowering trials/subtrials whose subjects all had diabetes and which included at least some elderly patients. Of the trials investigating statins for the primary prevention of cardiovascular disease in adults with diabetes, results from the collaborative atorvastatin diabetes study (CARDS) have been the most persuasive.[30] The study enrolled patients of age 40 to 75 years old, with a mean age of 62 years. Atorvastatin was associated with a 36% reduction in acute coronary events; as a result, the trial was terminated prematurely. Adjustment for baseline age made no difference to the estimate of the treatment effect, and tests for heterogeneity of effect were not significant for age. The anglo-scandinavian cardiac outcomes trial—lipid-lowering arm (ASCOT-LLA) diabetes substudy included adults 40 to 79 years old, with a mean age of 64 years. This trial found a nonsignificant reduction in cardiovascular events and procedures for adults 60 years and older.[35] However, the trial was terminated prematurely due to findings in the larger population sample, thereby underpowering the older adult subgroup analysis.

Several trials have investigated statins for the secondary prevention of cardiovascular disease in adults with diabetes.[36–60] In general, these trials demonstrated a beneficial effect of statins on lipid profiles and a reduction in cardiovascular events. The only 2 trials that included an analysis of older adults reported either no change in the magnitude of risk reduction after adjustment for age (cholesterol and recurrent events trial),[48,49] or an 18% reduction in major vascular events for adults age 65 years and older (heart protection study).[58–60]

Three large trials have investigated fibrates for primary and/or secondary prevention of cardiovascular disease in adults with diabetes. In each, fibrates had a favorable effect on the lipid profile. Two trials demonstrated reduction in cardiovascular events,[61–65] and the other found decreased progression of atherosclerosis on angiography.[66,67] Only one study, the fenofibrate intervention and event lowering in diabetes (FIELD) trial, included a subanalysis of older adults. This study found that there was no significant reduction in total cardiovascular disease events for adults 65 years and older; in contrast, there was a 20% reduction in events in subjects younger than 65 years ($P = .003$).[64]

In sum, trials investigating lipid-lowering agents, specifically the more recent statin trials, suggest benefit in older adults with diabetes. However, evidence is more limited

Table 3
Trials of lipid control in adults with type 2 diabetes mellitus: participation of older adults

Study	Year	Participants	Intervention	Cardiovascular Outcomes	Findings
Collaborative Atorvastatin Diabetes Study (CARDS)[30-32] N = 2838	1997–2001; trial terminated prematurely in 2003	40–75 y old, mean age 62 ± 8 y ≥1 CV risk factors: HTN, retinopathy, micro/ macroalbuminuria, current smoking LDL <4.14 mmol/L No known CVD	Atorvastatin 10 mg daily (vs placebo)	Acute CHD events, coronary revascularization	Reduction in acute coronary events (36%) and coronary revascularization (31%) Adjustment for baseline age made no difference to estimate of treatment effect
Anglo-Scandinavian Cardiac Outcomes Trial—Lipid-Lowering Arm (ASCOT-LLA), analysis of diabetes subgroup[33-35] N = 2532	1998–2000; trial terminated prematurely in 2002	40–79 y old, mean age 64 ± 8 y HTN ≥3 other risk factors, one of which was diabetes No known CHD	Atorvastatin 10 mg daily (vs placebo)	Total CV events and procedures	Reduction in major CV events and procedures (23%) Subgroup analysis of participants >60 y old: reduction in major CV events and procedures nonsignificant (hazard ratio 0.87, P = .30) (Note: subgroup analysis underpowered due to trial termination)
Treating to New Targets (TNT), analysis of diabetes subgroup[36-39] N = 1501	1998–1999; trial ended in 2004	35–75 y old, mean age: 63 ± 8 y CHD	Atorvastatin 80 mg daily (vs atorvastatin 10 mg daily)	CHD death, nonfatal MI, resuscitated cardiac arrest	Reduction in major CV events (25%) No older adult subgroup analysis

Study	Dates	Inclusion criteria	Intervention	Outcome	Results/Notes
Pravastatin or Atorvastatin Evaluation and Infection Therapy—Thrombolysis in Myocardial Infarction 22 (PROVE IT—TIMI 22), analysis of diabetes subgroup[40-42] N = 978 (3184 without diabetes)	2000–2001; trial ended in 2003	≥ 18 y old, mean age 60 ± 11 y Recent hospitalization for ACS Total cholesterol ≤240 mg/dL OR ≤200 mg/dL if on long-term lipid-lowering medication	Atorvastatin 80 mg daily (vs pravastatin 40 mg daily)	Death from any cause, MI, unstable angina, coronary revascularization	Absolute risk reduction in composite of acute cardiac events (5.5%) Note: Study may have included small numbers of participants with type 1 diabetes No older adult subgroup analysis
Lescol Intervention Prevention Study (LIPS), analysis of diabetes subgroup[43,44] N = 202 (1475 without diabetes)	1996–1998; follow-up was 3–4 y	18–80 y old, mean age 63 ± 8 y Total cholesterol 135–270 mg/dL Fasting triglycerides <400 mg/dL Undergoing first successful PCI	Fluvastatin 80 mg daily (vs placebo)	Major adverse cardiac events (MACE): cardiac death, nonfatal MI, reintervention procedure	Reduction in MACE (51%) No older adult subgroup analysis
Long-Term Intervention with Pravastatin in Ischemic Disease (LIPID), analysis of diabetes and IFG subgroup[45-47] N = 1077, diabetes N = 940, IFG (6997 without diabetes)	1990–1992; trial ended in 1997	31–75 y old, mean age 64 y Recent MI/unstable angina Total cholesterol 4.0–7.0 mmol/L and fasting triglycerides <5.0 mmol/L	Pravastatin 40 mg daily (vs placebo)	CHD death, nonfatal MI	Reduction in the composite of CHD death and nonfatal MI in both subgroups: diabetes (19%) and impaired fasting glucose (36%) No older adult subgroup analysis

(continued on next page)

Table 3
(continued)

Study	Year	Participants	Intervention	Cardiovascular Outcomes	Findings
Cholesterol and Recurrent Events (CARE), analysis of diabetes subgroup[48,49] N = 586 (3573 without diabetes)	1989–1991; trial ended in 1996	21–75 y old, mean age 61 ± 8 y MI 3–20 mo before study LDL 115–174 mg/dL Triglycerides <350 mg/dL	Pravastatin 40 mg daily (vs placebo)	CHD death, nonfatal MI	Reduction in composite of coronary events (25%) Adjustment for age did not alter magnitude of risk reduction
Post Coronary Artery Bypass Graft (CABG) Trial, analysis of diabetes subgroup[50,51] N = 116 (1235 without diabetes)	1989–1991; mean duration of follow-up was 4 y	21–74 y old, mean age 63 y CABG using saphenous vein grafts 1–11 y previously	Lovastatin (and cholestyramine as necessary) to LDL of 60–85 mg/dL (vs therapy to LDL of 130–140 mg/dL)	Clinical: death, MI, or repeat revascularization Angiographic: substantial progression of atherosclerosis in grafts	No significant reduction in clinical or angiographic outcomes (but trial not powered for clinical outcomes) Reduction in both clinical and angiographic outcomes similar in magnitude to adults without diabetes No older adult subgroup analysis

Study	Dates	Inclusion criteria	Intervention	Outcome	Results/Notes
Scandinavian Simvastatin Survival Study (4S), analysis of diabetes subgroup[52-56] N = 202 (4242 without diabetes)	1988–1989; trial ended in 1994	35–70 y old, mean age 60 ± 7 y History of MI or angina Total cholesterol 5.5–8.0 mmol/L Triglycerides ≤2.5 mmol/L	Simvastatin 20–40 mg daily (vs placebo)	Total mortality	No significant reduction in total mortality Reduction in major CHD events (45%) Note: Study may not have included subjects with more severe diabetes Study may have included small numbers of subjects with type 1 diabetes No older adult subgroup analysis
Atorvastatin Study for Prevention of Coronary Heart Disease Endpoints in Non-Insulin-Dependent Diabetes Mellitus (ASPEN)[57] N = 2410	1996–1999; median duration of follow-up was 4 y	40–75 y old, mean age 61 ± 8 y LDL ≤140 mg/dL (if MI or interventional procedure previously) OR LDL ≤160 mg/dL (if not) Triglycerides ≤600 mg/dL	Atorvastatin 10 mg daily (vs placebo)	CV death, nonfatal MI, CV procedures, worsening/unstable angina	No significant reduction in composite of cardiovascular outcomes No older adult subgroup analysis
Heart Protection Study (HPS), analysis of diabetes subgroup[58-60] N = 5963	1994–1997; trial ended in 2001	40–80 y old, mean age 62 ± 9 y Total cholesterol ≥135 mg/dL	Simvastatin 40 mg daily (vs placebo)	CHD death, nonfatal MI	Reduction in major coronary events (27%) Note: Study included subjects with type 1 diabetes Subgroup analysis of participants ≥65 y old: 18% reduction in major vascular events

(continued on next page)

Table 3
(continued)

Study	Year	Participants	Intervention	Cardiovascular Outcomes	Findings
Veterans Affairs HDL Intervention Trial (VA-HIT), analysis of diabetes subgroup[61–63] N = 627, diabetes N = 142, undiagnosed diabetes N = 323, IFG (1425 without diabetes)	1991–1993; trial ended in 1998	<74 y old, mean age 65 ± 6 y Male Coronary heart disease HDL ≤40 mg/dL LDL ≤140 mg/dL Triglycerides ≤300 mg/dL 4 study groups: diagnosed diabetes, undiagnosed diabetes, IFG, normal fasting glucose	Gemfibrozil 1200 mg daily (vs placebo)	CHD death, nonfatal MI	Reduction in major CV events (32%) and CHD death (41%) for subjects with diabetes No older adult subgroup analysis
Fenofibrate Intervention and Event Lowering in Diabetes (FIELD)[64,65] N = 9795	1998–2000; trial ended in 2005	50–75 y old, mean age 62 ± 7 y Total cholesterol 3.0–6.5 mmol/L Total cholesterol/HDL ≥4.0 OR triglycerides 1.0–5.0 mmol/L	Fenofibrate 200 mg daily (vs placebo)	CHD death, nonfatal MI	No significant reduction in composite of CHD death and nonfatal MI Reduction in total CV events (11%) Subgroup analysis of participants ≥65 y old: no reduction in total CV events ($P = .9$)

| Diabetes Atherosclerosis Intervention Study (DAIS)[66,67] N = 731 | Mid 1990s | 40–65 y old, mean age 57 ± 6 y Cholesterol/HDL ≥4.0 LDL 3.5–4.5 mmol/L AND triglyceride ≤5.2 mmol/L, OR LDL ≤4.5 mmol/L AND triglyceride 1.7–5.2 mmol/L Hemoglobin A1c ≤170% laboratory's upper limit | Fenofibrate 200 mg daily (vs placebo) | Angiographic: average mean segment diameter, average minimum lumen diameter, average percentage diameter stenosis | Significantly less progression in mean segment diameter (25%), minimum lumen diameter (40%), and percentage diameter stenosis (42%) No older adult subgroup analysis |

Abbreviations: ACS, acute coronary syndrome; CABG, coronary artery bypass graft; CHD, coronary heart disease; CV, cardiovascular; CVD, cardiovascular disease; HTN, hypertension; IFG, impaired fasting glucose; PCI, percutaneous coronary intervention.

Table 4
Trials of blood pressure control in adults with type 2 diabetes mellitus: participation of older adults

Study	Year	Participants	Intervention	Cardiovascular Outcomes	Findings
Anglo-Scandinavian Cardiac Outcomes Trial—Blood Pressure-Lowering Arm (ASCOT-BPLA), analysis of diabetes subgroup[68,69] N = 5137	1998–2000; trial terminated prematurely in 2004	40–79 y old, mean age 63 ± 8 y HTN ≥3 other risk factors, one of which was diabetes	Target BP <130/80 Amlodipine ± perindopril vs Atenolol ± bendroflumethiazide	Fatal CHD, nonfatal MI, total CV events and procedures	Reduction in total CV events and procedures (14%) in amlodipine arm (Trial terminated prematurely as a result) Reductions in systolic and diastolic BP: amlodipine to 136/75, atenolol to 137/76 Reduction in events was comparable in age groups above and below 60 y
Antihypertensive and Lipid-Lowering Treatment to Prevent Heart Attack Trial (ALLHAT)[70-74] N = 13101, diabetes N = 1399, IFG (17012 without diabetes)	1994–1998; trial ended in 2002	≥55 y old, mean age 67 ± 7 y HTN	Target BP <140/90 Chlorthalidone vs Amlodipine vs Lisinopril, followed by dose increase/ addition of other agents	Fatal CHD, nonfatal MI	Diabetes group: No significant differences in relative risk for fatal coronary heart disease/nonfatal MI Impaired fasting glucose group: Significantly higher risk for fatal CHD/ nonfatal MI for amlodipine vs chlorthalidone treatment No older adult subgroup analysis

Study	Duration	Population	Intervention	Outcome	Results
Hypertension Optimal Treatment (HOT)[75-77] N = 1501 (17289 without diabetes)	1992–1994; trial ended in 1997	50–80 y old, mean age 63 ± 7 y HTN Diastolic BP: 100–115	Target diastolic BP ≤90 vs ≤85 vs ≤80 Felodipine, followed by dose increase/addition of other agents	Major CV events (MI, CVD)	Reduction in CVD (67%, $P = .016$) and in major CV events (50%, $P = .005$) for target group ≤80 compared with target group ≤90 No older adult subgroup analysis
Appropriate Blood Pressure Control In Diabetes (ABCD)[78-83] N = 950	1991–1992; nisoldipine arm terminated prematurely in 1997; trial ended in 1998	40–74 y old, mean age 57 ± 8 y Noninsulin-dependent diabetes Diastolic BP ≥ 90 mm Hg (N = 470), OR diastolic BP 80–89 mm Hg (N = 480)	Target diastolic BP 75 vs 80–89 Stepwise Nisoldipine vs Enalapril (vs placebo)	CVD, nonfatal MI, HF	Hypertensive group: Reduction in fatal and nonfatal MI in enalapril group Adjusted risk ratio for nisoldipine group was 4.2 for MI No significant differences in BP control between intensive and moderate groups Normotensive group: No significant difference in CV events or deaths Note: Primary outcome measure was glomerular filtration rate. Not powered for CV outcome measures Risk ratios adjusted for age (and other covariates)

(continued on next page)

Table 4
(continued)

Study	Year	Participants	Intervention	Cardiovascular Outcomes	Findings
Systolic Hypertension in Europe (Syst-Eur) analysis of diabetes subgroup[84–88] N = 492 (4203 without diabetes)	1989–1997; trial terminated prematurely in 1997	≥60 y old Diabetes with adequate blood glucose control Systolic BP 160–219 (sitting) Diastolic BP <95 (sitting) Systolic BP ≥140 (standing)	Target to reduce systolic BP (sitting) by ≥20, to <150 Stepwise: Nitrendipine with/ replaced by Enalapril and/or hydrochlorothiazide (vs placebo)	HF, MI, sudden death	Reduction in overall mortality (55%), CVD (76%), all CV events (69%), and cardiac events (63%) Cox regression adjusted for age (and other covariates) Study limited to adults ≥60 y old
Systolic Hypertension in the Elderly Program (SHEP)[89] N = 583 (4149 without diabetes)	Late 1980s	≥60 y old Noninsulin treated diabetes only Systolic BP ≥160 mm Hg Diastolic BP <90 mm Hg	Chlorthalidone, with step up to Atenolol or Reserpine	Death from any cause, fatal CHD, nonfatal MI, major coronary heart events	Reduction in major CVD events (34%) Study limited to adults ≥60 y old

| United Kingdom Prospective Diabetes Study (UKPDS)/Hypertension in Diabetes Study (HDS), 10-year follow-up study[90]

N = 1148
(N = 884 for post-trial follow-up) | 1987–1991; trial ended in 1997; 10-y follow-up study ended in 2007 | 25–65 y old, mean age 63 ± 8, at beginning of 10-y follow-up Newly diagnosed diabetes HTN | Target BP <150/85 Captopril vs Atenolol (vs target <180/105, not using ACE-inhibitors or β-blockers) | Death from any cause, MI | Nonsignificant relative risk reductions seen during the trial for death from any cause and for MI diminished during post-trial follow-up

No significant differences between ACE-inhibitor and β-blocker groups in aggregate end points were seen during the trial or during post-trial follow-up, except for emerging increase in risk of death from any cause in the ACE-inhibitor group ($P = .047$)

Baseline differences between intensive- and moderate-control groups in mean systolic and diastolic BPs were lost by y 1 and y 2, respectively

No older adult subgroup analysis |

Abbreviations: ACE, angiotensin-converting enzyme; BP, blood pressure; CHD, coronary heart disease; CV, cardiovascular; CVD, cardiovascular disease; HF, heart failure; HTN, hypertension; IFG, impaired fasting glucose; MI, myocardial infarction.

Table 5
Trials of ACE inhibitor use in adults with type 2 diabetes mellitus: participation of older adults

Study	Year	Participants	Intervention	Cardiovascular Outcomes	Findings
Action in Diabetes and Vascular disease (ADVANCE)[91] N = 11140	2001–2003; trial ended in 2007	≥55 y old, mean age 66 ± 6 y Age at diabetes diagnosis ≥30 y old History of major CVD or ≥1 other CVD risk factors	Perindopril and indapamide, in addition to current therapy (vs placebo, in addition to current therapy)	CV death, nonfatal MI.	Nonsignificant reduction in major macrovascular events (hazard ratio 0.92, P = .16) Reduction in CV death (18%) and in death from any cause (14%) Reduction in combined major macrovascular or microvascular events (11%) in adults ≥65 y old No heterogeneity of treatment effects between subgroups for total mortality, CV death, and total coronary events
Bergamo Nephrologic Diabetes Complications Trial (BENEDICT), ECG-LVH subanalysis[92–94] N = 816	Early 2000s	≥40 y old, mean age 62 ± 8 y HTN Duration of type 2 diabetes ≤25 y Creatinine ≤1.5 mg/dL Normal urinary albumin excretion rate No ECG evidence of LVH at baseline	Trandolapril (vs non-ACE inhibitor therapy) Target BP <130/80	ECG-defined LVH	Reduction in incidence of LVH (adjusted hazard ratio 0.35, P = .0018) Small differences between groups in systolic and diastolic BPs Hazard ratio remained significant when adjusted for baseline characteristics, including age

Study	Dates/status	Population	Intervention	Composite end point	Results
Reduction of Endpoints in NIDDM with the Angiotensin II Antagonist Losartan (RENAAL)[95-99] N = 1513	1996–1998; trial terminated prematurely in 2001	31–70 y old, mean age 60 ± 7 y Nephropathy	Losartan, in addition to current therapy (vs placebo, in addition to current therapy)	Composite end point of morbidity and mortality from CV causes (secondary outcome)	No significant differences in composite end point Reduction in first hospitalization for HF (32%) Reduction in LVH and in risk conferred by LVH on CV outcomes Extensive analysis in adults >65 y old: no difference in benefits or risks of intervention compared with younger adults
Non-Insulin-Dependent Diabetes, Hypertension, Microalbuminuria or Proteinuria, Cardiovascular Events, and Ramipril (DIABHYCAR)[100,101] N = 4912	1995–1998; trial ended in 2001	>50 y old, mean age 65 ± 8 y Microalbuminuria or proteinuria	Ramipril (low dose), in addition to current therapy (vs placebo, in addition to current therapy)	CV death, nonfatal MI, HF requiring hospitalization	No effect on CV outcomes Minimal but significant reduction in systolic and diastolic BPs No older adult subgroup analysis
Heart Outcomes Prevention Evaluation (HOPE)[102-108] N = 3577	1993–1995; trial terminated prematurely in 1999	≥55 y old, mean age 65 ± 6 y Previous CV event or ≥1 CV risk factors (in addition to diabetes)	Ramipril, in addition to current therapy (vs placebo, in addition to current therapy)	CV death, MI	Reduction in major CV outcomes (25%) Minimal but significant reduction in systolic and diastolic BPs No older adult subgroup analysis in diabetics

Abbreviations: ACE, angiotensin-converting enzyme; BP, blood pressure; CV, cardiovascular; CVD, cardiovascular disease; ECG, electrocardiogram; HF, heart failure; HTN, hypertension; LVH, left ventricular hypertrophy; MI, myocardial infarction.

Table 6
Trials of aspirin use in adults with type 2 diabetes mellitus: participation of older adults

Study	Year	Participants	Intervention	Cardiovascular Outcomes	Findings
Japanese Primary Prevention of Atherosclerosis With Aspirin for Diabetes (JPAD)[109,110] N = 2539	2002–2005; trial ended in 2008	30–85 y old, mean age 65 ± 10 y No documented CVD	Aspirin 81–100 mg daily (vs placebo)	Any atherosclerotic event	No significant reduction in atherosclerotic events Significant reduction in combined secondary outcome of fatal coronary and cerebrovascular events (hazard ratio 0.10, P = .0037) In subgroup of 1363 adults ≥65 y old, atherosclerotic events were significantly lower in the aspirin group (hazard ratio 0.68, P = .047)
Primary Prevention Project (PPP), analysis of diabetes subgroup[111] N = 1031 (3753 without diabetes)	1994–1998; trial terminated prematurely in 1998	≥50 y old, mean age 64 ± 8 y No history of major CV events	Aspirin 100 mg daily (vs placebo)	CV death, nonfatal MI	Nonsignificant reduction in total CV events Main trial terminated prematurely due to efficacy of aspirin in entire population sample, causing diabetes substudy to be underpowered No older adult subgroup analysis

Abbreviations: CV, cardiovascular; CVD, cardiovascular disease.

for older adults, especially those older than 80 years, compared with middle-age people. Further, evidence for the efficacy of fibrates in preventing cardiovascular disease in older adults is lacking. None of the trials demonstrated major adverse effects for statins or for fibrates in older patients. In summary, the available evidence indicates that statin therapy seems to be warranted for most older adults with diabetes.[1]

Blood Pressure Control

Similar to dyslipidemia, multiple trials have investigated elevated blood pressure as a modifiable risk factor in the prevention of cardiovascular disease (see **Table 4**).[68–90] Benefit for older adults with diabetes has been drawn from trials of older adults including but not limited to those with diabetes and from trials of middle- and older-age adults with diabetes.

An early study, the systolic hypertension in the elderly program (SHEP) trial, found that lowering systolic blood pressure in older adults resulted in decreased coronary heart disease death and nonfatal myocardial infarction (27%) and in decreased cardiovascular events (32%).[89] A substudy of participants with diabetes demonstrated a 34% reduction in cardiovascular events.

Several trials and their substudies have investigated blood pressure as a modifiable risk factor in the prevention of cardiovascular disease in adults with diabetes.[68–88,90] However, older adult subgroup analyses have generally been limited in scope. Both the systolic hypertension in Europe trial (Syst-Eur) diabetes substudy[84–88] and the Appropriate Blood Pressure Control in Diabetes (ABCD) trial[78–83] found substantial reduction in cardiac events, findings that persisted when adjusted for age. The anglo-Scandinavian cardiac outcomes trial—Blood Pressure-Lowering Arm (ASCOT-BPLA) diabetes substudy included a subanalysis of older adults, and found that reduction in events was comparable in age groups older and younger than 60 years.[68,69]

A related group of prospective trials evaluated the role of renin-angiotensin system antagonism (via angiotensin-converting enzyme [ACE] inhibitors or angiotensin-II receptor antagonists [ARB]) in modifying cardiovascular risk in adults with diabetes, irrespective of their effect on blood pressure (see **Table 5**).[91–108] Again, older adult subgroup analyses were limited in these studies. When performed, findings for older adults were generally consistent with those for middle-age adults. The reduction of endpoints in NIDDM with the angiotensin II antagonist losartan (RENAAL) trial included extensive analysis in participants 65 years and older, and found no difference in benefits or risks of losartan for older compared with younger subjects.[95–99] More recently, the ADVANCE trial found an 11% reduction in the relative risk for combined major macrovascular or microvascular events in adults 65 years and older.[91] Further, no heterogeneity of treatment effects between older and younger subgroups was found for total coronary events, cardiovascular deaths, or total mortality.

Thus, evidence from clinical trials suggests substantial benefit from lowering blood pressure in reducing cardiovascular risk in older adults with diabetes. Of note, blood pressure intervention trials and ACE inhibitor/ARB trials generally lack outcomes data on risk and side effect profiles relevant to the older adult population, such as orthostatic hypotension and falls.

Antiplatelet Agents

There has been limited study of aspirin for primary prevention in older adults with diabetes. Despite evidence for the efficacy of aspirin in the primary prevention of cardiovascular disease in adults at high risk, there is no clear evidence for its efficacy in adults with diabetes. Some researchers theorize that aspirin-insensitive mechanisms of platelet activation and thrombus formation may predominate in diabetes patients.[109] The primary prevention project (PPP) was terminated prematurely due to the efficacy of aspirin in the entire population sample; as a result, the diabetes substudy was underpowered (see **Table 6**).[109,110] Further, no older adult subgroup analysis was performed. More recently, the Japanese primary prevention of atherosclerosis with aspirin for diabetes (JPAD) found no significant reduction in atherosclerotic events.[111] However, in the older adults subgroup, atherosclerotic events were significantly lower in the aspirin group (hazard ratio [HR] 0.68, $P = .047$), suggesting that older adults with diabetes may selectively benefit from its use.

There is a rich literature on the place of aspirin in the secondary prevention of cardiovascular disease. Numerous prospective trials and retrospective observational studies have examined the role of aspirin in patient populations with specific diagnoses (eg, acute myocardial infarction) or undergoing specific procedures (eg, coronary angioplasty). For example, the Antiplatelet Trialists' Collaboration concluded that aspirin reduced vascular events in adults with known cardiovascular disease in both diabetes and older adult subgroups.[118] The Israeli Bezafibrate Infarction Prevention Study Group examined the efficacy of aspirin in adults with diabetes and coronary artery disease. Participants were 45 to 74 years in age, with a mean age of 60 years.[119] After adjustment for possible confounders, including age, treatment with aspirin predicted reduced cardiac (HR 0.8, 95% confidence interval [CI] 0.6–1.0) and overall mortality (HR 0.8, 95% CI 0.7–0.9).

Lifestyle Factors

There are no large prospective trials demonstrating the efficacy of targeting lifestyle factors as modifiable risk factors for cardiovascular disease in older adults with diabetes. Several studies have demonstrated the effect of lifestyle interventions on intermediate outcomes, that is, cardiovascular risk factors (glucose levels, lipid levels, blood pressure). The Look AHEAD (action for health in diabetes) trial is currently in progress and has randomized 5145 adults aged 45 to 75 years (mean age 60 years) either to intensive lifestyle intervention or to diabetes support and education.[120–122] The primary outcome is time to first cardiovascular disease event, and the study will continue until 2012, allowing for over 10 years of follow-up.

Drawing on epidemiologic studies and on expert recommendations, the American Geriatrics Society currently recommends the following lifestyle interventions for older adults with diabetes: smoking cessation, dietary therapy, weight loss, and increased physical activity.[1]

CARE DELIVERY AND POLICY: MULTIMORBIDITY, GERIATRIC CONDITIONS, AND FUNCTIONAL STATUS

Older adults with diabetes are a heterogeneous group, including older patients with known long-standing diabetes, persons with undiagnosed long-standing diabetes, and individuals with new-onset diabetes. Older adults with diabetes consequently vary in age, age at onset, duration of diabetes, comorbidity burden, functional status, and, importantly, life expectancy.

Interventions that target the key modifiable risk factors for cardiovascular disease require the involvement of both the physician and the patient to devise a comprehensive but individualized strategy for decreasing cardiovascular risk. In patients with complex health status, it may be difficult to integrate and prioritize interventions designed to decrease cardiovascular risk. Boyd and colleagues[123] suggested that for patients with multiple chronic diseases, adherence to multiple guidelines for individual diseases can be difficult. However, a recent study showed that those with multiple diseases were more likely to meet individual disease guidelines, as these patients had greater contact with physicians.[124]

It is important to recognize, however, that older adult health status goes beyond multiple diseases. Older adults with diabetes have increased prevalence of geriatric conditions. Cognitive impairment and falling affect the ability of these patients to implement regimens that target blood glucose and blood pressure. Individualizing and prioritizing interventions in the heterogeneous older adult group is a key health care priority. A substantial portion of the population has low or moderate health burden and should not be denied effective interventions due to age alone. The ADA and the American Geriatrics Society recommend that older adults who are cognitively and functionally intact and who have substantial life expectancy should follow standard recommendations to decrease cardiovascular risk. For older adults with reduced functional capacity or decreased life expectancy, weighing the benefit versus risk and associated burden of individual interventions is warranted.

SUMMARY

Cardiovascular disease is the major cause of death, and a leading cause of disability and impaired quality of life in older adults with diabetes. Therefore, preventing cardiovascular events in this population is an important goal of care. Available evidence supports the use of lipid-lowering agents and treatment of hypertension as effective measures to reduce cardiovascular risk in older adults with diabetes. Glucose control, smoking cessation, weight control, regular physical activity, and a prudent diet are also recommended, although data supporting the efficacy of these interventions are limited. While reducing cardiovascular morbidity and mortality remains a primary objective of preventive cardiology in older adults with diabetes, the impact of these interventions on functional well-being, cognition, and other geriatric syndromes requires further study.[125]

REFERENCES

1. Brown AF, Mangione CM, Saliba D, et al. Guidelines for improving the care of the older person with diabetes mellitus. J Am Geriatr Soc 2003;51(Suppl 5): S265–80.
2. Standards of medical care in diabetes—2009. Diabetes Care 2009;32(Suppl 1): S13–61.
3. Percentage of civilian, noninstitutionalized population with diagnosed diabetes, by age, United States, 1980–2006. Available at: http://www.cdc.gov/diabetes/statistics/prev/national/figbyage.htm; 2009. Accessed May 10, 2009.
4. Centers for Disease Control and Prevention. National Diabetes Fact Sheet, 2007;2008.
5. Incidence of diagnosed diabetes per 1,000 population aged 18–79 years, by age, United States, 1980–2007. Available at. http://www.cdc.gov/diabetes/statistics/incidence/fig3.htm. Accessed May 10, 2009.
6. Scranton RE, Dave JK, Gaziano JM. Macrovascular complication of diabetes in older adults. In: Munshi MN, Lipsitz LA, editors. Geriatric diabetes. New York: Informa Healthcare USA, Inc; 2007. p. 169–82.
7. Barzilay JI, Spiekerman CF, Kuller LH, et al. Prevalence of clinical and isolated subclinical cardiovascular disease in older adults with glucose disorders: the Cardiovascular Health Study. Diabetes Care 2001;24(7):1233–9.

8. Kuller LH, Arnold AM, Psaty BM, et al. 10-year follow-up of subclinical cardiovascular disease and risk of coronary heart disease in the Cardiovascular Health Study. Arch Intern Med 2006;166(1):71–8.

9. Chiasson JL, Josse RG, Gomis R, et al. Acarbose for prevention of type 2 diabetes mellitus: the STOP-NIDDM randomised trial. Lancet 2002;359(9323): 2072–7.

10. Gerstein HC, Yusuf S, Bosch J, et al. Effect of rosiglitazone on the frequency of diabetes in patients with impaired glucose tolerance or impaired fasting glucose: a randomised controlled trial. Lancet 2006;368(9541):1096–105.

11. Knowler WC, Barrett-Connor E, Fowler SE, et al. Reduction in the incidence of type 2 diabetes with lifestyle intervention or metformin. N Engl J Med 2002; 346(6):393–403.

12. Kosaka K, Noda M, Kuzuya T. Prevention of type 2 diabetes by lifestyle intervention: a Japanese trial in IGT males. Diabetes Res Clin Pract 2005;67(2): 152–62.

13. Pan XR, Li GW, Hu YH, et al. Effects of diet and exercise in preventing NIDDM in people with impaired glucose tolerance. The Da Qing IGT and Diabetes Study. Diabetes Care 1997;20(4):537–44.

14. Ramachandran A, Snehalatha C, Mary S, et al. The Indian Diabetes Prevention Programme shows that lifestyle modification and metformin prevent type 2 diabetes in Asian Indian subjects with impaired glucose tolerance (IDPP-1). Diabetologia 2006;49(2):289–97.

15. Torgerson JS, Hauptman J, Boldrin MN, et al. XENical in the prevention of diabetes in obese subjects (XENDOS) study: a randomized study of orlistat as an adjunct to lifestyle changes for the prevention of type 2 diabetes in obese patients. Diabetes Care 2004;27(1):155–61.

16. Tuomilehto J, Lindstrom J, Eriksson JG, et al. Prevention of type 2 diabetes mellitus by changes in lifestyle among subjects with impaired glucose tolerance. N Engl J Med 2001;344(18):1343–50.

17. Crandall J, Schade D, Ma Y, et al. The influence of age on the effects of lifestyle modification and metformin in prevention of diabetes. J Gerontol A Biol Sci Med Sci 2006;61(10):1075–81.

18. Nathan DM, Davidson MB, DeFronzo RA, et al. Impaired fasting glucose and impaired glucose tolerance: implications for care. Diabetes Care 2007;30(3): 753–9.

19. Gaede P, Vedel P, Parving HH, et al. Intensified multifactorial intervention in patients with type 2 diabetes mellitus and microalbuminuria: the Steno type 2 randomised study. Lancet 1999;353(9153):617–22.

20. Gaede P, Vedel P, Larsen N, et al. Multifactorial intervention and cardiovascular disease in patients with type 2 diabetes. N Engl J Med 2003;348(5):383–93.

21. Gaede P, Lund-Andersen H, Parving HH, et al. Effect of a multifactorial intervention on mortality in type 2 diabetes. N Engl J Med 2008;358(6):580–91.

22. Gerstein HC, Miller ME, Byington RP, et al. Effects of intensive glucose lowering in type 2 diabetes. N Engl J Med 2008;358(24):2545–59.

23. Goff DC Jr, Gerstein HC, Ginsberg HN, et al. Prevention of cardiovascular disease in persons with type 2 diabetes mellitus: current knowledge and rationale for the Action to Control Cardiovascular Risk in Diabetes (ACCORD) trial. Am J Cardiol 2007;99(12A):4i–20i.

24. Patel A, MacMahon S, Chalmers J, et al. Intensive blood glucose control and vascular outcomes in patients with type 2 diabetes. N Engl J Med 2008; 358(24):2560–72.

25. Abraira C, Duckworth W, McCarren M, et al. Design of the cooperative study on glycemic control and complications in diabetes mellitus type 2: Veterans Affairs Diabetes Trial. J Diabet Complications 2003;17(6):314–22.

26. Duckworth W, Abraira C, Moritz T, et al. Glucose control and vascular complications in veterans with type 2 diabetes. N Engl J Med 2009;360(2):129–39.

27. Holman RR, Paul SK, Bethel MA, et al. 10-year follow-up of intensive glucose control in type 2 diabetes. N Engl J Med 2008;359(15):1577–89.

28. Dormandy JA, Charbonnel B, Eckland DJ, et al. Secondary prevention of macrovascular events in patients with type 2 diabetes in the PROactive Study (PROspective pioglitAzone Clinical Trial In macroVascular Events): a randomised controlled trial. Lancet 2005;366(9493):1279–89.

29. Erdmann E, Dormandy JA, Charbonnel B, et al. The effect of pioglitazone on recurrent myocardial infarction in 2,445 patients with type 2 diabetes and previous myocardial infarction: results from the PROactive (PROactive 05) Study. J Am Coll Cardiol 2007;49(17):1772–80.

30. Colhoun HM, Betteridge DJ, Durrington PN, et al. Primary prevention of cardiovascular disease with atorvastatin in type 2 diabetes in the Collaborative Atorvastatin Diabetes Study (CARDS): multicentre randomised placebo-controlled trial. Lancet 2004;364(9435):685–96.

31. Neil HA, DeMicco DA, Luo D, et al. Analysis of efficacy and safety in patients aged 65-75 years at randomization: collaborative atorvastatin diabetes study (CARDS). Diabetes Care 2006;29(11):2378–84.

32. Plummer CJ. What's in the CARDS? Diabet Med 2006;23(7):711–4.

33. Sever PS, Dahlof B, Poulter NR, et al. Prevention of coronary and stroke events with atorvastatin in hypertensive patients who have average or lower-than-average cholesterol concentrations, in the Anglo-Scandinavian Cardiac Outcomes Trial—Lipid Lowering Arm (ASCOT-LLA): a multicentre randomised controlled trial. Lancet 2003;361(9364):1149–58.

34. Sever PS, Dahlof B, Poulter NR, et al. Rationale, design, methods and baseline demography of participants of the Anglo-Scandinavian Cardiac Outcomes Trial. ASCOT investigators. J Hypertens 2001;19(6):1139–47.

35. Sever PS, Poulter NR, Dahlof B, et al. Reduction in cardiovascular events with atorvastatin in 2,532 patients with type 2 diabetes: Anglo-Scandinavian Cardiac Outcomes Trial—lipid-lowering arm (ASCOT-LLA). Diabetes Care 2005;28(5):1151–7.

36. Deedwania P, Barter P, Carmena R, et al. Reduction of low-density lipoprotein cholesterol in patients with coronary heart disease and metabolic syndrome: analysis of the Treating to New Targets study. Lancet 2006;368(9539):919–28.

37. LaRosa JC, Grundy SM, Waters DD, et al. Intensive lipid lowering with atorvastatin in patients with stable coronary disease. N Engl J Med 2005;352(14):1425–35.

38. Shepherd J, Barter P, Carmena R, et al. Effect of lowering LDL cholesterol substantially below currently recommended levels in patients with coronary heart disease and diabetes: the Treating to New Targets (TNT) study. Diabetes Care 2006;29(6):1220–6.

39. Waters DD, Guyton JR, Herrington DM, et al. Treating to New Targets (TNT) Study: does lowering low-density lipoprotein cholesterol levels below currently recommended guidelines yield incremental clinical benefit? Am J Cardiol 2004;93(2):154–8.

40. Ahmed S, Cannon CP, Murphy SA, et al. Acute coronary syndromes and diabetes: is intensive lipid lowering beneficial? Results of the PROVE IT-TIMI 22 trial. Eur Heart J 2006;27(19):2323–9.

41. Cannon CP, Braunwald E, McCabe CH, et al. Intensive versus moderate lipid lowering with statins after acute coronary syndromes. N Engl J Med 2004; 350(15):1495–504.

42. Cannon CP, McCabe CH, Belder R, et al. Design of the pravastatin or atorvastatin evaluation and infection therapy (PROVE IT)-TIMI 22 trial. Am J Cardiol 2002;89(7):860–1.

43. Arampatzis CA, Goedhart D, Serruys PW, et al. Fluvastatin reduces the impact of diabetes on long-term outcome after coronary intervention—a Lescol Intervention Prevention Study (LIPS) substudy. Am Heart J 2005;149(2):329–35.

44. Serruys PW, de Feyter P, Macaya C, et al. Fluvastatin for prevention of cardiac events following successful first percutaneous coronary intervention: a randomized controlled trial. JAMA 2002;287(24):3215–22.

45. Design features and baseline characteristics of the LIPID (long-term intervention with pravastatin in ischemic disease) study: a randomized trial in patients with previous acute myocardial infarction and/or unstable angina pectoris. Am J Cardiol 1995;76(7):474–9.

46. Prevention of cardiovascular events and death with pravastatin in patients with coronary heart disease and a broad range of initial cholesterol levels. The Long-Term Intervention with Pravastatin in Ischaemic Disease (LIPID) Study Group. N Engl J Med 1998;339(19):1349–57.

47. Keech A, Colquhoun D, Best J, et al. Secondary prevention of cardiovascular events with long-term pravastatin in patients with diabetes or impaired fasting glucose: results from the LIPID trial. Diabetes Care 2003;26(10):2713–21.

48. Goldberg RB, Mellies MJ, Sacks FM, et al. Cardiovascular events and their reduction with pravastatin in diabetic and glucose-intolerant myocardial infarction survivors with average cholesterol levels: subgroup analyses in the cholesterol and recurrent events (CARE) trial. The Care Investigators. Circulation 1998; 98(23):2513–9.

49. Sacks FM, Pfeffer MA, Moye LA, et al. The effect of pravastatin on coronary events after myocardial infarction in patients with average cholesterol levels. Cholesterol and Recurrent Events Trial investigators. N Engl J Med 1996; 335(14):1001–9.

50. The effect of aggressive lowering of low-density lipoprotein cholesterol levels and low-dose anticoagulation on obstructive changes in saphenous-vein coronary-artery bypass grafts. The Post Coronary Artery Bypass Graft Trial Investigators. N Engl J Med 1997;336(3):153–62.

51. Hoogwerf BJ, Waness A, Cressman M, et al. Effects of aggressive cholesterol lowering and low-dose anticoagulation on clinical and angiographic outcomes in patients with diabetes: the Post Coronary Artery Bypass Graft Trial. Diabetes 1999;48(6):1289–94.

52. Randomised trial of cholesterol lowering in 4444 patients with coronary heart disease: the Scandinavian Simvastatin Survival Study (4S). Lancet 1994; 344(8934):1383–9.

53. Haffner SM. The Scandinavian Simvastatin Survival Study (4S) subgroup analysis of diabetic subjects: implications for the prevention of coronary heart disease. Diabetes Care 1997;20(4):469–71.

54. Kjekshus J, Pedersen TR. Reducing the risk of coronary events: evidence from the Scandinavian Simvastatin Survival Study (4S). Am J Cardiol 1995;76(9):64C–8C.

55. Pedersen TR, Wilhelmsen L, Faergeman O, et al. Follow-up study of patients randomized in the Scandinavian simvastatin survival study (4S) of cholesterol lowering. Am J Cardiol 2000;86(3):257–62.

56. Pyorala K, Pedersen TR, Kjekshus J, et al. Cholesterol lowering with simvastatin improves prognosis of diabetic patients with coronary heart disease. A subgroup analysis of the Scandinavian Simvastatin Survival Study (4S). Diabetes Care 1997;20(4):614–20.

57. Knopp RH, d'Emden M, Smilde JG, et al. Efficacy and safety of atorvastatin in the prevention of cardiovascular end points in subjects with type 2 diabetes: the atorvastatin study for prevention of coronary heart disease endpoints in non-insulin-dependent diabetes mellitus (ASPEN). Diabetes Care 2006;29(7): 1478–85.

58. Heart Protection Study Collaborative Group. MRC/BHF heart protection study of cholesterol-lowering therapy and of antioxidant vitamin supplementation in a wide range of patients at increased risk of coronary heart disease death: early safety and efficacy experience. Eur Heart J 1999;20(10):725–41.

59. Heart Protection Study Collaborative Group. MRC/BHF Heart Protection Study of cholesterol lowering with simvastatin in 20,536 high-risk individuals: a randomised placebo-controlled trial. Lancet 2002;360(9326):7–22.

60. Collins R, Armitage J, Parish S, et al. MRC/BHF heart protection study of cholesterol-lowering with simvastatin in 5963 people with diabetes: a randomised placebo-controlled trial. Lancet 2003;361(9374):2005–16.

61. Robins SJ, Rubins HB, Faas FH, et al. Insulin resistance and cardiovascular events with low HDL cholesterol: the veterans affairs HDL intervention trial (VA-HIT). Diabetes Care 2003;26(5):1513–7.

62. Rubins HB, Robins SJ, Collins D, et al. Gemfibrozil for the secondary prevention of coronary heart disease in men with low levels of high-density lipoprotein cholesterol. Veterans Affairs High-Density Lipoprotein Cholesterol Intervention Trial Study Group. N Engl J Med 1999;341(6):410–8.

63. Rubins HB, Robins SJ, Collins D, et al. Diabetes, plasma insulin, and cardiovascular disease: subgroup analysis from the department of veterans affairs high-density lipoprotein intervention trial (VA-HIT). Arch Intern Med 2002;162(22): 2597–604.

64. Keech A, Simes RJ, Barter P, et al. Effects of long-term fenofibrate therapy on cardiovascular events in 9795 people with type 2 diabetes mellitus (the FIELD study): randomised controlled trial. Lancet 2005;366(9500):1849–61.

65. Scott R, Best J, Forder P, et al. Fenofibrate Intervention and Event Lowering in Diabetes (FIELD) study: baseline characteristics and short-term effects of fenofibrate [ISRCTN64783481]. Cardiovasc Diabetol 2005;4:13.

66. Effect of fenofibrate on progression of coronary-artery disease in type 2 diabetes: the diabetes atherosclerosis intervention study, a randomised study. Lancet 2001;357(9260):905–10.

67. Steiner G. The Diabetes Atherosclerosis Intervention Study (DAIS): a study conducted in cooperation with the World Health Organization. The DAIS Project Group. Diabetologia 1996;39(12):1655–61.

68. Dahlof B, Sever PS, Poulter NR, et al. Prevention of cardiovascular events with an antihypertensive regimen of amlodipine adding perindopril as required versus atenolol adding bendroflumethiazide as required, in the Anglo-Scandinavian Cardiac Outcomes Trial—Blood Pressure Lowering Arm (ASCOT-BPLA): a multicentre randomised controlled trial. Lancet 2005;366(9489): 895–906.

69. Ostergren J, Poulter NR, Sever PS, et al. The Anglo-Scandinavian Cardiac Outcomes Trial: blood pressure-lowering limb: effects in patients with type II diabetes. J Hypertens 2008;26(11):2103–11.

70. The ALLHAT Officers and Coordinators for the ALLHAT Collaborative Research Group. Major outcomes in high-risk hypertensive patients randomized to angiotensin-converting enzyme inhibitor or calcium channel blocker vs diuretic: The Antihypertensive and Lipid-Lowering Treatment to Prevent Heart Attack Trial (ALLHAT). JAMA 2002;288(23):2981–97.

71. Davis BR, Cutler JA, Gordon DJ, et al. Rationale and design for the antihypertensive and lipid lowering treatment to prevent heart attack trial (ALLHAT). ALLHAT Research Group. Am J Hypertens 1996;9(4 Pt 1):342–60.

72. Davis BR, Furberg CD, Wright JT Jr, et al. Setting the record straight. Ann Intern Med 2004;141(1):39–46.

73. Varughese GI, Lip GY. Antihypertensive therapy in diabetes mellitus: insights from ALLHAT and the Blood Pressure-Lowering Treatment Trialists' Collaboration meta-analysis. J Hum Hypertens 2005;19(11):851–3.

74. Whelton PK, Barzilay J, Cushman WC, et al. Clinical outcomes in antihypertensive treatment of type 2 diabetes, impaired fasting glucose concentration, and normoglycemia: Antihypertensive and Lipid-Lowering Treatment to Prevent Heart Attack Trial (ALLHAT). Arch Intern Med 2005;165(12):1401–9.

75. Hansson L, Zanchetti A. The Hypertension Optimal Treatment (HOT) Study—patient characteristics: randomization, risk profiles, and early blood pressure results. Blood Press 1994;3(5):322–7.

76. Hansson L, Zanchetti A, Carruthers SG, et al. Effects of intensive blood-pressure lowering and low-dose aspirin in patients with hypertension: principal results of the Hypertension Optimal Treatment (HOT) randomised trial. HOT Study Group. Lancet 1998;351(9118):1755–62.

77. Zanchetti A, Hansson L, Dahlof B, et al. Effects of individual risk factors on the incidence of cardiovascular events in the treated hypertensive patients of the Hypertension Optimal Treatment Study. HOT Study Group. J Hypertens 2001;19(6):1149–59.

78. Estacio RO, Jeffers BW, Hiatt WR, et al. The effect of nisoldipine as compared with enalapril on cardiovascular outcomes in patients with non-insulin-dependent diabetes and hypertension. N Engl J Med 1998;338(10):645–52.

79. Estacio RO, Schrier RW. Antihypertensive therapy in type 2 diabetes: implications of the appropriate blood pressure control in diabetes (ABCD) trial. Am J Cardiol 1998;82(9B):9R–14R.

80. Havranek EP, Esler A, Estacio RO, et al. Differential effects of antihypertensive agents on electrocardiographic voltage: results from the Appropriate Blood Pressure Control in Diabetes (ABCD) trial. Am Heart J 2003;145(6):993–8.

81. Savage S, Johnson Nagel N, Estacio RO, et al. The ABCD (Appropriate Blood Pressure Control in Diabetes) trial. Rationale and design of a trial of hypertension control (moderate or intensive) in type II diabetes. Online J Curr Clin Trials 1993; 2. Doc No 104:[6250 words; 6128 paragraphs].

82. Schrier RW, Estacio RO. Additional follow-up from the ABCD trial in patients with type 2 diabetes and hypertension. N Engl J Med 2000;343(26):1969.

83. Schrier RW, Estacio RO, Mehler PS, et al. Appropriate blood pressure control in hypertensive and normotensive type 2 diabetes mellitus: a summary of the ABCD trial. Nat Clin Pract Nephrol 2007;3(8):428–38.

84. Amery A, Birkenhager W, Bulpitt CJ, et al. Syst-Eur. A multicentre trial on the treatment of isolated systolic hypertension in the elderly: objectives, protocol, and organization. Aging (Milano) 1991;3(3):287–302.

85. Gasowski J, Birkenhager WH, Staessen JA, et al. Benefit of antihypertensive treatment in the diabetic patients enrolled in the Systolic Hypertension in Europe (Syst-Eur) trial. Cardiovasc Drugs Ther 2000;14(1):49–53.

86. Staessen JA, Fagard R, Thijs L, et al. Randomised double-blind comparison of placebo and active treatment for older patients with isolated systolic hypertension. The Systolic Hypertension in Europe (Syst-Eur) Trial Investigators. Lancet 1997;350(9080):757–64.

87. Staessen JA, Fagard R, Thijs L, et al. Subgroup and per-protocol analysis of the randomized European Trial on Isolated Systolic Hypertension in the Elderly. Arch Intern Med 1998;158(15):1681–91.

88. Tuomilehto J, Rastenyte D, Birkenhager WH, et al. Effects of calcium-channel blockade in older patients with diabetes and systolic hypertension. systolic hypertension in Europe Trial Investigators. N Engl J Med 1999;340(9): 677–84.

89. Prevention of stroke by antihypertensive drug treatment in older persons with isolated systolic hypertension. Final results of the Systolic Hypertension in the Elderly Program (SHEP). SHEP Cooperative Research Group. JAMA 1991; 265(24):3255–64.

90. Holman RR, Paul SK, Bethel MA, et al. Long-term follow-up after tight control of blood pressure in type 2 diabetes. N Engl J Med 2008;359(15):1565–76.

91. Patel A, MacMahon S, Chalmers J, et al. Effects of a fixed combination of perindopril and indapamide on macrovascular and microvascular outcomes in patients with type 2 diabetes mellitus (the ADVANCE trial): a randomised controlled trial. Lancet 2007;370(9590):829–40.

92. The BENEDICT Group. The BErgamo NEphrologic DIabetes Complications Trial (BENEDICT): design and baseline characteristics. Control Clin Trials 2003;24(4): 442–61.

93. Ruggenenti P, Fassi A, Ilieva AP, et al. Preventing microalbuminuria in type 2 diabetes. N Engl J Med 2004;351(19):1941–51.

94. Ruggenenti P, Iliev I, Costa GM, et al. Preventing left ventricular hypertrophy by ACE inhibition in hypertensive patients with type 2 diabetes: a prespecified analysis of the Bergamo Nephrologic Diabetes Complications Trial (BENEDICT). Diabetes Care 2008;31(8):1629–34.

95. Boner G, Cooper ME, McCarroll K, et al. Adverse effects of left ventricular hypertrophy in the reduction of endpoints in NIDDM with the angiotensin II antagonist losartan (RENAAL) study. Diabetologia 2005;48(10):1980–7.

96. Brenner BM, Cooper ME, de Zeeuw D, et al. The losartan renal protection study—rationale, study design and baseline characteristics of RENAAL (Reduction of Endpoints in NIDDM with the Angiotensin II Antagonist Losartan). J Renin Angiotensin Aldosterone Syst 2000;1(4):328–35.

97. Brenner BM, Cooper ME, de Zeeuw D, et al. Effects of losartan on renal and cardiovascular outcomes in patients with type 2 diabetes and nephropathy. N Engl J Med 2001;345(12):861–9.

98. Kowey PR, Dickson TZ, Zhang Z, et al. Losartan and end-organ protection—lessons from the RENAAL study. Clin Cardiol 2005;28(3):136–42.

99. Winkelmayer WC, Zhang Z, Shahinfar S, et al. Efficacy and safety of angiotensin II receptor blockade in elderly patients with diabetes. Diabetes Care 2006; 29(10):2210–7.

100. Lievre M, Marre M, Chatellier G, et al. The non-insulin-dependent diabetes, hypertension, microalbuminuria or proteinuria, cardiovascular events, and ramipril (DIABHYCAR) study: design, organization, and patient recruitment. DIABHYCAR Study Group. Control Clin Trials 2000;21(4):383–96.

101. Marre M, Lievre M, Chatellier G, et al. Effects of low dose ramipril on cardiovascular and renal outcomes in patients with type 2 diabetes and raised excretion

of urinary albumin: randomised, double blind, placebo controlled trial (the DIABHYCAR study). BMJ 2004;328(7438):495.

102. The HOPE (Heart Outcomes Prevention Evaluation) Study: the design of a large, simple randomized trial of an angiotensin-converting enzyme inhibitor (ramipril) and vitamin E in patients at high risk of cardiovascular events. The HOPE study investigators. Can J Cardiol 1996;12(2):127–37.

103. Effects of ramipril on cardiovascular and microvascular outcomes in people with diabetes mellitus: results of the HOPE study and MICRO-HOPE substudy. Heart Outcomes Prevention Evaluation Study Investigators. Lancet 2000;355(9200): 253–9.

104. Dagenais GR, Yusuf S, Bourassa MG, et al. Effects of ramipril on coronary events in high-risk persons: results of the Heart Outcomes Prevention Evaluation Study. Circulation 2001;104(5):522–6.

105. Gerstein HC. Reduction of cardiovascular events and microvascular complications in diabetes with ACE inhibitor treatment: HOPE and MICRO-HOPE. Diabetes Metab Res Rev 2002;18(Suppl 3):S82–5.

106. Salehian O, Healey J, Stambler B, et al. Impact of ramipril on the incidence of atrial fibrillation: results of the Heart Outcomes Prevention Evaluation study. Am Heart J 2007;154(3):448–53.

107. Sleight P. The HOPE Study (Heart Outcomes Prevention Evaluation). J Renin Angiotensin Aldosterone Syst 2000;1(1):18–20.

108. Yusuf S, Sleight P, Pogue J, et al. Effects of an angiotensin-converting-enzyme inhibitor, ramipril, on cardiovascular events in high-risk patients. The Heart Outcomes Prevention Evaluation Study Investigators. N Engl J Med 2000; 342(3):145–53.

109. Sacco M, Pellegrini F, Roncaglioni MC, et al. Primary prevention of cardiovascular events with low-dose aspirin and vitamin E in type 2 diabetic patients: results of the Primary Prevention Project (PPP) trial. Diabetes Care 2003; 26(12):3264–72.

110. de Gaetano G. Low-dose aspirin and vitamin E in people at cardiovascular risk: a randomised trial in general practice. Collaborative Group of the Primary Prevention Project. Lancet 2001;357(9250):89–95.

111. Ogawa H, Nakayama M, Morimoto T, et al. Low-dose aspirin for primary prevention of atherosclerotic events in patients with type 2 diabetes: a randomized controlled trial. JAMA 2008;300(18):2134–41.

112. Dluhy RG, McMahon GT. Intensive glycemic control in the ACCORD and ADVANCE trials. N Engl J Med 2008;358(24):2630–3.

113. Skyler JS, Bergenstal R, Bonow RO, et al. Intensive glycemic control and the prevention of cardiovascular events: implications of the ACCORD, ADVANCE, and VA Diabetes Trials: a position statement of the American Diabetes Association and a scientific statement of the American College Of Cardiology Foundation and the American Heart Association. J Am Coll Cardiol 2009;53(3):298–304.

114. Downs JR, Beere PA, Whitney E, et al. Design & rationale of the Air Force/Texas Coronary Atherosclerosis Prevention Study (AFCAPS/TexCAPS). Am J Cardiol 1997;80(3):287–93.

115. Downs JR, Clearfield M, Weis S, et al. Primary prevention of acute coronary events with lovastatin in men and women with average cholesterol levels: results of AFCAPS/TexCAPS. Air Force/Texas Coronary Atherosclerosis Prevention Study. JAMA 1998;279(20):1615–22.

116. Influence of pravastatin and plasma lipids on clinical events in the West of Scotland Coronary Prevention Study (WOSCOPS). Circulation 1998;97(15):1440–5.

117. Shepherd J, Blauw GJ, Murphy MB, et al. Pravastatin in elderly individuals at risk of vascular disease (PROSPER): a randomised controlled trial. Lancet 2002;360(9346):1623–30.
118. Collaborative overview of randomised trials of antiplatelet therapy—I: Prevention of death, myocardial infarction, and stroke by prolonged antiplatelet therapy in various categories of patients. Antiplatelet Trialists' Collaboration. BMJ 1994; 308(6921):81–106.
119. Harpaz D, Gottlieb S, Graff E, et al. Effects of aspirin treatment on survival in non-insulin-dependent diabetic patients with coronary artery disease. Israeli Bezafibrate Infarction Prevention Study Group. Am J Med 1998;105(6):494–9.
120. Bray G, Gregg E, Haffner S, et al. Baseline characteristics of the randomised cohort from the Look AHEAD (Action for Health in Diabetes) study. Diab Vasc Dis Res 2006;3(3):202–15.
121. Pi-Sunyer X, Blackburn G, Brancati FL, et al. Reduction in weight and cardiovascular disease risk factors in individuals with type 2 diabetes: one-year results of the look AHEAD trial. Diabetes Care 2007;30(6):1374–83.
122. Ryan DH, Espeland MA, Foster GD, et al. Look AHEAD (Action for Health in Diabetes): design and methods for a clinical trial of weight loss for the prevention of cardiovascular disease in type 2 diabetes. Control Clin Trials 2003;24(5): 610–28.
123. Boyd CM, Darer J, Boult C, et al. Clinical practice guidelines and quality of care for older patients with multiple comorbid diseases: implications for pay for performance. JAMA 2005;294(6):716–24.
124. Higashi T, Wenger NS, Adams JL, et al. Relationship between number of medical conditions and quality of care. N Engl J Med 2007;356(24):2496–504.
125. Blaum CS. Descriptive epidemiology of diabetes. In: Munshi MN, Lipsitz LA, editors. Geriatric diabetes. New York: Informa Healthcare USA, Inc; 2007. p. 1–9.

The Obesity Paradox in the Elderly: Potential Mechanisms and Clinical Implications

Antigone Oreopoulos, MSc[a],*, Kamyar Kalantar-Zadeh, MD, MPH, PhD[b],
Arya M. Sharma, MD, PhD[c], Gregg C. Fonarow, MD, FACC[d]

KEYWORDS

- Obesity • Body composition • Elderly
- Mortality • Epidemiology

Obesity is a well-established and independent risk factor for cardiovascular disease and mortality in the general population.[1] Obesity is related to several diseases including diabetes mellitus, hypertension, dyslipidemia, coronary artery disease, and chronic heart failure.[2] An independent association between obesity and all-cause mortality exists in adults.[3] According to the Framingham Heart Study, increased life span can be achieved by reducing the prevalence and severity of obesity.[4] Recent data from the National Health and Nutrition Examination Survey indicate that approximately 32% of adults in the United States are obese.[5] In Canada, 20% of adults are obese.[6] The prevalence of obesity increases up to age 60 to 69 years in men and women, and then declines (**Table 1**).[7] At the same time, the prevalence of obesity is increasing among older age groups in both developed[8] and developing countries.[9] Those over 65 years of age account for approximately 12% to 13% of the population in Canada and the United States,[10] and that proportion is expected to grow to approximately 21%[11] and 18%,[12] respectively, by the year 2025.

The prevalence of overweight and obesity in the elderly has become a growing concern. It is a common presumption that older adults with higher body mass index (BMI) are at risk of shortened survival. Recent evidence, however, indicates that in

[a] Department of Clinical Epidemiology, School of Public Health, University of Alberta, 2F1.26 Walter C Mackenzie HSC, 8440-112 St, Edmonton, Alberta, Canada T6G 2B7
[b] Division of Nephrology and Hypertension, Harbor-UCLA Medical Center, UCLA Schools of Medicine and Public Health, 1124 West Carson Street, Box 406, Torrance, CA 90502, USA
[c] Division of Endocrinology, Royal Alexandra Hospital, University of Alberta, Edmonton, Alberta, Canada T6G 2S2
[d] UCLA Division of Cardiology, David Geffen School of Medicine at UCLA, Ahmanson-UCLA Cardiomyopathy Center, Los Angeles, CA 90095, USA
* Corresponding author.
E-mail address: antigone@ualberta.ca (A. Oreopoulos).

Clin Geriatr Med 25 (2009) 643–659
doi:10.1016/j.cger.2009.07.005
0749-0690/09/$ – see front matter © 2009 Elsevier Inc. All rights reserved.

geriatric.theclinics.com

Table 1		
Obesity prevalence in older adults (NHANES 1999–2000)		
Age (Years)	% Men	% Women
40–49	26.3	35.4
50–59	32.2	41.2
60–69	38.1	42.5
70–79	28.9	31.9
≥80	9.6	19.5

Data from Flegal KM, Carroll MD, Ogden CL, et al. Prevalence and trends in obesity among US adults, 1999–2000. JAMA 2002;288:1723–7.

the elderly, obesity is paradoxically associated with a lower, not higher, mortality risk. In contrast to younger individuals, numerous studies[13–38] and several systematic[39,40] and critical reviews[41–44] do not support the view that being overweight (ie, BMI in the range of 25–30 kg/m^2) is a risk factor for all-cause and cardiovascular mortality among elderly men or women. Most studies show this BMI range to be associated with the lowest mortality risk in older adults, and report an inverse or U-shaped association between BMI and all-cause mortality. These seemingly counterintuitive observations have been termed the "obesity paradox"[45] or "reverse epidemiology."[46] Although it is true that obesity in the general adult population is associated with higher mortality, this relationship is unclear for persons of advanced age and has led to great controversy regarding the relationship between obesity and mortality in the elderly, the definition of obesity in the elderly, and the need for its treatment in this population. This article examines the evidence on these controversial issues, explores potential explanations for these findings, discusses the clinical implications, and provides recommendations for further research in this area.

METHODS

An extensive electronic search was conducted in MEDLINE (1966–January 2009), EMBASE (1988–January 2009), the Cochrane Library (1990–January 2009), and Web of Science (1900–January 2009) to retrieve research articles on obesity in older adults. Primary studies, review articles, letters, and commentaries were included. Reference lists of primary studies and review articles were also scanned. Key search terms were used: obesity, body mass, body mass index, body weight, weight, weight change, waist circumference, waist-to-hip ratio, body fat, adiposity, and body composition in combination with elderly, older adults, older people, old age, geriatric, oldest old, older men, older women, octogenarians, nonagenarians, veterans, nursing home residents, and aging. Search strategies were limited to publications in English.

DEFINITIONS AND MEASUREMENTS

Several classifications of obesity exist. Some methods for measuring body composition, such as hydrostatic densitometry (underwater weighing), dual-energy x-ray absorptiometry, and near-infrared interactance, although accurate, require technologies and expertise that are not readily available.

BMI, calculated as body weight in kilograms divided by the square of the height in meters, is the most commonly used measure of obesity. Current American College of Cardiology and American Heart Association guidelines[47] suggest using BMI at all ages to define obesity, and recommend the same cut-off values of BMI in the elderly as in younger adults. A BMI under 18.5 kg/m^2 is almost universally considered underweight and a BMI between 18.5 and 24.9 kg/m^2 is usually, but not always, viewed as normal or ideal weight.[48] Individuals with a BMI in the 25 to 30 kg/m^2 range are considered overweight, and those with a BMI 30 kg/m^2 or greater are considered obese. This index is based on the assumption that most of the variation in weight among individuals of the same height is caused by fat mass. Because BMI calculations do not differentiate between weight because of fat versus lean muscle, age-related body composition changes, such as decreased lean tissue and height and increased fat deposits, make the use of BMI less valid in determining obesity in older adults. There is an age-related decline in height because of thinning of the intervertebral disks and loss of vertebral body height, and the cumulative height loss from age 30 to 80 years averages about 5 cm for men and 8 cm for women.[49] Age-dependent height decreases may induce a false BMI increase of 1.5 to 2.5 kg/m^2 in the elderly despite minimal changes in body weight. Furthermore, beginning in the third decade lean body mass declines at a rate of 0.3 kg per year.[50] At the same time, there is an increase in body fat, which continues up to age 70.[51] As a result, the total body weight tends to peak in the fifth to sixth decade, remains stable until age 65 to 70 years, and then slowly declines. This is in contrast to young adults where an increase in total body mass is also associated with an increase in skeletal muscle acquired to support the extra weight. The combination of increased fat mass and decreased lean body mass in the elderly is termed "sarcopenic obesity" and has been associated with decreased muscular strength and frailty.[52] Elderly persons may seem to have a stable "healthy" BMI despite excess fat and low muscle mass.

Not only do older adults have more body fat than young adults, but the fat is also distributed differently. Aging is associated with a greater proportion of visceral (intra-abdominal) fat.[53] An increase in visceral fat has been associated with increased cardiovascular risk in the general population.[54] In the past few years, waist circumference (WC) has been proposed as a surrogate of abdominal obesity.[55] WC is strongly related to both visceral and total fat as measured by CT.[56] A WC of greater than or equal to 88 cm in women and greater than or equal to 102 cm in men has been suggested as an indicator of obesity and increased health risk.[48] Waist-to-hip ratio (WHR) is another alternative metric: women with ratios greater than or equal to 0.8 and men with ratios greater than or equal to 1 are considered high risk for obesity-related diseases.[57] In 1985, Andres and colleagues[58] published tables of ideal weight standardized by age, suggesting an age-related increase of 5 kg per decade. Clearly, if BMI is to be used as the primary clinical measure of obesity in the elderly, the current definition and target healthy range need to be revised.

PATHOPHYSIOLOGY

The results from most studies demonstrate that energy intake does not change, or even declines with age.[59] The age-related increase in fat mass is most likely caused by a decrease in energy expenditure. A decline in the resting metabolic rate and thermal effect of food (the rise in metabolic rate during digestion of food) and reduced physical activity contribute to the decrease in energy expenditure.[60] This, combined with a stable energy intake, results in gradual fat accumulation. Hormonal changes also play a role in the amount of fat and its distribution. These changes include reduced production of growth hormone and testosterone,[61] and decreased responsiveness to thyroid[62] and leptin hormones.[63]

ASSOCIATION BETWEEN BMI AND MORTALITY AFTER AGE 65

In younger adults, there is strong evidence that obesity shortens the life span.[64] Data from the American Cancer Society's Cancer Prevention Study[65] have shown, however, that the relative mortality risk decreases with age (**Fig. 1**). This was also demonstrated in a 12-year prospective study of over 1 million Korean men and women (**Fig. 2**).[66] An assessment of 13 observational studies from 1966 to 1999 by Heiat and colleagues,[41] in which nonhospitalized people over 65 years were followed for at least 3 years, found a lower relative mortality risk in obese older persons compared with

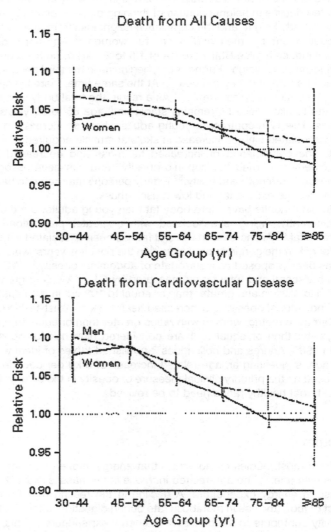

Fig. 1. The effect of age on the association between BMI and mortality. 62, 116 men and 262, 091 women never smoked followed over 12 years. *Data from* Stevens J, Cai J, Pamuk ER, et al. The effect of age on the association between body-mass index and mortality. N Engl J Med 1998;338:1–7; with permission. Copyright © 2006, Massachusetts Medical Society.

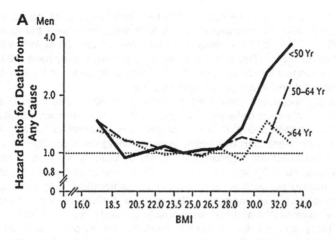

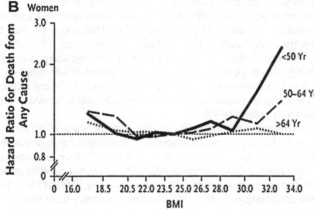

Fig. 2. BMI and mortality in men and women by age groups. 12-year prospective cohort study of 1,213,829 individuals between the ages of 30 and 95 years examining 82,372 deaths. *From* Jee SH, Sull JW, Park J, et al. Body-mass index and mortality in Korean men and women. N Engl J Med 2006;355:779–87; with permission. Copyright © 2006, Massachusetts Medical Society.

young and middle-aged obese persons after adjustment for smoking and baseline health status. There was a positive association between mortality and being overweight or obese (BMI ≥ 27 kg/m^2) only in 3 out of the 13 studies among 65 to 74 year olds, with little or no increase in all-cause or cardiovascular mortality for people with BMI greater than or equal to 30 kg/m^2 compared with those with normal BMI among people over 75 years of age. Results were generally consistent between males and females.

There is evidence that the relationship between BMI and mortality in the elderly may be U-shaped or reverse J-shaped, whereby the risk of mortality begins to rise again with extreme BMI values over 35 to 40 kg/m^2;[14–18,21–23,25–27,31,37,38,67] however, in most studies the increased risk was not significant.[16,17,67] Similarly, a systematic review and meta-analysis by Janssen and Mark[68] showed that whereas elderly individuals with a BMI in the overweight range were not at higher risk for all-cause mortality, a BMI in the moderately obese range was associated with a 10% increase in mortality risk, independent of gender, disease status, and smoking status.

Where studies examining the relationship between BMI and all-cause mortality in older adults identified an optimum BMI (the BMI associated with the lowest risk of death),[13–18,20–23,25–27,30,31,38] the range was between 24 and 35 kg/m^2, with most in the range 27 to 30 kg/m^2 (**Table 2**). Older women, however, may have a 2 to 5 kg/m^2 higher optimal range than older men.[16,23,27] Optimal targets for BMI in the elderly have yet to be validated in a large prospective trial.

Zamboni and colleagues[42] reviewed the findings of 20 studies from 1997 to 2004 examining the relationship between BMI and mortality with at least 4.5 years follow-up. The authors concluded that body composition (abdominal fat and lean body mass) is more important than BMI alone in determining the mortality risk associated with obesity in older adults. A prospective study by Wannamethee and colleagues[69] in 4107 men aged 60 to 79 years and followed for a mean of 6 years found that lean body mass, measured by mid arm muscle circumference, was significantly and inversely associated with mortality. The authors further demonstrated that the combined measure of WC and mid arm muscle circumference provided an effective measure of body composition to assess mortality risk in older men. Janssen and colleagues[70] showed that after controlling for WC, increased BMI was protective against mortality, whereas after controlling for BMI, increased WC was linearly associated with mortality in persons 65 years and older. This suggests that BMI reflects lean body mass for individuals with equivalent WC, whereas WC reflects fat mass for individuals with equal BMI.[71] The authors recommend using both measures in the clinical setting. Other studies have shown a similar linear positive relationship between WHR and mortality in older adults.[15,34,37,72] In the clinical setting, however, WC has the advantage of requiring only one measurement, whereas two measurements are required to calculate WHR.

Obesity and cardiovascular mortality in the elderly were examined in a recent systematic review by McTigue and colleagues.[39] There was no consistent relationship between cardiovascular mortality and BMI. In one study[65] that excluded underweight individuals from the normal BMI reference group, a significant positive association was reported in men and women up to age 74. In two studies,[15,73] WC and WHR showed stronger positive associations with cardiovascular mortality than BMI.

Longitudinal studies have examined the impact of midlife BMI on survival in the elderly.[13,36,74–76] These studies have consistently shown that current and midlife BMI have independent effects on mortality in the elderly. Although mortality risk is increased in obese older adults who were already obese at midlife, this is not the case for newly obese older adults. In addition, Janssen and Bacon[36] observed that compared with 70 year olds who were nonobese at both 50 and 70 years of age, mortality risk was increased by 47% in those who were obese at both 50 and 70 years of age, increased by 56% in those who were obese at 50 years of age and nonobese at 70 years of age, but not significantly different in those who were nonobese at 50 years of age and obese at 70 years of age.

POTENTIAL EXPLANATIONS FOR AGE DIFFERENCES IN THE RELATIONSHIP BETWEEN BMI AND MORTALITY

Several explanations have been offered for the reverse epidemiology of obesity in the elderly (**Table 3**). Overweight and obese individuals who survive to old age may have characteristics that protect them from the adverse effects of being overweight or obese. This is known as the "survival effect." Individuals who are susceptible to the complications of obesity may have already died, leaving behind those who are more resistant.

Another possible explanation for the obesity paradox is that the higher the age, the shorter is the remaining life span, regardless of the presence of obesity. Because most

Table 2
Summary of studies with large sample sizes (>1000 subjects), mean follow-up time of at least 5 years, and mean age of ≥65 indicating a reverse epidemiology of obesity in older adults

Reference	Sample Size	Mean Age and Range	Follow-up Period (Y)	Findings and Source of Data
Losonczy et al,[13] 1995, USA	2449 men, 3938 women	≥70	5	Inverse BMI-mortality association, lowest mortality at BMI 26.3–28.3 in men and ≥29.2 in women; data from the Established Populations for Epidemiologic Studies of the Elderly
Allison et al,[23] 1997, USA	2769 men, 4491 women	77 (70–99)	6	U-shaped BMI-mortality association, lowest mortality risk at BMI 27–30 for men and 30–35 for women; data from the Longitudinal Study of Aging
Wassertheil-Smoller et al,[27] 2000, USA	3975 men and women	71	5	No relationship between death or stroke and BMI in the placebo group, a U- or J-shaped BMI-mortality association in the treatment group. Lowest risk of death for men at BMI of 26 and for women at BMI of 29.6 in the treatment group; data from the Systolic Hypertension in the Elderly Program trial
Dey et al,[18] 2001, Sweden	1225 men, 1403 women	70	15	U-shaped BMI-mortality association, lowest mortality risk at BMI 27–29 for men and 25–27 for women, weight loss increased mortality; cohort study in Sweden
Grabowski and Ellis,[20] 2001, USA	2860 men, 4667 women	77 (≥70)	8	Inverse association between BMI and mortality, lowest mortality risk in subjects with obesity (BMI >28.5) compared with subjects with normal BMI (19.5–28.4); data from the Longitudinal Study of Aging
Janssen et al,[70] 2005, Canada	2262 men, 2938 women	(65–90+)	9	Inverse relationship between BMI and mortality after adjustment of WC, linear positive relationship between WC and mortality after adjustment of BMI; participants of the Cardiovascular Health Study
Price et al,[34] 2006, UK	7892 men, 13,667 women	80 (≥75)	5.9	Inverse association between BMI and mortality, linear positive association between WHR and mortality; data from 53 family practices in United Kingdom
Corrada et al,[38] 2006, USA	8609 women, 4842 men	73 (44–101)	23	U-shaped BMI-mortality association among persons >80, lowest mortality risk at BMI 25–29.9 in persons >80; data from the Leisure World Cohort Study in California
Dolan et al,[31] 2007, USA	8029 women	72 (65–77)	8	U-shaped BMI-mortality and WC-mortality associations, lowest mortality risk at BMI 23.4–29.8; data from Community-based study in Baltimore, Maryland
Al Snih et al,[26] 2007, USA	4870 men, 3489 women	73	7	U-shaped BMI-mortality association, lowest mortality risk at BMI 25–35; 5 sites of the Established Populations for Epidemiologic Studies of the Elderly
Mazza et al,[32] 2007, Italy	1275 men, 1982 women	74 (65–95)	12	Inverse association between BMI and mortality; participants from the Cardiovascular Study in the Elderly

Abbreviations: BMI, body mass index; WC, waist circumference; WHR, waist-to-hip ratio.

Table 3 Possible mechanisms leading to the observed associations between obesity and improved survival in the elderly	
Potential Biases	**Potential Beneficial Effects**
Survival effect	Prevention or delay in cognitive decline
Time discrepancy of competitive risk factors	Protection from bone mineral density loss and osteoporotic fractures
Reverse causation	Reduction in oxidative stress and inflammation
Confounding variables	Energy reserve and prevention of malnutrition
Cohort effect	

obesity-related consequences take years to develop, those who become obese in old age may die of other conditions before the adverse effects of obesity become manifest. This is known as "time discrepancy of competing risk factors," and could potentially explain the finding by Janssen and Bacon[36] that nonobese older adults who were obese in midlife had an increased mortality risk compared with those who were not obese either at midlife or in old age.

A major challenge in analyzing the obesity-mortality association in epidemiologic studies is the phenomenon of reverse causation. It has been observed repeatedly that weight loss and being underweight are strong predictors of mortality, especially in the elderly.[77] Unintentional weight loss caused by unrecognized systemic illness can affect BMI–mortality analyses if the weight loss occurs before the BMI measurement. This can lead to an overestimation of the mortality risk of the "healthy" weight reference group, thereby making the obese group seem protected.

Obesity requires many years to show its harmful effects on health. Studies with short follow-up times generally do not show associations between obesity and mortality, whereas studies with longer follow-up show significant associations.[42] With longer follow-up, it becomes increasingly important to account for the effects of confounding factors, such as smoking, comorbid conditions, socioeconomic status, health insurance, medication compliance, and especially the effect of voluntary versus involuntary weight loss.

A cohort effect occurs when a study compares different cohorts (or groups) of people that are not actually comparable. BMI-mortality associations are often determined for various age groups using different cohorts who have grown up at different time periods. Cohorts may have been exposed to different lifestyles, environments, and risk factors (eg, infections) that were a much more common cause of death before the introduction of antibiotics.

It is also possible that obesity or a high BMI provide beneficial effects later in life. In contrast with younger adults, obesity has not been found to be associated with depression in older adults.[78] Cognitive function is also a major determinant of disability in the elderly population.[79] In one study, being underweight (BMI <18.5 kg/m^2) was associated with cognitive decline in elderly adults as measured by the Mini Mental State Examination, whereas obesity (BMI ≥30 kg/m^2) was not associated with cognitive decline.[80] In addition, Deschamps and colleagues[81] found that subjects with a BMI less than 23 kg/m^2 had a 3.6-fold higher risk of cognitive decline as assessed by the Mini Mental State Examination at 5 years follow-up. This relationship, however, may be different for males and females. For example, Han and colleagues[82] found that increases in BMI and WC in elderly men were associated with improvement in cognitive function, whereas for elderly women, they were associated with cognitive decline.

Another important benefit of a higher BMI later in life is the protection from osteoporotic fractures. A higher BMI is associated with greater bone mineral density (BMD) in both weight-bearing and non–weight-bearing bones.[83] The increase in BMD and the extra cushioning effect of fat surrounding areas, such as the hip, may provide protection against hip fracture during a fall in older obese persons.[84]

Weight loss and sarcopenia in the elderly may also be associated with reduced skeletal muscle oxidative metabolism, leading to oxidative stress and inflammation.[85] Obesity later in life might improve antioxidant defense.

Another potential benefit of excess adiposity later in life could be to serve as an energy reserve. Malnutrition and the inability to maintain weight and protein status are common problems in elderly nursing home residents.[86] Obesity may protect against this protein-energy malnutrition in the elderly.

The "obesity paradox" is not unique to the elderly population; there is considerable evidence supporting the survival benefit of an increased BMI in chronic wasting diseases, such as AIDS,[87] cancer,[88] heart failure,[89] and in patients on hemodialysis.[90] This "reverse epidemiology" may be partially explained by a larger amount of energy stored as fat and the somewhat larger stores of lean mass, but also by the influence of body fat on fuel selection during negative energy balance.[40] During starvation, the proportion of energy expenditure derived from protein metabolism is lower and lean tissue is better preserved in persons with larger fat stores.[91]

EFFECT OF OBESITY ON MORBIDITY, FUNCTIONAL STATUS, AND QUALITY OF LIFE IN THE ELDERLY

Both cross-sectional and longitudinal studies have shown that a high BMI and increased abdominal fat are associated with metabolic changes even in older age.[39] These changes include insulin resistance, dyslipidemia, and hypertension, which directly contribute to the development of metabolic syndrome, diabetes mellitus, and cardiovascular disease.[92] In the systematic review by McTigue and colleagues,[39] most studies reported a significantly increased risk of incident cardiovascular morbidity (myocardial infarction or stroke) with increasing BMI. The studies that used WC or WHR as the measure of obesity produced similar results. An elevated BMI was also associated with some cancers, including breast, uterine, colon, and leukemia. Studies examining WC or WHR and cancer incidence yielded similar findings. An increase in lean body mass, however, has not been associated with an increase in cardiovascular disease or diabetes mellitus,[93] and has been associated with a neutral[93] or decreased cancer risk.[94] Obesity measured by BMI or WC has also been associated with increased long-term medication use in elderly individuals.[39] The finding of a relationship between higher BMI values and increased cardiovascular morbidity, but a neutral or inverse relationship between higher BMI and total and cardiovascular mortality, seems contradictory and merits further study.

There is a progressive decrease in physical function and mobility with aging because of the loss of lean body mass, strength, and balance, and an increase in joint dysfunction and arthritis.[95] This decrease in physical function is linked to poorer health-related quality of life in older adults.[52] Several studies have shown an inverse association between BMI and physical function in older adults despite no greater risk in mortality.[26,96,97] It is less clear, however, whether it is the increase in body fat or the age-related decline in lean body mass that plays the major role in causing this functional decline, with studies supporting both hypotheses.[98,99] The optimal BMI for the maintenance of functional capacity may be above the normal range; some authors have found that the BMI range associated with the lowest rate of decline in physical function is between 23 and 30 kg/m^2.[26,81]

RELATIONSHIP BETWEEN PHYSICAL FITNESS, OBESITY, AND MORTALITY IN THE ELDERLY

Physical inactivity and a low level of physical fitness are risk factors for all-cause and cardiovascular mortality.[100] Low levels of physical activity and fitness have also been associated with obesity.[100] A study of 831 male veterans[101] showed a strong inverse relationship between exercise capacity (evaluated on a maximal exercise treadmill test) and mortality, independent of BMI. Another study of 35 middle-aged and elderly men and women[102] showed that perceived physical fitness, but not BMI, was an independent risk factor for all-cause or cardiovascular mortality at 16 years follow-up. In the Yale Health and Aging Study, Dziura and colleagues[103] found that even modest levels of physical activity (measured by a physical activity questionnaire) can attenuate age-related weight loss in older adults with chronic disease, independent of smoking and mobility status.

EFFECT OF INTENTIONAL WEIGHT LOSS ON MORTALITY IN THE ELDERLY

Because of the potential benefits associated with being overweight or obese in old age, including prevention or delay in cognitive decline, protection from bone fractures, an increase in antioxidant defense, a reserve of fat and energy stores, and possibly an increase in longevity, there has been hesitation to recommend weight reduction in older adults. A recent systematic review by Bales and Buhr[40] identified 16 studies on the effect of weight loss interventions in subjects 60 years of age or older with baseline BMI of at least 27 kg/m^2, weight loss greater than or equal to 3% or greater than or equal to 2 kg, and trial duration 6 months or longer. The weight loss interventions led to significant benefits for those with osteoarthritis, coronary heart disease, and type II diabetes mellitus, whereas having slightly negative effects on BMD and lean body mass. Markers of inflammation, including interluekin-6, C-reactive protein, and tumor necrosis factor, were reduced with weight loss, and improvements in WC, blood pressure, serum levels of low-density lipoprotein cholesterol, and fasting glucose were evident. One study[104] found that an average weight loss of 3 kg was associated with a 30% reduction in a composite cardiovascular end point (cardiovascular events, poorly controlled blood pressure, and the need to reinitiate antihypertensive medications) at 2.5 years follow-up. In patients with osteoarthritis, significant improvements were seen in the physical function components of the Short Form 36 Health Survey and the Western Ontario and McMaster Universities Osteoarthritis Index.[105,106] An increase in the 6-minute walk time, decrease in stair climb time, and decrease in knee pain were also noted. Two trials[107,108] evaluated BMD changes in response to weight loss. Although significant effects on total body BMD were observed, there was no effect on regional BMD at common sites of fractures, such as the hip or spine. With regard to the loss of lean body mass associated with weight loss reported in some trials, this is a common finding in weight loss trials of any age group, but it is more of a concern in the elderly population. The best way to avoid loss of lean body mass is to couple the weight reduction intervention with a resistance training exercise program.[108] Resistance exercises are beneficial for preserving bone density and for maintaining lean mass and muscular strength.[40] To date, no clinical trials have evaluated the effect of intentional weight loss on mortality in elderly individuals.

These are conflicting findings: intervention trials show clinically important benefits of weight reduction with regard to osteoarthritis, physical function, and possibly diabetes and coronary heart disease, yet longitudinal studies suggest that maintaining weight is favorable in older persons who become obese after age 60. It is clear that evidence-based recommendations for weight loss in obese elderly persons cannot currently be made, and that decisions about whether or not to advise weight loss must be individualized, with particular attention to the patient's weight history and coexisting medical conditions.[40] Additionally, a focus on physical fitness, muscular strength, and improvement of physical function may be more productive than weight loss in many cases.

Table 4 summarizes the associations between measures of body composition (BMI, abdominal fat, lean body mass), intentional weight loss, and morbidity and mortality outcomes in the elderly.

CLINICAL IMPLICATIONS

A summary of clinical implications follows:

1. Obesity, as defined by BMI greater than or equal to 30 kg/m², does not carry the same mortality risk in older adults (>60 years of age) as in younger adults. The association between BMI and mortality in older individuals is neutral or inverse. The current targets for normal BMI derived from epidemiologic studies of younger and middle-aged populations (BMI 18.5–24.9) do not seem to apply to the elderly. BMI should be used in

Table 4
Associations between BMI, abdominal fat, and intentional weight loss with outcomes in the elderly

	High BMI	High Abdominal Fat	Increased Lean Muscle	Effect of Intentional Weight Loss
All cause mortality	↓ or neutral	↑	↓	Unknown
Cardiovascular mortality	↓ or neutral	↑ or neutral	Unknown	Unknown
Cardiovascular morbidity (myocardial infarction or stroke)	↑	↑	Neutral	↓
Cancer incidence	↑	↑	↓ or neutral	Unknown
Diabetes mellitus/ insulin sensitivity	↑	↑	Neutral	↓
Blood pressure	↑	↑	Unknown	↓
Physical function	↓ but higher than normal	↓	↑	↑
Quality of life	↓	↓	↑	↑
Cognitive function	↑ or neutral (may be different for females)	↑ or neutral (may be different for females)	Unknown	Unknown
Long-term medication use	↑	↑	Unknown	Potential ↓ for antihypertensives
Bone mineral density	↑	↑	↑	Slight ↓
Dyslipidemia	↑	↑	Unknown	↓

↓: decreased; ↑: increased.

conjunction with indices of lean body mass and fat distribution, such as waist circumference and mid arm muscle circumference, to assess mortality risk.
2. The ideal BMI target in the elderly may be closer to 25 to 35 kg/m^2 (lower range for males and upper range for females). This and other indices of body composition, however, should be validated in prospective clinical trials in the population to which they are going to be applied.
3. Increased weight or a high BMI in advanced age may provide benefits, such as protection from bone loss and fractures, malnutrition, and cognitive decline.
4. Obesity, especially abdominal obesity, in older age may confer adverse health risks, such as metabolic syndrome, diabetes, and cancer risk.
5. Physical activity and physical fitness are important determinants of mortality risk in the elderly, independent of obesity, and may attenuate age-related weight loss. Physical fitness and functional independence may be a more productive focus than weight loss in older adults with obesity.
6. Being underweight in any age group is associated with substantially increased risk of mortality. In the elderly, underweight status by BMI poses far greater threat than being overweight or obese.
7. Unintentional weight loss is never normal and requires clinical investigation for the underlying cause.
8. Elderly subjects with obesity in conjunction with decreased lean body mass (sarcopenic obesity) are at increased mortality risk. There is no consensus, however, on the definition of sarcopenic obesity or guidelines for management.

SUMMARY

The prevalence of obesity is increasing at all ages, including the elderly. The complexity of measuring body fat and fat distribution in the clinical setting makes it difficult to determine the most valid, practical definition of obesity in the elderly population. In contrast to younger people, an overweight BMI is associated with lower mortality risk in the elderly. Similarly, an obese BMI does not confer increased risk of mortality in the elderly, although it is related to cardiovascular morbidity and physical disability. A greater emphasis should be placed on preventing functional decline and muscle loss in older adults through increased physical activity, including resistance training. More research is needed to determine the optimal BMI and other potential indices of body composition to guide therapeutic decisions.

REFERENCES

1. Bray GA, Macdiarmid J. The epidemic of obesity. West J Med 2000;172:78–9.
2. Must A, Spadano J, Coakley EH, et al. The disease burden associated with overweight and obesity. JAMA 1999;282:1523–9.
3. Calle E, Thun MJ, Petrelli JM, et al. Body mass index and mortality in a prospective cohort of U.S. adults. N Engl J Med 1999;341:1097–105.
4. Pardo Silva MC, De Laet C, Nusselder WJ, et al. Adult obesity and number of years lived with and without cardiovascular disease. Obesity (Silver Spring) 2006;14:1264–73.
5. Ogden CL, Carroll MD, Curtin LR, et al. Prevalence of overweight and obesity in the United States, 1999–2004. JAMA 2006;295:1549–55.
6. Sokar-Todd HB, Sharma AM. Obesity research in Canada: literature overview of the last 3 decades. Obes Res 2004;12:1547–53.
7. Flegal KM, Carroll MD, Ogden CL, et al. Prevalence and trends in obesity among US adults, 1999–2000. JAMA 2002;288:1723–7.

8. Yusuf S. The global problem of cardiovascular disease. Int J Clin Pract Suppl 1998;94:3–6.
9. Haslam DW, James WP. Obesity. Lancet 2005;366:1197–209.
10. Organization for Economic Co-operation and Development (OECD) Factbook 2008. Economic, environmental and social statistics. Paris (France): OECD Publishing; 2008.
11. Moore E, Rosenberg M. Canada's elderly population: the challenges of diversity. Can Geogr 2001;45:145.
12. Projections of the population by selected age groups and sex for the United States: 2010 to 2050. Available at: http://www.census.gov/population/www/projections/summarytables.html. Accessed April 1, 2009.
13. Losonczy K, Harris T, Coroni-Huntley J, et al. Does weight loss from middle age to old age explain the inverse weight mortality relation in old age? Am J Epidemiol 1995;141:312–21.
14. Thorpe R, Ferraro K. Aging, obesity and mortality. Res Aging 2004;26:108–29.
15. Folsom AR, Kushi LH, Anderson KE, et al. Associations of general and abdominal obesity with multiple health outcomes in older women: the Iowa Women's Health Study. Arch Intern Med 2000;160:2117–28.
16. Reuser M, Bonneux L, Willekens F. The burden of mortality of obesity at middle and old age is small: a life table analysis of the US Health and Retirement Survey. Eur J Epidemiol 2008;23:601–7.
17. Bender R, Jockel KH, Trautner C, et al. Effect of age on excess mortality in obesity. JAMA 1999;281:1498–504.
18. Dey DK, Rothenberg E, Sundh V, et al. Body mass index, weight change and mortality in the elderly: a 15 y longitudinal population study of 70 y olds. Eur J Clin Nutr 2001;55:482–92.
19. Diehr P, O'Meara ES, Fitzpatrick A, et al. Weight, mortality, years of healthy life, and active life expectancy in older adults. J Am Geriatr Soc 2008;56:76–83.
20. Grabowski D, Ellis J. High body mass index does not predict mortality in older people: an analysis of the Longitudinal Study of Aging. J Am Geriatr Soc 2001;49:968–79.
21. Grabowski DC, Campbell CM, Ellis JE. Obesity and mortality in elderly nursing home residents. J Gerontol A Biol Sci Med Sci 2005;60:1184–9.
22. Landi F, Onder G, Gambassi G, et al. Body mass index and mortality among hospitalized patients. Arch Intern Med 2000;160:2641–4.
23. Allison D, Gallagher D, Heo M, et al. Body mass index and all-cause mortality among people age 70 and over: the Longitudinal Study of Aging. Int J Obes 1997;21:424–31.
24. McAuley P, Myers J, Abella J, et al. Body mass, fitness and survival in veteran patients: another obesity paradox? Am J Med 2007;120:518–24.
25. Menotti A, Kromhout D, Nissinen A, et al. Short-term all-cause mortality and its determinants in elderly male populations in Finland, The Netherlands, and Italy: the FINE Study. Finland, Italy, Netherlands Elderly Study. Prev Med 1996;25:319–26.
26. Al Snih S, Ottenbacher KJ, Markides KS, et al. The effect of obesity on disability vs mortality in older Americans. Arch Intern Med 2007;167:774–80.
27. Wassertheil-Smoller S, Fann C, Allman RM, et al. Relation of low body mass to death and stroke in the systolic hypertension in the elderly program. The SHEP Cooperative Research Group. Arch Intern Med 2000;160:494–500.
28. Kinney E, Caldwall J. Relationship between body weight and mortality in men aged 75 years and older. South Med J 1990;83:1256–8.

29. Weiss A, Beloosesky Y, Boaz M, et al. Body mass index is inversely related to mortality in elderly subjects. J Gen Intern Med 2007;23:19–24.

30. Takata Y, Ansai T, Soh I, et al. Association between body mass index and mortality in an 80-year-old population. J Am Geriatr Soc 2007;55:913–7.

31. Dolan C, Kraemer H, Browner W, et al. An intermediate body mass index (23 to 30 kg/m²) was associated with the most favorable mortality in older women. Am J Public Health 2007;97:93–8.

32. Mazza A, Zamboni S, Tikhonoff V, et al. Body mass index and mortality in elderly men and women from general population: the experience of Cardiovascular Study in the Elderly (CASTEL). Gerontology 2007;53:36–45.

33. Woo J, Ho S, Yu A, et al. Is waist circumference a useful measure in predicting health outcomes in the elderly? Int J Obes 2002;26:1349–55.

34. Price GM, Uauy R, Breeze E, et al. Weight, shape, and mortality risk in older persons: elevated waist-hip ratio, not high body mass index, is associated with a greater risk of death. Am J Clin Nutr 2006;84:449–60.

35. Heitmann BL, Erikson H, Ellsinger BM, et al. Mortality associated with body fat, fat-free mass and body mass index among 60-year-old Swedish men-a 22-year follow-up. The study of men born in 1913. Int J Obes Relat Metab Disord 2000; 24:33–7.

36. Janssen I, Bacon E. Effect of current and midlife obesity status on mortality risk in the elderly. Obesity (Silver Spring) 2008;16:2504–9.

37. Lahmann PH, Lissner L, Gullberg B, et al. A prospective study of adiposity and all-cause mortality: the Malmo Diet and Cancer Study. Obes Res 2002;10:361–9.

38. Corrada MM, Kawas CH, Mozaffar F, et al. Association of body mass index and weight change with all-cause mortality in the elderly. Am J Epidemiol 2006;163: 938–49.

39. McTigue KM, Hess R, Ziouras J. Obesity in older adults: a systematic review of the evidence for diagnosis and treatment. Obesity (Silver Spring) 2006;14:1485–97.

40. Bales C, Buhr G. Is obesity bad for older persons? A systematic review of the pros and cons of weight reduction in later life. J Am Med Dir Assoc 2008;9:302–12.

41. Heiat A, Vaccarino V, Krumholz HM. An evidence-based assessment of federal guidelines for overweight and obesity as they apply to elderly persons. Arch Intern Med 2001;161:1194–203.

42. Zamboni M, Mazzali G, Zoico E, et al. Health consequences of obesity in the elderly: a review of four unresolved questions. Int J Obes 2005;29:1011–29.

43. Heiat A. Impact of age on definition of standards for ideal weight. Prev Cardiol 2003;6:104–7.

44. Villareal DT, Apovian CM, Kushner RF, et al. Obesity in older adults: technical review and position statement of the American Society for Nutrition and NAASO, the Obesity Society. Obes Res 2005;13:1849–63.

45. Kalantar-Zadeh K, Horwich TB, Oreopoulos A, et al. Risk factor paradox in wasting diseases. Curr Opin Clin Nutr Metab Care 2007;10:433–42.

46. Kalantar-Zadeh K, Kilpatrick RD, Kuwae N, et al. Reverse epidemiology: a spurious hypothesis or a hardcore reality? Blood Purif 2005;23(1):57–63.

47. Smith SC Jr, Allen J, Blair SN, et al. AHA/ACC guidelines for secondary prevention for patients with coronary and other atherosclerotic vascular disease: 2006 update endorsed by the National Heart, Lung, and Blood Institute. J Am Coll Cardiol 2006;47:2130–9.

48. Pi-Sunyer FX. Clinical guidelines on the identification, evaluation, and treatment of overweight and obesity in adults. Bethesda (MD): National Institutes of Health; 1998. Publication NIH 98-4083.

49. Sorkin JD, Muller DC, Andres R. Longitudinal change in height of men and women: implications for interpretation of the body mass index: the Baltimore Longitudinal Study of Aging. Am J Epidemiol 1999;150:969–77.
50. Elia M. Organ and tissue contribution to metabolic rate. New York: Raven Press; 1992.
51. Baumgartner RN, Heymsfield SB, Roche AF. Human body composition and the epidemiology of chronic disease. Obes Res 1995;3:73–95.
52. Villareal DT, Banks M, Siener C, et al. Physical frailty and body composition in obese elderly men and women. Obes Res 2004;12:913–20.
53. Zamboni M, Armellini F, Harris T, et al. Effects of age on body fat distribution and cardiovascular risk factors in women. Am J Clin Nutr 1997;66:111–5.
54. Bjorntorp P. Portal adipose tissue as a generator of risk factors for cardiovascular disease and diabetes. Arteriosclerosis 1990;10:493–6.
55. Turcato E, Bosello O, Di Francesco V, et al. Waist circumference and abdominal sagittal diameter as surrogates of body fat distribution in the elderly: their relation with cardiovascular risk factors. Int J Obes Relat Metab Disord 2000;24:1005–10.
56. Harris TB, Visser M, Everhart J, et al. Waist circumference and sagittal diameter reflect total body fat better than visceral fat in older men and women. The Health, Aging and Body Composition Study. Ann N Y Acad Sci 2000;904:462–73.
57. Segal K, Dunaif A, Gutin B, et al. Body composition, not body weight, is related to cardiovascular disease risk factors and sex hormone levels in men. J Clin Invest 1987;80:1050–5.
58. Andres R, Elahi D, Tobin JD, et al. Impact of age on weight goals. Ann Intern Med 1985;103:1030–3.
59. Hallfrisch J, Muller D, Drinkwater D, et al. Continuing diet trends in men: the Baltimore Longitudinal Study of Aging (1961–1987). J Gerontol 1990;45:M186–91.
60. Elia M, Ritz P, Stubbs RJ. Total energy expenditure in the elderly. Eur J Clin Nutr 2000;54(Suppl 3):S92–103.
61. Corpas E, Harman SM, Blackman MR. Human growth hormone and human aging. Endocr Rev 1993;14:20–39.
62. Matsumoto AM. Andropause: clinical implications of the decline in serum testosterone levels with aging in men. J Gerontol A Biol Sci Med Sci 2002;57:M76–99.
63. Moller N, O'Brien P, Nair KS. Disruption of the relationship between fat content and leptin levels with aging in humans. J Clin Endocrinol Metab 1998;83:931–4.
64. Fontaine K, Redden D, Wang C, et al. Years of life lost due to obesity. JAMA 2003;289:187–93.
65. Stevens J, Cai J, Pamuk ER, et al. The effect of age on the association between body-mass index and mortality. N Engl J Med 1998;338:1–7.
66. Jee SH, Sull JW, Park J, et al. Body-mass index and mortality in Korean men and women. N Engl J Med 2006;355:779–87.
67. Su D. Body mass index and old-age survival: a comparative study between the Union Army Records and the NHANES-I Epidemiological Follow-Up Sample. Am J Hum Biol 2005;17:341–54.
68. Janssen I, Mark AE. Elevated body mass index and mortality risk in the elderly. Obes Rev 2007;8:41–59.
69. Wannamethee SG, Shaper AG, Lennon L, et al. Decreased muscle mass and increased central adiposity are independently related to mortality in older men. Am J Clin Nutr 2007;86:1339–46.
70. Janssen I, Katzmarzyk P, Ross R. Body mass index is inversely related to mortality in older people after adjustment for waist circumference. J Am Geriatr Soc 2005;52:2112–8.

71. Bigaard J, Tjonneland A, Thomsen BL, et al. Waist circumference, BMI, smoking, and mortality in middle-aged men and women. Obes Res 2003;11: 895–903.
72. Kalmijn S, Curb JD, Rodriguez BL, et al. The association of body weight and anthropometry with mortality in elderly men: the Honolulu Heart Program. Int J Obes Relat Metab Disord 1999;23:395–402.
73. Baik I, Ascherio A, Rimm EB, et al. Adiposity and mortality in men. Am J Epidemiol 2000;152:264–71.
74. Taylor DH Jr, Ostbye T. The effect of middle- and old-age body mass index on short-term mortality in older people. J Am Geriatr Soc 2001;49:1319–26.
75. Yan LL, Daviglus ML, Liu K, et al. Midlife body mass index and hospitalization and mortality in older age. JAMA 2006;295:190–8.
76. Adams KF, Schatzkin A, Harris TB, et al. Overweight, obesity, and mortality in a large prospective cohort of persons 50 to 71 years old. N Engl J Med 2006; 355:763–78.
77. Newman AB, Yanez D, Harris T, et al. Weight change in old age and its association with mortality. J Am Geriatr Soc 2001;49:1309–18.
78. Heo M, Pietrobelli A, Fontaine KR, et al. Depressive mood and obesity in US adults: comparison and moderation by sex, age, and race. Int J Obes (Lond) 2006;30:513–9.
79. Barberger-Gateau P, Fabrigoule C. Disability and cognitive impairment in the elderly. Disabil Rehabil 1997;19:175–93.
80. Sakakura K, Hoshide S, Ishikawa J, et al. Association of body mass index with cognitive function in elderly hypertensive Japanese. Am J Hypertens 2008;21: 627–32.
81. Deschamps V, Astier X, Ferry M, et al. Nutritional status of healthy elderly persons living in Dordogne, France, and relation with mortality and cognitive or functional decline. Eur J Clin Nutr 2002;56:305–12.
82. Han C, Jo SA, Seo JA, et al. Adiposity parameters and cognitive function in the elderly: application of "Jolly Fat" hypothesis to cognition. Arch Gerontol Geriatr 2009;49:e133–8.
83. Felson DT, Zhang Y, Hannan MT, et al. Effects of weight and body mass index on bone mineral density in men and women: the Framingham study. J Bone Miner Res 1993;8:567–73.
84. Schoptt A, Cormier C, Hans D, et al. How hip and whole-body bone mineral density predict hip fracture in elderly women: the EPIDOS prospective study. Osteoporos Int 1998;8:247–54.
85. Imbeault P, Tremblay A, Simoneau JA, et al. Weight loss-induced rise in plasma pollutant is associated with reduced skeletal muscle oxidative capacity. Am J Physiol Endocrinol Metab 2002;282:E574–9.
86. Nelson KJ, Coulston AM, Sucher KP, et al. Prevalence of malnutrition in the elderly admitted to long-term-care facilities. J Am Diet Assoc 1993;93:459–61.
87. Chlebowski RT, Grosvenor M, Lillington L, et al. Dietary intake and counseling, weight maintenance, and the course of HIV infection. J Am Diet Assoc 1995; 95:428–32 [quiz 433–435].
88. Yeh S, Wu SY, Levine DM, et al. Quality of life and stimulation of weight gain after treatment with megestrol acetate: correlation between cytokine levels and nutritional status, appetite in geriatric patients with wasting syndrome. J Nutr Health Aging 2000;4:246–51.
89. Horwich T, Fonarow GC, Hamilton MA, et al. The relationship between obesity and mortality in patients with heart failure. J Am Coll Cardiol 2001;38:789–95.

90. Kalantar-Zadeh K, Block G, Humphreys MH, et al. Reverse epidemiology of cardiovascular risk factors in maintenance dialysis patients. Kidney Int 2003; 63:793–808.
91. Elia M. Hunger disease. Clin Nutr 2000;19:379–86.
92. DeFronzo RA, Ferrannini E. Insulin resistance: a multifaceted syndrome responsible for NIDDM, obesity, hypertension, dyslipidemia, and atherosclerotic cardiovascular disease. Diabetes Care 1991;14:173–94.
93. Ramsay SE, Whincup PH, Shaper AG, et al. The relations of body composition and adiposity measures to ill health and physical disability in elderly men. Am J Epidemiol 2006;164:459–69.
94. Oppert JM, Charles MA, Thibult N, et al. Anthropometric estimates of muscle and fat mass in relation to cardiac and cancer mortality in men: the Paris Prospective Study. Am J Clin Nutr 2002;75:1107–13.
95. Ensrud KE, Nevitt MC, Yunis C, et al. Correlates of impaired function in older women. J Am Geriatr Soc 1994;42:481–9.
96. Lang IA, Llewellyn DJ, Alexander K, et al. Obesity, physical function, and mortality in older adults. J Am Geriatr Soc 2008;56:1474–8.
97. Reynolds SL, Saito Y, Crimmins EM. The impact of obesity on active life expectancy in older American men and women. Gerontologist 2005;45:438–44.
98. Sternfeld B, Ngo L, Satariano WA, et al. Associations of body composition with physical performance and self-reported functional limitation in elderly men and women. Am J Epidemiol 2002;156:110–21.
99. Janssen I, Heymsfield SB, Ross R. Low relative skeletal muscle mass (sarcopenia) in older persons is associated with functional impairment and physical disability. J Am Geriatr Soc 2002;50:889–96.
100. DiPietro L. Physical activity, body weight, and adiposity: an epidemiologic perspective. Exerc Sport Sci Rev 1995;23:275–303.
101. McAuley PA, Myers JN, Abella JP, et al. Exercise capacity and body mass as predictors of mortality among male veterans with type 2 diabetes. Diabetes Care 2007;30:1539–43.
102. Haapanen-Niemi N, Miilunpalo S, Pasanen M, et al. Body mass index, physical inactivity and low level of physical fitness as determinants of all-cause and cardiovascular disease mortality: 16 y follow-up of middle-aged and elderly men and women. Int J Obes Relat Metab Disord 2000;24:1465–74.
103. Dziura J, Leon C, Kasl S, et al. Can physical activity attenuate aging-related weight loss in older people. Am J Epidemiol 2004;159:759–67.
104. Whelton PK, Appel LJ, Espeland MA, et al. Sodium reduction and weight loss in the treatment of hypertension in older persons: a randomized controlled trial of nonpharmacologic interventions in the elderly (TONE). TONE Collaborative Research Group. JAMA 1998;279:839–46.
105. Rejeski WJ, Focht BC, Messier SP, et al. Obese, older adults with knee osteoarthritis: weight loss, exercise, and quality of life. Health Psychol 2002;21:419–26.
106. Messier SP, Loeser RF, Miller GD, et al. Exercise and dietary weight loss in overweight and obese older adults with knee osteoarthritis: the Arthritis, Diet, and Activity Promotion Trial. Arthritis Rheum 2004;50:1501–10.
107. Chao D, Espeland MA, Farmer D, et al. Effect of voluntary weight loss on bone mineral density in older overweight women. J Am Geriatr Soc 2000;48:753–9.
108. Daly R, Dunstan D, Owen N, et al. Does high-intensity resistance training maintain bone mass during moderate weight loss in older overweight adults with type 2 diabetes? Osteoporos Int 2005;16:1703–12.

Physical Activity and Prevention of Cardiovascular Disease in Older Adults

David M. Buchner, MD, MPH

KEYWORDS

• Aged • Exercise • Cardiovascular disease
• Primary prevention • Guideline

Regular physical activity is essential for healthy aging. Physical activity reduces the risk of premature mortality and many age-related chronic diseases[1]; it provides therapeutic benefits for many common chronic diseases. Physical activity provides mental health benefits important for healthy aging, for example, by reducing risk of depressive illness and cognitive impairment.[1] Physical activity improves physical fitness in older adults. In part because of higher fitness, physically active older adults have less risk of functional limitations and fall-related injuries.[1] Physically active and fit older adults are more likely to live independently in the community.

The purpose of this article is to discuss the types and amounts of physical activity recommended for the primary prevention of cardiovascular disease (CVD) in older adults. The preventive benefits of physical activity in CVD have been extensively studied. Public health guidelines have recently been updated to reflect new research in this area, and in other areas of research on the health benefits of physical activity. The discussion builds on the first national physical activity guidelines recently released by the US Department of Health and Human Services—the 2008 *Physical Activity Guidelines for Americans* (or "the *Guidelines*").[2] A systematic evidence review laid the scientific basis for the *Guidelines* that included a separate article on cardiovascular health.[1] The review was conducted by the Physical Activity Guidelines Advisory Committee (PAGAC), and is referred to as the PAGAC report. As the PAGAC report is comprehensive and long (683 pages not including all the tables), this article seeks to make its content more accessible, and put key findings of the report in a clinical context dealing with prevention of CVD in older adults.

This work was supported in part by a Shahid and Ann Carlson Khan Professorship in Applied Health Sciences.
Department of Kinesiology and Community Health, University of Illinois at Urbana-Champaign, 129 Huff Hall, MC-588, 1206 S. Fourth Street, Champaign IL 61820, USA
E-mail address: dbuchner@illinois.edu

The article is organized into 4 sections. After reviewing terminology, the first section discusses the *Guidelines* and the scientific consensus on the dose-response relationship between physical activity and risk of CVD and other chronic diseases. The second section focuses on issues and evidence specific to CVD. The third section deals with the effects of physical activity on functional limitations and health-related quality of life in older adults. The final section deals with gaps in knowledge and provides recommendations for future research.

DOSE-RESPONSE RELATIONSHIP BETWEEN PHYSICAL ACTIVITY AND HEALTH
Terminology

The *Guidelines* divide daily activity into 2 types. *Baseline activity* refers to light-intensity activities of daily life (eg, standing and walking slowly) and very short bouts of moderate- and vigorous-intensity activity. *Health-enhancing physical activity* refers to the types and amounts of moderate- and vigorous-intensity activity that provide substantial health benefits, and count toward meeting guidelines. In common usage, the term "physical activity" is used inconsistently. Sometimes it refers to any bodily movement produced by skeletal muscles that expends energy. Sometimes the term refers to only health-enhancing physical activity. In this article, as in the *Guidelines*, physical activity refers only to health-enhancing physical activity.

Intensity refers to the level of effort during physical activity. The *absolute intensity* of activity refers to the rate of energy expenditure during activity, and is measured in metabolic equivalents (METs). One MET is the rate of energy expenditure at rest, usually estimated to be 3.5 ml O_2/kg/min. For example, a task with an intensity of 4 METs expends energy at 4 times the resting rate. **Table 1** describes how the range of absolute intensity is divided into light-, moderate-, and vigorous-intensity levels. For example, walking at 3.0 miles per hour requires on average 3.3 METs of energy expenditure, and is a moderate-intensity activity. Running a mile in 10 minutes requires about 10 METs of energy expenditure, and is a vigorous-intensity activity. The *relative intensity* of activity refers to level of effort relative to a person's fitness.

Table 1
Definitions of absolute intensity and relative intensity of aerobic physical activity used in the *2008 Physical Activity Guidelines for Americans*

Absolute intensity measured in METs (metabolic equivalents)
   Light-intensity: <3.0 METs
   Moderate-intensity: 3.0–5.9 METs
   Vigorous-intensity: >6.0 METs
Relative intensity measured on an 11-point scale[a]
   0 = sitting
   1–4 = light-intensity
   5 & 6 = moderate-intensity
   7 & 8 = vigorous-intensity
   9 = near maximal effort
   10 = maximal effort

[a] In the framework of an exercise prescription based on oxygen uptake reserve or heart rate reserve (HRR), moderate-intensity is activity performed at 45% to 64% of HRR, and vigorous-intensity is activity performed at 65% to 84% of HRR. See Appendix 1 of the Guidelines for how these definitions compare with others.

Data from Department of Health and Human Services. 2008 Physical Activity Guidelines for Americans. Available at: http://www.health.gov/paguidelines/guidelines/default.aspx. Accessed August 17, 2009.

The *Guidelines* use an 11-point scale to communicate the concept of relative intensity (see **Table 1**). On this scale "0" is sitting, and "10" is maximal level of effort.

The total amount of physical activity in a period of time (typically a week) is referred to as the *volume* of physical activity. Volume is the product of frequency × duration × intensity. Volume is commonly measured in MET-minutes (or MET-hours). For example, doing a 4.0 MET task for 15 minutes is 60 MET-minutes of activity. Volume can also be measured as energy expenditure during physical activity.

Health Benefits of Physical Activity

The major health benefits of physical activity identified by the PAGAC report are listed in **Table 2**. Regular physical activity decreases risk of many forms of CVD. However, the evidence is inconclusive as to whether activity prevents incident peripheral vascular disease.

The evidence for the health benefits of physical activity depends on both randomized trials and prospective observational studies. Physical activity produces acute, short-term, and long-term effects on health. Acute benefits occur with a single bout of exercise and include reduction in blood pressure. Short-term benefits occur after several months of regular physical activity and include improved physical fitness,

---

Table 2
Health benefits of physical activity in adults and older adults

Lower risk of chronic conditions and of premature mortality
  Strong evidence
    Premature mortality
    Coronary heart disease
    Stroke
    Type 2 diabetes
    Colon cancer
    Breast cancer
    Hypertension
    Adverse blood lipid profile
    Metabolic syndrome
    Weight gain and obesity
    Weight loss (especially when combined with reduced calorie intake)
    Depressive illness
  Moderate evidence
    Hip fracture
    Lung cancer
    Endometrial cancer
    Weight maintenance after weight loss
    Abdominal obesity
Beneficial effects of physical activity on fitness and function
  Strong evidence
    Improved cardiorespiratory and muscular fitness
    Improved cognitive function (in older adults)
    Reduced risk of falls (in older adults)
  Moderate evidence
    Improved functional health (in older adults)
    Increased bone density
    Improved sleep quality

Data from PAGAC (Physical Activity Guidelines Advisory Committee). Physical Activity Guidelines Advisory Committee Report 2008. Available at: http://www.health.gov/paguidelines/committeereport.aspx. Accessed August 17, 2009.

fewer symptoms of depression, and reduction in risk of falls. Generally speaking, conclusions about the acute and short-term benefits of physical activity are based mainly on data from randomized controlled trials. However, prospective observational studies (cohort studies) remain the only cost-effective approach to studying the long-term effects of many years of regular physical activity on major health outcomes, such as risk of coronary heart disease and cardiovascular mortality.

Dose-Response Relationship

The main determinant of the health benefits of physical activity is volume.[1] For most important health benefits of physical activity, including prevention of coronary artery disease and stroke, a dose-response relationship exists between volume and disease risk. **Fig. 1** illustrates the dose-response relationship between volume of activity and risk of premature mortality. The figure is based on an analysis of 73 studies, of which 71 were prospective cohort studies, and 67 reported a significant inverse relationship between level of activity and mortality risk.[1] The exact shape of the dose-response curve varies by health outcome. For example, evidence suggests that a larger volume of physical activity is required to substantially reduce risk of breast cancer than to substantially reduce risk of coronary heart disease.[1] There are several notable features to the dose-response relationship in **Fig. 1**:

- Even relatively low levels of physical activity (60 minutes of moderate-intensity activity per week) provide some health benefits compared with inactivity.
- The curvilinear relationship indicates that most of the benefits of physical activity occur by the time a person participates in the range of 150 to 300 minutes of moderate-intensity activity per week.
- Additional benefits of physical activity accrue through participation in high amounts of physical activity—above the equivalent of 300 minutes of moderate-intensity activity per week. However, there is decreasing marginal health benefit from each additional minute per week.
- There is no known upper limit, at which an additional minute per week of physical activity provides no additional health benefit.

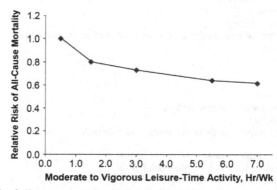

Fig. 1. Relative risk of all-cause mortality by level of physical activity. This figure from the Physical Activity Guidelines Advisory Committee report presents a summary of the "median" shape of the dose-response curve synthesized from 11 studies (out of 73 studies identified in the evidence review), which used 5 categories of physical activity. Hr/Wk, hours per week. (*Data from* PAGAC [Physical Activity Guidelines Advisory Committee]. Physical Activity Guidelines Advisory Committee Report 2008. Available at: http://www.health.gov/paguidelines/committeereport.aspx. Accessed August 17, 2009.)

Medium Amounts of Physical Activity Provide Substantial Health Benefits

The PAGAC report concluded that 500 to 1000 MET-minutes per week, when accumulated from moderate- to vigorous-intensity activity, provide substantial health benefits.[1] The PAGAC report indicated that 500 to 1000 MET-minutes is roughly the same as 150 to 300 minutes of moderate-intensity physical activity. The *Guidelines* regard this amount as a *medium amount* of activity. Reflecting the evidence for a dose-response effect, the report concluded that *high amounts* of activity (in excess of 1000 MET-minutes) provide even more health benefits.

Whereas 500 MET-minutes is a medium amount of activity in terms of health benefits, it is a small amount relative to what humans are capable of doing. Consider a recent study of 98 old order Amish adults, who accomplish the work of farming using manual labor and draft animals.[3] In this study, men performed an average of about 18,000 MET-minutes per week, and women about 12,500 MET-minutes per week.

Physical Activity Guidelines for Older Adults

The *Guidelines* contain 8 key recommendations for older adults (**Table 3**). These guidelines represent the core public health recommendations on the types and amounts of physical activity required for the primary prevention of CVD, emphasizing the dose-response relationship between activity and health benefits. Some benefits occur even at low amounts of activity, so it is important to avoid inactivity. Substantial health benefits occur with 150 to 300 minutes of moderate-intensity aerobic activity (or an equivalent amount of vigorous-intensity activity). Greater health benefits occur with high amounts of activity. There is now sufficient evidence to recommend muscle strengthening activity for its health benefits, not just for its fitness benefit. For example, there is reasonably strong evidence that muscle strengthening activities reduce blood pressure.[1] Other guidelines deal with fall prevention and with the importance of physical activity in older adults who have chronic conditions (even conditions that reduce a person's ability to lead an active lifestyle). The *Guidelines* specify that older adults should monitor the relative intensity (as opposed to absolute intensity) of their activity. The purpose of this recommendation is to reduce risk of activity-related adverse events in people with low fitness. Whereas the key guidelines emphasize attainment of at least a medium amount of activity each week, they also stipulate a minimum intensity and duration for activity, and comment on the frequency of activity.

Intensity

Only moderate-intensity and vigorous-intensity bouts count toward meeting the guidelines for aerobic activity and muscle strengthening activity. Evidence is insufficient whether vigorous-intensity aerobic activity has greater health benefits than moderate activity, after controlling for volume. As a result, the *Guidelines* do not state that vigorous-intensity activity is preferable. However, vigorous-intensity activity is clearly more effective at improving cardiorespiratory fitness. Studies consistently report that higher fitness is associated with lower risk of CVD (see later discussion).

Duration

To count toward meeting guidelines, bouts of aerobic activity must last at least 10 minutes. This recommendation is not based on observational studies, as these studies have provided little insight into the minimum bout duration required for meaningful health benefits. Bouts of at least 10 minutes are recommended, based on evidence from randomized trials showing that bouts of 10+ minutes have beneficial effects on cardiovascular health indicators, such as lipoprotein profile, blood pressure, and insulin sensitivity.[1]

Table 3
Summary of key physical activity guidelines for adults and older adults in the *2008 Physical Activity Guidelines for Americans*

Guidelines that apply to adults and older adults
1. All adults should avoid inactivity. Some physical activity is better than none.
2. For substantial health benefits, adults should do a medium amount of aerobic physical activity each week:
   • At least 150 min of moderate-intensity aerobic activity
OR
   • At least 75 min of vigorous-intensity aerobic activity
OR
   • A combination of moderate- and vigorous-intensity, where 1 vigorous minute = 2 moderate-intensity minutes
3. For additional and more extensive health benefits, adults should do the equivalent of 300 or more minutes per week of moderate-intensity physical activity
4. Adults should also do muscle strengthening activities at least 2 days each week, of moderate or high intensity, and which involve all major muscle groups

Guidelines that apply only to older adults
5. When older adults cannot do 150 min of moderate-intensity activity a week because of chronic conditions, they should be as active as abilities and conditions allow
6. Older adults at risk of falls should do exercises that maintain or improve balance
7. Older adults should monitor their level of effort of physical activity relative to their level of fitness (ie, should use relative intensity to guide level of effort)
8. Older adults with chronic conditions should understand whether and how the conditions affect ability to do regular physical activity safely

Data from Department of Health and Human Services. 2008 Physical Activity Guidelines for Americans. Available at: http://www.health.gov/paguidelines/guidelines/default.aspx. Accessed August 17, 2009.

Frequency

The PAGAC report found insufficient information on how frequency affects health benefits. Hence, in a departure from most previous recommendations, the *Guidelines* do not specify a minimum frequency (minimum number of active days per week). However, the previous recommendation for at least 30 minutes of moderate-intensity activity on 5 or more days per week is not wrong, as it prescribes 150+ minutes per week of moderate-intensity activity. Rather, it is too specific. The evidence is insufficient to conclude, for example, that the health benefits of 50 minutes of activity 3 times a week differs from the benefits of 30 minutes of activity 5 times a week. The *Guidelines* do advise that dividing activity among 3 or more days per week is *preferable*, as high volumes of activity on only 1 or 2 days per week probably increase risk of injury. The flexibility in the guidelines as to frequency should appeal to older adults. For example, older adults can now meet guidelines by attending a combined aerobics and muscle-strengthening exercise class 3 days a week (assuming sufficient amounts of activity during class).

Health Benefits and Health Risks of Walking

Walking is the most prevalent type of activity performed by older adults. Whereas slow walking is light-intensity and race walking is vigorous-intensity, walking as commonly performed is the best example of a moderate-intensity physical activity. There is strong evidence that a medium volume of walking provides substantial health benefits.[1] The evidence includes studies reporting that walking decreases risk of CVD in a dose-response manner. In 3 studies of CVD risk in women, women who walked the most reduced risk of CVD by 35%,[4] 32%,[5] and 52%[6] compared with women who walked the least. A significant dose-response relationship was reported in each study.

Walking is particularly appropriate for older adults because the risk of injury while walking is very low. A community-based study from Finland estimated that walking for transportation had a risk of 20 injuries per 100,000 hours of walking.[7] The same study estimated that running (as a sport) had a risk of 360 injuries per 100,000 hours of running. Because running is a vigorous activity, it provides more health benefit per minute of activity than does moderate-intensity walking. After adjusting for volume of activity, the PAGAC report estimated that the difference in injury rates between walking and running is less dramatic, but still walking has lower injury risk: risk for walking was 0.8 injuries per 100,000 MET-minutes, versus 6.0 injuries per 100,000 MET-minutes for running. Of course, the *net* health benefit is determined by both the benefits and risks of physical activity.

Objective Assessment of Physical Activity

With one exception, cohort studies of the long-term effects of physical activity have measured physical activity by self-report using questionnaires. Objective measures provide a more accurate assessment of physical activity. The 3 most commonly used objective measures are doubly labeled water, pedometers, and accelerometers. Doubly labeled water assesses the total activity energy expenditure from light, moderate, and vigorous activity combined. Pedometers primarily measure the amount of walking and running. Accelerometers measure movement, and can be used to assess the intensity, duration, frequency, and total volume of most types of activity.

The agreement between self-report and accelerometer measures of physical activity is usually modest. For example, a study of older adults reported a correlation in the range of $R = 0.14$ to 0.25 between activity counts in the moderate- to vigorous-intensity range (obtained from accelerometers) and various subscores of the CHAMPS Activities Questionnaire for Older Adults.[8] The concern about reliance on self-report from questionnaire is dramatically illustrated by data from national surveillance systems that provide estimates of the percentage of older adults who meet the 1995 Centers for Disease Control and Prevention/American College of Sports Medicine physical activity recommendation. Based on questionnaire data from the Behavioral Risk Factor Surveillance System (BRFSS),[9] about 40% of older adults obtained recommended amounts of physical activity in 2007. However, based on accelerometer data collected in the National Health and Nutrition Examination Survey (NHANES), only 2.4% of older adults met recommendations.[10]

Cohort studies that include objective assessments of physical activity could provide important new insights into how physical activity influences health. The only prospective cohort study to date that used an objective assessment of physical activity was the Dynamics of Health, Aging and Body Composition (Health ABC) study.[11] Of note, this study reported a stronger relationship between level of activity and premature mortality than generally found in other studies. The study measured total activity energy expenditure using doubly labeled water in 302 older adults. The relationship between activity energy expenditure and risk of premature mortality is shown in **Fig. 2**. The study included a physical activity questionnaire to measure self-reported moderate- to vigorous-intensity physical activity, allowing estimation of energy expended in reported versus unreported activity. Several aspects of the data in **Fig. 2** are notable:

- The data show a clear dose-response relationship across tertiles of physical activity.

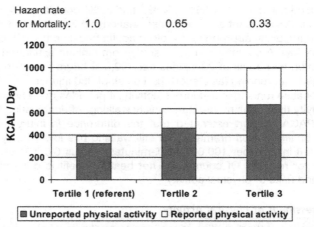

Hazard rate
for Mortality: 1.0   0.65   0.33

Fig. 2. Risk of all-cause mortality by tertile of activity energy expenditure in adults age 70 to 82 years. Energy expenditure was measured using doubly labeled water. Energy expenditure (kcal) estimated from self-reported physical activity was subtracted from total activity energy expenditure to derive energy expenditure from unreported physical activity. (*Data from* Manini TM, Everhart JE, Patel KV, et al. Daily activity energy expenditure and mortality among older adults. JAMA 2006:296:171–9.)

- The most active tertile of older adults had a 67% reduction in risk of premature mortality—a larger risk reduction than reported in most studies that used questionnaires to assess physical activity.
- The data affirm the health benefits of medium amounts of physical activity, as the percentage of older adults who do high amounts of activity is relatively small.
- Both reported and unreported physical activity increased across the tertiles. The study raises the possibility that health benefits attributed to reported activity may be partly due to unreported physical activity (most of which is baseline physical activity).

PHYSICAL ACTIVITY AND CARDIOVASCULAR HEALTH
Importance of Physical Activity for Prevention of Cardiovascular Disease

A recent study calculated the number of deaths that would be prevented or postponed with perfect prevention and treatment of heart disease.[12] A model was created to simulate the risk factor and event rate profile of United States adults aged 30 to 84 years. The study identified 6 interventions known to reduce risk of heart disease in individuals without apparent disease: physical activity, prudent diet, abstaining from tobacco, ω-3 fatty acids, control of hypertension, and avoiding environmental tobacco smoke. As shown in **Fig. 3**, the model estimated the largest reduction in premature mortality would accrue from increasing population levels of physical activity.

This large estimated impact of increasing physical activity is consistent with the breadth of effects of physical activity in CVD. Most of the effects of physical activity CVD have been well studied, and published reviews and meta-analyses are available.[1] Here, each of the major effects is briefly discussed, based mainly on the review in the PAGAC report.

Cardiovascular morbidity and mortality

There is strong evidence of an inverse relationship between level of physical activity and risk of cardiovascular morbidity and mortality. The median risk reduction in

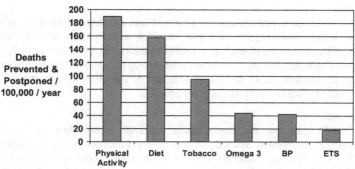

Fig. 3. Estimated effect of 6 interventions on deaths prevented or postponed due to heart disease per 100,000 adults per year, age 30 to 84 years. The estimates depend on a model of heart disease occurrence in the United States population, and assume perfect care for the prevention of heart disease in the United States. Physical Activity, engaging in adequate physical activity; Diet, following dietary guidelines; Tobacco, abstaining from tobacco; Omega 3, consuming adequate amounts of ω-3 fatty acids; BP, controlling hypertension; ETS, avoiding environmental tobacco smoke. (*Data from* Kottke TE, Faith DA, Jordan CO, et al. The comparative effectiveness of heart disease prevention and treatment strategies. Am J Prev Med 2009;36:82–8.)

CVD and coronary heart disease among the most active adults was 30% and 32%, respectively. Benefits were observed in both men and women, and in all ethnic groups studied. However, existing studies have not had sufficient statistical power to test whether the benefit differs among ethnic groups.

Cerebrovascular disease and stroke
There is strong evidence for an inverse relationship between level of physical activity and risk of stroke. More active adults have about a 25% to 30% lower risk of stroke. The relationship is not influenced by sex or age.

Peripheral artery disease
Evidence is insufficient to conclude that regular physical activity prevents peripheral vascular disease. There is some evidence that physical activity is correlated with the ankle-brachial index, an indicator of the severity of lower extremity arterial disease. There is strong evidence that exercise training is effective treatment for adults with peripheral artery disease.

Hypertension
The PAGAC evidence review identified 10 published meta-analyses of the relationship of aerobic exercise with resting blood pressure. The most recent and inclusive analysis included 72 studies, and reported that exercise reduced resting systolic blood pressure by 3 mm Hg and resting diastolic blood pressure by 2 mm Hg.[13] Effects of exercise on blood pressure were greater in adults with hypertension, reducing systolic pressure by about 7 mm Hg and diastolic pressure by about 5 mm Hg. The meta-analysis concluded that aerobic training reduces blood pressure by reducing vascular resistance, due at least in part to effects of activity on the sympathetic nervous system and the renin-angiotensin system. In the analysis, exercise caused a 7.1% reduction in vascular resistance, a 29% reduction in plasma norepinephrine, and a 20% reduction in plasma renin activity.[13] Other research shows that resistance training reduces blood pressure, although the evidence is stronger for aerobic exercise.

Dyslipidemia
The effect of exercise on blood lipids has also been extensively studied, and there is generally a direct relationship between level of activity and serum high-density lipoprotein (HDL) cholesterol and an inverse relationship between activity level and triglycerides. Evidence is less consistent and strong for an effect of activity on serum low-density lipoprotein (LDL) cholesterol, possibly because it may require a higher dose of activity to significantly reduce serum LDL.

Vascular health
Vascular health can be assessed using brachial artery flow-mediated dilation (BAFMD), which correlates with coronary artery function measures and predicts CVD events. The PAGAC evidence review located 22 randomized trials of exercise and BAFMD, with most trials reporting that exercise caused beneficial changes in BAFMD.

Cardiorespiratory fitness
It is well documented that regular aerobic exercise improves measures of cardiorespiratory fitness, such as peak rate of oxygen consumption during exercise testing. There is strong evidence that higher cardiorespiratory fitness reduces risk of many chronic diseases, including CVD. For example, a cohort study in 906 women reported that each 1 MET increase in maximal aerobic capacity was associated with an 8% decrease in risk of major adverse events during follow-up.[14]

Independence of Effects of Physical Activity on Cardiovascular Disease

Of note, physical activity reduces the risk of heart disease independent of the status of other CVD risk factors. A person can reduce their risk of heart disease by engaging in physical activity, and the beneficial effect does not depend, for example, on whether they smoke or are obese. A study of older adults in the Aerobics Center Longitudinal Study reported that each additional MET of exercise capacity significantly reduced risk of CVD.[15] The effect of fitness was similar in smokers and nonsmokers, and similar in overweight/obese adults and normal weight adults. Overall, subjects with high fitness had lower risk of CVD mortality (hazard rate = 0.57, 95% confidence interval [CI] = 0.41–0.80) compared with those with low fitness.

Physiologic Mechanisms by Which Physical Activity Reduces Cardiovascular Disease Risk

The mechanisms by which physical activity reduces risk of heart disease are only partly understood. The Women's Health Study provided an opportunity to examine how the effect of physical activity on heart disease in women could be explained by its effects on cardiovascular risk factors.[16] Known risk factors for heart disease explained only about 40% of the observed association between MET-hours of physical activity per week and risk of coronary heart disease events. The effect of physical activity on blood pressure, lipids (total, LDL, and HDL cholesterol), body mass index, and inflammatory/hemostatic factors (high-sensitivity C-reactive protein, fibrinogen, soluble intracellular adhesion molecule-1) were most important in explaining the reduction in risk. The effects of physical activity on novel lipid biomarkers (lipoprotein(a), apolipoprotein A1, apolipoprotein B-100), glycosylated hemoglobin (HbA1c), and homocysteine were relatively less important mechanisms for reducing risk of heart disease.

There is growing evidence that physical activity reduces CVD risk partly because of its anti-inflammatory effects.[17] For example, an interesting randomized trial compared regular exercise to percutaneous angioplasty in 101 men with coronary artery disease

(CAD).[18] The study reported at 2-year follow-up a significantly higher event-free survival rate in the exercise group (78%) compared with the angioplasty group (62%). In this trial, exercise significantly reduced high-sensitivity C-reactive protein by 41% and interleukin-6 by 18% at 2-year follow-up, whereas angioplasty had no effect on these inflammatory markers.

PHYSICAL ACTIVITY AND FUNCTIONAL LIMITATIONS

Older adults place a high value on the ability to live independently. By preventing chronic diseases such as CVD, and by improving physical and mental fitness, physical activity should promote independent living. Evidence that the amounts and types of activity that are effective in preventing CVD also reduce the risk of functional limitations in older adults is summarized here.

Observational studies consistently report that regular physical activity reduces risk of functional limitations, particularly mobility limitations.[1] The PAGAC review located 28 prospective cohort studies, and essentially all studies reported a lower risk of functional limitations in active older adults. The data suggest a dose-response effect, as illustrated in **Fig. 4**, for the effect of physical activity on mobility limitations. Of course, there is concern that observational studies cannot adequately adjust for confounding due to chronic conditions. No large randomized trial has been done to determine whether regular physical activity in relatively healthy older adults prevents incident functional limitations. The PAGAC report concluded there was only limited evidence from randomized trials that exercise has beneficial effects on function in adults with existing functional limitations. In particular, there is a lack of data on dose response, in part because trials typically test roughly the amount of activity necessary to just meet physical activity guidelines, so there is little variation in dose across trials. One recent randomized trial with 3 different doses is an exception.[19] This trial showed

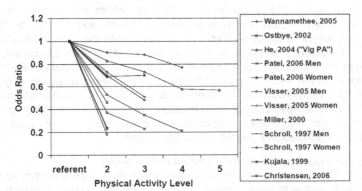

Fig. 4. Risk of mobility limitations in older adults by level of physical activity. This figure from the Physical Activity Guidelines Advisory Committee Report summarizes data from 12 analyses from prospective cohort studies. In each study, the category for the lowest level of physical activity was identified as the referent. The figure plots the odds ratios for the other categories in the study. Overall, the studies show a dose-response relationship, with higher levels of activity associated with lower risk. (*Data from* PAGAC [Physical Activity Guidelines Advisory Committee]. Physical Activity Guidelines Advisory Committee Report 2008. Available at: http://www.health.gov/paguidelines/committeereport.aspx. Accessed August 17, 2009.)

that higher doses of activity produced greater effects on functional limitations and quality of life.

RECOMMENDATIONS FOR RESEARCH
Research on Sedentary Behavior in Older Adults

There is growing interest in how sedentary behavior per se affects the risk of chronic conditions. In the framework of the guidelines, baseline activity comprises time spent in light activity (standing, slow walking, and so forth) and sedentary behavior comprises time spent in periods of little or no movement while awake (which nowadays is mainly sitting). This area of research addresses how variation in the amount of baseline activity affects health—an issue not addressed in the Guidelines. Research is currently investigating the hypothesis that large amounts of sedentary behavior have an adverse effect on the risk of chronic disease, and that this effect is independent of the amount of time spent in moderate- to vigorous-intensity physical activity (MVPA). A corollary hypothesis is that longer bouts of sedentary behavior have greater adverse effects.

The issue of sedentary behavior is particularly relevant to older adults. Accelerometer data from NHANES show that older adults spend more time in sedentary behavior than any age group.[20] Adults aged 60 to 69 years spend about 8.4 hours per day in sedentary behavior, whereas those aged 70 to 85 spend about 9.3 hours per day in sedentary behavior. In these age groups, women have slightly less sedentary behavior than men. The NHANES accelerometer data show that older adults spend little time in 10-minute bouts of MVPA that counts toward meeting guidelines.[10] Men aged 60 to 69 spent an average of about 7 minutes per day doing MVPA. Men aged 70 or older and women aged 60 or older did even less MVPA.

Obesity and sedentary behavior

Less sedentary time theoretically should reduce the risk of obesity by increasing total daily activity energy expenditure. Most energy expenditure (eg, as measured by doubly labeled water) is not due to MVPA but to light activity.[21] Data from the Health ABC study shown in **Fig. 2** illustrate this finding. Adults show wide variability in amounts of activity-related energy expenditure.[21] Energy expenditure of "standing workers" is reported as about 1400 kcal/d, compared with about 700 kcal/d for seated workers.[21] "Fidgeting" can produce substantial amounts of caloric expenditure.[22] As a rough rule of thumb, a person expends 100 kcal when walking a mile. It is thus possible for a person who sits most of the day, but meets physical activity guidelines by walking 25 minutes each day, to have a lower total daily caloric expenditure than an inactive person who does substantial amounts of light activity. Epidemiologic studies report that, in adults who are physically active, the amount of time spent watching television is an independent predictor of body weight.[23]

Sedentary behavior, chronic disease, and metabolic health

It is possible that sedentary time has an independent effect on risk of chronic disease. Using a questionnaire to assess sedentary behaviors, the Women's Health Initiative found that sedentary behavior had an independent effect on CVD risk.[5] The relative risk of CVD was 1.38 (95% CI = 1.01–1.87) among women who reported spending 12 to 15 hours per day lying down or sleeping, and 1.68 (95% CI = 1.07–2.64) for women who reported at least 16 hours per day sitting. The Health ABC data also show that total energy expenditure (not simply energy expenditure from MVPA) predicts premature mortality (see **Fig. 2**).

Sedentary muscle appears less metabolically active. For example, muscle lipoprotein lipase activity is decreased with prolonged sedentary behavior.[21] Due to this and other mechanisms, sedentary behavior could affect metabolic health. In one epidemiologic study, sedentary time was independently associated with waist circumference and metabolic risk.[24] Further, independent of total sedentary time and amount of MVPA, fewer breaks during sedentary time was associated with greater waist circumference, and higher serum triglycerides and 2-hour plasma glucose.[25]

Research Recommendations

The following recommendations are based on the PAGAC report and the discussion presented in this article:

- What is the time course of acquisition of the cardiovascular health benefits of activity, when an inactive adult adopts an active lifestyle?
- Why do the effects of physical activity on known risk factors for CVD explain less than 50% of the effect of physical activity on CVD risk?
- What are the independent effects on CVD risk attributable to variations in intensity, frequency, and duration of activity, while controlling for total volume of activity? In particular, is vigorous-intensity activity more effective than moderate-intensity activity in prevention of CVD?
- To what extent does the relationship between amount of physical activity and CVD risk depend on the method of measurement of physical activity? Is a stronger relationship found when physical activity is assessed using objective measures such as accelerometers, as opposed to questionnaires?
- To what extent is the effect of physical activity on CVD risk due to the total volume of moderate- to vigorous-intensity activity, versus the total volume of light, moderate, and vigorous activity as assessed by total activity energy expenditure? In particular, does sedentary behavior have adverse health effects and increase CVD risk, independent from the amount of MVPA?
- What are the effects of muscle-strengthening activities on cardiovascular health, and what is the nature of dose-response relationship (eg, how does the effect vary by intensity of resistance training)?
- Do the benefits of physical activity on cardiovascular health vary significantly by ethnic group or by gender, after controlling for total volume of activity?
- Does regular physical activity reduce risk of incident peripheral vascular disease? Does regular physical activity reduce age-related changes in biomarkers of vascular health, such as BAFMD?
- In older adults with existing functional limitations, does regular physical activity reduce these limitations, and if so, what combination of aerobic activity and muscle strengthening activity is optimal for producing these effects? What is the dose-response relationship between volume of activity and benefit?

SUMMARY

There is strong scientific evidence that regular physical activity reduces risk of CVD and other chronic illnesses in older adults. Consistent with these preventive effects, observational studies consistently report that active older adults have lower risk of functional limitations and higher health-related quality of life. The *2008 Physical Activity Guidelines for Americans* provide guidance on the types and amounts of physical activity in older adults that reduce the risk of chronic diseases. The guidelines reflect the scientific consensus that volume of moderate to vigorous aerobic physical activity is the main determinant of health benefits. A medium amount of physical activity substantially reduces the risk of cardiovascular and other chronic diseases. A medium amount of aerobic activity is characterized by 150 to 300 minutes of moderate-intensity activity, or 75 to 150 minutes of vigorous-intensity activity each week, accumulated from discrete activity bouts of at least 10 minutes. In particular, a medium amount of walking each week provides substantial health benefits for older adults, with relatively low risk of injury.

For most chronic diseases, physical activity reduces the risk of disease in a dose-response fashion, with even low amounts of activity having some benefit. High amounts of physical activity provide further reductions in the risk of cardiovascular disease. In addition to aerobic activity, muscle strengthening activities are also recommended for cardiovascular health. Research is needed to address several important gaps in knowledge, including how amounts of sedentary behavior influence the risk of CVD, independent of the amount of MVPA.

REFERENCES

1. PAGAC (Physical Activity Guidelines Advisory Committee). Physical Activity Guidelines Advisory Committee Report 2008. Available at: http://www.health. gov/paguidelines/committeereport.aspx. Accessed August 17, 2009.
2. Department of Health and Human Services. 2008. Physical activity guidelines for Americans. Available at: http://www.health.gov/paguidelines/guidelines/default. aspx. Accessed August 17, 2009.
3. Bassett DR, Schneider PL, Huntington GE. Physical activity in an old order Amish community. Med Sci Sports Exerc 2004;36:79–85.
4. Manson JE, Hu FB, Rich-Edwards JW, et al. A prospective study of walking as compared with vigorous exercise in the prevention of coronary heart disease in women. N Engl J Med 1999;341:650–8.
5. Manson JE, Greenland P, LaCroix AZ, et al. Walking compared with vigorous exercise for the prevention of cardiovascular events in women. N Engl J Med 2002; 347:716–25.
6. Lee IM, Rexrode KM, Cook NR, et al. Physical activity and coronary heart disease in women: is "no pain, no gain" passé? JAMA 2001;295:1447–54.
7. Parkkari J, Kannus P, Natri A, et al. Active living and injury risk. Int J Sports Med 2004;25(3):209–16.
8. Pruitt LA, Glynn NW, King AC, et al. Use of accelerometry to measure physical activity in older adults at risk for mobility disability. J Aging Phys Act 2008;16:416–34.
9. Centers for Disease Control and Prevention. U.S. physical activity statistics. Available at: http://apps.nccd.cdc.gov/PASurveillance/DemoComparev.asp. Accessed September 20, 2009.
10. Troiano RP, Berrigan D, Dodd KW, et al. Physical activity in the United States measured by accelerometer. Med Sci Sports Exerc 2007;40:181–8.
11. Manini TM, Everhart JE, Patel KV, et al. Daily activity energy expenditure and mortality among older adults. JAMA 2006;296:171–9.
12. Kottke TE, Faith DA, Jordan CO, et al. The comparative effectiveness of heart disease prevention and treatment strategies. Am J Prev Med 2009;36:82–8.
13. Cornelissen VA, Fagard RH. Effects of endurance training on blood pressure, blood pressure regulating mechanisms, and cardiovascular risk factors. Hypertension 2005;46:667–75.
14. Wessel TR, Arant CB, Olson MB, et al. Relationship of physical fitness vs. body mass index with coronary artery disease and cardiovascular disease events in women. JAMA 2004;292:1179–87.
15. Sui X, Laditka JN, Hardin JW, et al. Estimated functional capacity predicts mortality in older adults. J Am Geriatr Soc 2007;55:1940–7.

16. Mora S, Cook N, Buring JE, et al. Physical activity and reduced risk of cardiovascular events. Circulation 2007;116:2110–8.
17. Gielen S, Walther C, Schuler G, et al. Anti-inflammatory effects of physical exercise. A new mechanism to explain the benefits of cardiac rehabilitation? J Cardiopulm Rehabil 2005;25:339–42.
18. Walther C, Mobius-Winkler S, Linke A, et al. Regular exercise training compared with percutaneous intervention leads to a reduction in inflammatory markers and cardiovascular events in patients with coronary artery disease. Eur J Cardiovasc Prev Rehabil 2008;15:107–12.
19. Martin CK, Church TS, Thompson AM, et al. Exercise dose and quality of life. Arch Intern Med 2009;169:269–78.
20. Matthews CD, Chen KY, Freedson PS, et al. Amount of time sent in sedentary behaviors in the United States, 2003–2004. Am J Epidemiol 2008;167:875–81.
21. Hamilton MT, Hamilton DG, Zderic TW. Role of low energy expenditure and sitting in obesity, metabolic syndrome, type 2 diabetes, and cardiovascular disease. Diabetes 2007;56:2655–67.
22. Johannsen DL, Ravussin E. Spontaneous physical activity: relationship between fidgeting and body weight control. Curr Opin Endocrinol Diabetes Obes 2008;15:409–15.
23. Healy GN, Dunstan DW, Salmon J, et al. Television time and continuous metabolic risk in physically active adults. Med Sci Sports Exerc 2008;40:639–45.
24. Healy GN, Wijndaele K, Dunstan DW, et al. Objectively measured sedentary time, physical activity, and metabolic risk. Diabetes Care 2008;31:369–71.
25. Healy GN, Dunstan DW, Salmon J, et al. Breaks in sedentary time. Diabetes Care 2008;31:661–6.

Effects of Physical Activity on Cardiovascular and Noncardiovascular Outcomes in Older Adults

Jacob R. Sattelmair, MSc[a], Jeremy H. Pertman, MS[a],
Daniel E. Forman, MD[b,c,*]

KEYWORDS

• Aging • Cardiovascular • Elderly • Exercise • Physical activity

Although physical activity benefits adults of all ages, its advantages to older adults are especially noteworthy. Aging is associated with a cascade of morphologic and physiologic changes that naturally predispose older adults to progressive weakening, functional decline, morbidity, disability, poor quality of life, and increased mortality.[1] Physical activity moderates such insidious aging patterns, and exercise training, therefore, is vital therapy that can be used to resume or maintain active, healthful lifestyle patterns.[2] Physical activity not only brings about physiologic benefits but also reduces risk of disease outcomes (eg, cardiovascular events and falls) and triggers important psychological gains (eg, vitality, self-efficacy, mood, and quality of life). Advanced age, however, presents distinctive obstacles to physical activity and exercise training.[3] Multiple chronic medical conditions, limited access to appropriate programs, and fear of injury and logistic obstacles are among the common hindrances to initiating and sustaining active lifestyle patterns.[4]

This review begins by focusing on specific age-related physiologic gains associated with exercise and some of the diseases and affective implications. The spectrum of

[a] Department of Epidemiology, Harvard School of Public Health, 677 Huntington Avenue, Kresge Building, Boston, MA 02115, USA
[b] Cardiovascular Division, Brigham and Women's Hospital, 75 Francis Street, Boston, MA 02115, USA
[c] Geriatric Research, Education, and Clinical Center, VA Boston Healthcare System-JP Campus, 150 South Huntington Avenue, Jamaica Plain, Boston, MA 02130, USA
* Corresponding author. Cardiovascular Division, Brigham and Women's Hospital, 75 Francis Street, Boston, MA 02115.
E-mail address: deforman@partners.org (D.E. Forman).

Clin Geriatr Med 25 (2009) 677–702
doi:10.1016/j.cger.2009.07.004
0749-0690/09/$ – see front matter © 2009 Elsevier Inc. All rights reserved.

geriatric.theclinics.com

elderly individuals is considered, from those who are relatively robust to those who are frail and debilitated, and how physical activity may be useful in relation to each condition. Furthermore, given the notorious obstacles to physical activity among the elderly, this review also provides some recommendations to help facilitate activity-enhancing lifestyle changes.

PHYSIOLOGY OF AGING

To appreciate the utility of physical activity to older adults, it is important to first understand some of the aspects of normal aging and the common vulnerabilities that result. Aging is associated with pervasive changes to all physiologic systems, which are broadly categorized in this article as cardiovascular and noncardiovascular changes.

Cardiovascular Physiology of Aging

Vascular

Typical age-related cardiovascular changes include transformations of the large central arteries from pulsatile, dynamic vessels in most young adults to stiff, pipe-like cylinders in most elderly.[5] The pulsatile character of youthful arterial function serves to propel blood forward as vessels distend and recoil. The stiffer vessels of older adults lose this capacity, and the burden of pushing blood forward rests more completely on the heart.

In addition to constitutional changes in vessel media and intimal layers that lead to stiffening, the capacity of endothelial cells aligning vessel lumen to synthesize vital vasodilating peptides diminishes with age.[6] This compounds declines in vascular distensibility and adds to the tendency for cardiac workload to increase with age. Such changes also contribute to reduced cardiac reserve, increased vulnerability to instability in the midst of any clinical perturbation (eg, illness or physical stress), and erosion of exercise tolerance.

Cardiac

As the senescent central vasculature stiffens, the hearts of older adults must pump against increased afterload—a physiologic property that is independent of blood pressure (ie, blood pressure is contingent on flow dynamics of smaller resistance vessels). Therefore, even in normotensive elderly, myocytes in the left ventricle typically hypertrophy to moderate the resultant myocardial wall stress. Such myocyte growth stimulation, however, also increases the likelihood of apoptosis with associated fibrosis and stiffening of the ventricular walls. The hearts of most elderly have mild hypertrophy but the ventricles are distinctively stiff and particularly prone to diastolic filling abnormalities and arrhythmias.[7] All these factors increase the likelihood of reduced cardiac output and increased functional impairment.[8] In addition, aging is associated with diminished autonomic regulation of cardiac rhythm with a predominant down-regulation of β-adrenergic responsiveness,[9] less favorable indices of heart rate variability, and additional susceptibility to arrhythmias.[10]

Noncardiovascular Physiology of Aging

Skeletal muscle

Sarcopenia is a term used to describe age-related atrophy of skeletal muscle mass and strength, and it entails reduced number and size of skeletal muscle cells and intrinsic declines in their contractile performance. Changes in muscle mass are considerable, with 0.5% to 1% of muscle mass usually lost per year from ages 20 to 50 and accelerating in the years thereafter.[11] Such declines in muscle mass and performance predispose to several types of risk.[12] Resultant functional limitations are common: data from the Framingham Disability Study show that 65% of women aged 75 to 84 years were unable to lift 4.5 lb,[13] and cross-sectional studies indicate that muscle strength declines 15% per decade in the sixth and seventh decades and 30% per decade thereafter.[14] As strength erodes, daily physical tasks require a higher proportion of maximal functional capacity such that activities that were once routine become progressively more difficult, even overwhelming. Beyond risks concerning over-exertion, apprehension from such limitations is a risk itself and often predisposes to constrictive life patterns with less activity, progressive fearfulness, depression, and diminished quality of life.

Inflammation and oxidative stress

Increased oxidative stress and progressive inflammation are fundamental determinants of age-related propensity to frailty and disease. Detrimental mitochondrial and cellular derangements occur as do insidious changes to molecular signaling patterns that impair physiology and accelerate atrophy through processes of apoptosis and proteolysis.[15] Reactive oxygen species (ROS) are metabolites of molecular oxygen that, although normally generated as byproducts of aerobic metabolism, tend to accumulate abnormally in old age. Such increases in ROS can alter critical regulatory proteins, disrupting normal cellular function, and inducing changes in lipids, leading to increased oxidized low-density lipoprotein (LDL) and greater atherosclerotic risk. Potent antioxidant systems normally guard against ROS excesses, but these homeostatic capacities diminish with age.[15]

Levels of inflammatory peptides (eg, interleukin 1, tumor necrosis factor α, and inducible nitric oxide synthase) also increase with normal aging[16] whereas levels of anabolic peptides (eg, insulin-like growth factor I [IGF-I]) decrease, particularly in association with a sedentary lifestyle.[17] A complex age-related physiology involves increases in inflammatory cytokines combined with ROS that exacerbates risks for sarcopenia and many of the other disease and physiologic factors that are commonly attributed to age (eg, vascular stiffening).[18–20]

Telomeres, repeated DNA sequences that cap the ends of chromosomes, progressively shorten with age—changes that are believed principally mediated by oxidative stress and inflammation. Telomere shortening is now often used as a marker for biologic aging and has been found to correlate negatively with mortality.[21]

Body fat

Increases in total body fat with age contribute to the inflammatory physiologic processes (discussed previously).[22] Accumulation of abdominal visceral fat and fat between skeletal muscle fibers is common, predisposing to overall weakening and metabolism-based morbidities, such as insulin resistance, diabetes, dyslipidemia, and hypertension. Fat accumulation and overall weakness are components of a vicious cycle, as many adults respond to initial weakening by becoming even less inclined to engage in physical activities, thereby accelerating their vulnerabilities to muscle atrophy, fat accumulation, and systemic inflammation.[23]

Bone density

Osteoporosis results from increased osteoclast activity wherein the rate of bone resorption is greater than the rate of osteoblast-mediated bone deposition. Such bone loss is accelerated with increasing age, and the prevalence of osteoporosis and incidence of bone fracture increases dramatically.[24] The two primary concerns pertaining to osteoporosis are loss of bone mineral density and a marked increase in the risk of fracture, the chief clinical manifestation of osteoporosis, which invariably leads to a loss of independence and function and increased mortality.[25,26]

Functional capacity

Overall functional capacity predictably decreases with age. Although functional decrements are often attributed to age-related declines in maximal heart rate and cardiac output, the cardiac component only accounts for a small portion of functional decline.[27] Age-related changes in blood delivery to peripheral tissue, altered cellular biomechanics, and reduced lean body mass are also among the more significant contributors to functional changes.[28]

KEY BENEFITS OF PHYSICAL ACTIVITY IN MODERATING THE PHYSIOLOGIC CHANGES OF AGING
Cardiovascular Benefits

Vascular

Although progressive stiffening of the central vasculature is likely after age 40, evidence from cross-sectional analyses indicates that individuals who engage in habitual aerobic exercise exhibit less progression of central arterial stiffening over time compared with their sedentary counterparts.[29,30] Although the use of a wide array of techniques to gauge vascular distensibility adds to the complexity of the literature, regular aerobic-type activity has been consistently shown to preserve vascular compliance and the associated physiologic advantages.[29,30] In particular, short-term moderate and vigorous intensity aerobic exercise interventions have led to significant improvements in measures of central stiffness across sex and age ranges in healthy populations.[31–34]

Similarly, habitual physical activity among older adults helps moderate age-related declines in vascular endothelial function. Many studies demonstrate significantly better endothelial flow-mediated vascular responses among those who exercise regularly, mediated primarily by increased nitric oxide synthesis.[29,35] Secondary prevention trials have also demonstrated the utility of exercise training in improving endothelial health among those who initially demonstrate abnormal function.[36]

Cardiac

Physical activity has multiple direct and indirect effects on cardiac function. Activity-related vascular benefits serve not only to reduce cardiac afterload, thereby moderating typical patterns of age-related ventricular myocyte hypertrophy and apoptosis, but also to intrinsically improve myocyte mechanics. Such enhanced energy mechanics in myocytes helps facilitate improvements in ventricular diastolic filling. Increased cardiac output and functional benefits have both been attributed to improved diastolic filling mechanics in older adults who are physically active.[37,38] Other intrinsic cardiovascular exercise benefits include increased atherosclerotic plaque stability (mediated predominantly by an anti-inflammatory effect of regular activity) and enhanced autonomic balance[10,39] (decreasing vulnerability to both ventricular[40] and atrial arrhythmia[41]). A related body of literature indicates that regular physical activity attenuates age-related deterioration in heart rate variability,[42–45] a measure of autonomic regulation of cardiac rhythm.[10]

Noncardiovascular Benefits

Skeletal muscle

With increasing age, skeletal muscle undergoes progressive weakening and atrophy, and habitual physical activity plays a decisive role in preserving skeletal muscle mass and function in old age, increasing strength and muscle function even among very old individuals. Physical activity, in particular strength training, has been demonstrated to increase key anabolic peptides, such as IGF-I,[46,47] promoting myocyte health and function and counterbalancing inflammation and oxidative stress, which underlie much of age-related muscle deterioration. Strength-training studies have demonstrated increased fiber size, muscle mass, and muscle strength even in frail elderly.[28,29]

Inflammation and oxidative stress

Acute exercise leads to transient increases in oxidative stress and inflammation, although habitual physical activity is associated with lower levels of both. Among middle-aged[48–51] and elderly[52,53] individuals, more frequent engagement in physical activity is associated with lower levels of C-reactive protein, white blood cell count, fibrinogen levels, and other key markers of inflammation. Similarly, long-term physical activity favorably modifies the balance between antioxidant and pro-oxidant activity. Leisure time physical activity is cross-sectionally associated with higher levels of the antioxidant enzyme activity markers, superoxide dismutase and glutathione peroxidase.[54] Moreover, some short-term physical activity interventions have led to an increase in several markers of endogenous antioxidant activity, such as glutathione peroxidase in whole blood and glutathione reductase in plasma and a decrease in oxidized LDL.[55,56]

Physical activity has also been shown to consistently attenuate age-related telomere shortening. In a study comparing telomere length relative to exercise, the average telomere length among the most active subjects was 200 nucleotides longer than that among the least active. Given an average loss of 21 nucleotides per year, active individuals may have a "biologic age" that is 10 years younger than those who are inactive.[57]

Body fat

Habitual physical activity is an important component of energy expenditure that helps achieve fat and weight stability over time. Physical activity tends to decline with increasing age[4] and, in the absence of commensurate decline in calorie intake, a net positive caloric balance results, leading to excess adiposity and increased risk of cardiovascular and metabolic morbidities and related mortality.[58–60]

A dose-response relationship exists between physical activity and weight maintenance/weight loss. Physical activity of moderate to vigorous intensity or volume has been shown to reduce body weight and body fat while increasing lean muscle mass in middle-aged and older adults.[61,62] Physical activity of higher intensity or volume results in a several times greater reduction in adiposity, specifically intra-abdominal adiposity.[62]

Resistance training provides a synergistic benefit. Not only does resistance training augment activity and potential for energy expenditure by increasing muscle mass and neural responsiveness, it also leads to direct anti-inflammatory benefits and moderates the pro-inflammatory effects of body fat.[63]

Bone density

The bone weakening or osteopenia that develops as a predictable consequence of aging is exacerbated by sedentary lifestyle and is especially pronounced among post-menopausal women.[64,65] Weight-bearing physical activity, in particular (especially strength training), has been demonstrated to improve bone mineral density and strength.[66,67] Nelson and colleagues conducted a randomized controlled trial of high-intensity strength training for postmenopausal women aged 50 to 70 to study its benefits on bone.[68] It was shown that high-intensity strength training 2 days per week for 45-minute sessions was an adequate stimulus to preserve bone mineral density. Furthermore, the exercise regimen led to improved muscle mass and strength, reflecting the overlapping benefits to skeletal muscle health.

Functional capacity

Normal aging is associated with a vicious cycle of functional decline: decreasing heart rate, cardiac output, and sarcopenia predispose to a progressively more sedentary lifestyle that in turn increases inflammation, ROS, atherosclerosis, and other factors that curtail activity even further. Maintaining a lifestyle characterized by regular physical activity into old age significantly attenuates the rate of functional decline.[69,70] Furthermore, exercise training provides a means to resume a physically active lifestyle pattern for those who have already become sedentary. Intensive aerobic exercise programs have been shown to augment Vo_{2peak} by as much as 30%,[71] and strength training programs have been demonstrated to be synergistic, restoring muscle mass and intrinsic muscle strength.[28]

KEY BENEFITS OF PHYSICAL ACTIVITY IN MODERATING CARDIOVASCULAR RISK FACTORS AND CLINICAL OUTCOMES IN OLDER ADULTS
Risk Factors

Physical activity moderates multiple risk factors that underlie cardiovascular disease. Three of these risk factors—atherogenic dyslipidemia, high blood pressure (hypertension), and diabetes—are reviewed later.

Lipids

Atherogenic dyslipidemia is characterized by the presence of abnormally low levels of serum concentrations of high-density lipoprotein cholesterol (HDL-C) and elevated concentrations of triglycerides (TGs)[72] and LDL cholesterol (LDL-C). Overall evidence suggests that habitual physical activity favorably affects HDL-C and serum TG levels, with increases in HDL-C and decreases in serum TG related to the total volume of physical activity performed.[29] Although effects of exercise have not consistently demonstrated reductions of LDL, some studies demonstrate increased LDL particle size after exercise, suggesting that exercise reduces the proportion of oxidized LDL (a particle of smaller size), thereby moderating atherosclerotic risk. A recent 24-week aerobic exercise training trial involving 40 minutes of moderate aerobic exercise, 3 times per week among 100 sedentary, healthy middle-aged to older adults (aged 50–75), led to broad favorable changes in lipid levels. Subjects experienced a significant reduction in total cholesterol, TGs, and LDL-C, a significant increase in several HDL-C subfractions, and favorable changes in particle concentration and size for LDL-C.[73] A threshold volume of 10 to 12 metabolic equivalent (MET)-hours per week is required to achieve these benefits[29] (where a MET defines an intensity of exercise: leisurely walking is a mild exercise that generates approximately 2.5 METS/hour; 10–12 MET-hours is approximately 4 to 5 hours of walking a week).

Blood pressure

Diastolic blood pressure tends to decrease after age 60, whereas systolic blood pressure generally rises with increasing age as the large central arteries gradually stiffen. A meta-analysis of randomized controlled trials involving older adults between 50 and 87 years of age demonstrated that 6 months of moderate-intensity aerobic exercise led to a 2% decrease in resting systolic blood pressure but had no effect on diastolic blood pressure.[74]

Beyond the issues of measurable blood pressure changes, however, vascular stiffening is an insidious process that can progress in a subtle manner. Aging-related stiffening of the larger central vessels typically leads to increases in vascular impedance that are disproportionately greater than might be inferred from mild changes in blood pressure. Although the population mean systolic blood pressure tends to rise approximately 20% (from 120 to 145 mm Hg between 20 and 80 years) and mean diastolic blood pressure tends to fall (from 80 to 75 mm Hg) as a function of aging, brachial pulse pressure (the difference of systolic and diastolic pressures), an index of vascular stiffening, increases approximately 70% and aortic pulse pressure increases approximately 200% with normal aging.[75] Therefore, major increases in vascular impedance (and corresponding increases in cardiac afterload) typically occur with age. Moderate physical activity, however, can delay central-vascular stiffening or mitigate stiffening that has already occurred.[31,76]

Diabetes

Observational studies, randomized trials, and physiologic studies provide evidence that physical activity is important for the prevention and treatment of type 2 diabetes and the prevention of macrovascular and microvascular complications associated with diabetes. Although most studies have considered vigorous physical activity, moderate activities, such as walking, have also been found to reduce risk,[77] and there does not seem to be a minimal level of activity required to demonstrate some benefit in terms of reducing diabetes risk. An inverse relation between type 2 diabetes and leisure physical activity,[78] vigorous physical activity,[79] walking,[80] occupational and commuting activity,[81] and physical fitness[82] has been demonstrated in observational studies. In several randomized trials,[83–85] physical activity interventions greatly reduced the risk of developing diabetes (by approximately 45%) among healthy subjects and those with impaired glucose tolerance—that is, those at higher risk of diabetes. This association between physical activity and risk of diabetes is consistent in middle aged and older adults.[86,87] The physiologic rationale for this effect is robust, as exercise has significant effects on insulin sensitivity, glucose transporters, glycemic control, and carbohydrate/fat metabolism.[88,89]

Aerobic and resistance exercise have been shown to be beneficial in diabetes treatment, with combined exercise programs showing even greater benefit.[90] Among the elderly, moderate-intensity aerobic activity has been shown to improve glucose tolerance (but not insulin resistance).[91,92] Although added safety concerns exist for exercising diabetics with respect to acutely fluctuating glucose levels in response to an exercise session, cumulative benefits have been shown to far outweigh the risks.[29] Among persons who have impaired glucose tolerance or type 2 diabetes, a minimum of 4—but preferably 3 or more—hours of moderate-intensity physical activity per week reduces the risk of macrovascular complications, such as cardiovascular disease and mortality.[93–95] Physical activity may also prevent microvascular complications, such as diabetic neuropathy.[96]

CLINICAL OUTCOMES

There is strong evidence for an inverse dose-response relationship between habitual physical activity and risk of coronary heart disease (CHD) morbidity and mortality for middle-aged and older men and women. A moderate level of physical activity is associated with an approximately 20% lower risk of CHD, whereas a high amount or intensity of physical activity is associated with an approximately 30% lower risk.[29,97,98] Many exercise modalities, including total physical activity; vigorous activity, such as running; moderate activity, such as walking; and weight training have been shown to protect against risk in men[99] and women.[100] Total physical activity[101] and walking[102] have also been shown to protect against CHD among older individuals. Consistently, physical activity has also been shown to be beneficial in secondary prevention among older adults with known CHD,[103] increasing ischemic threshold, improving quality of life, and reducing mortality.[104]

Physical activity also has a prominent benefit for heart failure (HF) in older adults. HF is a common end-stage condition of advancing age,[105–107] arising almost predictably owing to age-related increases in prevalence of CHD, hypertension, arrhythmia, renal insufficiency, vascular stiffening, and many other predisposing factors. Not only can exercise help to modify vulnerability to age-related atherosclerosis, hypertension, diastolic filling abnormalities, and arrhythmias that commonly lead to HF,[108] but the use of exercise as a means of secondary prevention after developing HF is also safe and beneficial.[109] The large multicenter HF-ACTION trial recently demonstrated all cause mortality and hospitalization benefit (after factoring in 5 prespecified prognostic variables) of aerobic training for systolic HF patents who were already receiving optimal medical therapy. Beneficial effects were observed in the 640 HF patients aged 60 to 69 years and in the 477 patients aged 70 years and older. Other trials in elderly systolic HF patients show that exercise produces predominant peripheral benefits (eg, skeletal muscle and vascular flow dynamics), improved autonomic balance, and other improvements.[110] Aerobic and resistance regimens are beneficial, with most studies using low- and moderate-intensity regimens for patients who are typically frail and deconditioned at the onset.[111]

KEY BENEFITS OF PHYSICAL ACTIVITY IN MODERATING NONCARDIAC DISEASE AND OVERALL MORTALITY IN OLDER ADULTS
Sarcopenia

Lack of physical activity is a significant risk factor for sarcopenia, whereas habitual physical activity is effective in the prevention and mitigation of age-related loss of muscle mass and can increase strength and muscle function even among very old individuals. In particular, high-intensity/velocity progressive resistance exercise holds the potential to preserve and even increase skeletal muscle mass, strength, power, and intrinsic neuromuscular activation in men and women throughout the lifespan, including those at high risk for sarcopenia (eg, those who are sedentary or obese).[28,29] Multiple studies demonstrate the usefulness of resistance training in also increasing muscle mass even among frail older men and women.[68,112–114] Nelson and colleagues showed an increase in muscle mass of 1.2 kg in strength-trained women aged 50 to 70 after 1 year of resistance training versus a decrease of 0.5 kg among controls.[68] Similarly, a 12-week, high-intensity, resistance training program in older men (mean age 65.4 years) showed an 11.8% increase in muscle cross-sectional area of the midthigh and increases in muscle strength of greater than 100%.[72]

Osteoporosis

Habitual physical activity over a lifetime decreases the risk of hip and total body fractures at older ages, particularly by increasing peak bone mass attained during earlier skeletal development. Regular physical activity initiated in older adulthood has also been shown to improve bone mineral density among males and postmenopausal women.[115,116] No clear dose-response relationship between physical activity and fracture risk has been found.[29] Vogel and colleagues describe a U-shaped relationship wherein moderate physical activities reduce risk of fracture, but more intense activities may increase risk.[117] Moreover, a regimen of different types of moderate physical activity provides therapeutic synergy: weight-bearing endurance and resistance activities improve bone density,[66,67] whereas resistance, balance, and flexibility activities reduce risk of falling.[118]

Balance and Stability

The risk of falls increases with advancing age, and declines in muscular strength, reaction speed, and balance common to older adulthood are considered key determinants of these risks.[119,120] Physical activities that involve balance, strength, and flexibility are associated with a reduced risk of falls among older individuals.[121] The benefits of physical activity on improving balance are less conclusive.[122,123] The most successful reduction in risk of falls is achieved using multimodal physical activity interventions, which include a combination of simultaneous strength/resistance, aerobic/endurance, and balance/stability training regimens.[124] Such programs have led to as much as a 35% reduction in the number of falls, with the greatest benefit accruing in those aged 80 or more years.[125] Tai chi is a prime example of a multimodal activity that has demonstrated a positive effect on balance and physical performance among the elderly in some[126] but not all[127,128] trials.

Cognition

Progressive decline in cognitive function and risk of neurodegenerative disorders, such as Alzheimer's disease and other forms of dementia (ie, cognitive decline beyond that which might be expected with normal aging), are associated with advancing age. Evidence from prospective cohort studies indicates that physical activity over the life-course delays the onset of aging-related cognitive decline and the onset of dementia.[129-134] Randomized trials among older individuals indicate that participation in regular physical activity improves cognitive function and reduces symptoms of dementia regardless of disease status.[29,129,135] No firm conclusions can be made at this time, however, regarding whether or not these benefits differ significantly by particular features of physical activity.[29] Evidence supports many plausible mechanisms for these effects, including increased cerebral blood flow and neocortical activation in the prefrontal cortex and hippocampus;[136,137] stimulation of growth factors, such as brain-derived neurotrophic factor,[138] neurogenesis[139] and capillarization;[140] and prevention of reductions in brain volume, synaptic plasticity, and neuronal cell loss.[129] Physical activity, in conjunction with an active and engaged lifestyle, including social and intellectual stimulation, is an important behavioral intervention to optimize cognitive function and prevent cognitive decline and dementia with increasing age.

Mortality

A significant inverse relation between physical activity and risk of all-cause mortality (measured over a discrete follow-up period) reflects the vital importance of an active lifestyle. Data from a multitude of prospective cohort studies demonstrate significant mortality benefits associated with increased physical activity, pertaining to healthy elders and to those with chronic diseases, such as diabetes[141] and CHD.[102,142] Likewise, benefits extend to those who are normal weight, overweight, or obese, and to those who are frail.[143] The relation described between physical activity and mortality is more significant in adults aged 65 or more than in younger adults. Regular physical activity has been associated with an approximately 45% lower risk of death[29] among elderly individuals, where an inverse relation has been found with leisure energy expenditure,[144] occasional and frequent activity,[145] and distance walked[146] for total, cardiovascular, and cancer mortality.[147]

KEY BENEFITS OF PHYSICAL ACTIVITY IN MODERATING PSYCHOLOGICAL DIMENSIONS OF AGING

Quality of Life and Psychological Well-being

Psychological well-being and self-perceived quality of life are associated with reduced psychiatric risk and are critical components of overall health status.[148] Cross-sectional analyses demonstrate that physically active individuals often have higher levels of self-perceived well-being than their sedentary counterparts.[149–151] Although the cross-sectional design prohibits a direct causal interpretation, physical activity is also associated with life satisfaction, well-being, positive affect, and reduced depressive symptoms among elderly individuals,[152–155] lending strong support to the potential role of regular physical activity as a viable strategy for improving and maintaining quality of life among the elderly.

Progressive decline in physical activity with increasing age is believed to contribute to increased age-related prevalence of sleep disorders among elderly adults.[4] Initial evidence supports the assertion that increased physical activity improves sleep quality.[29,156] Physical activity has been associated with nearly 40% lower odds of insomnia;[157] likewise, the probability of insufficient or interrupted sleep is significantly lower among elderly individuals engaged in a high level of physical activity compared with their less active peers.[158–160]

AGING-RELATED CONSIDERATIONS FOR ACHIEVING INCREASED PHYSICAL ACTIVITY

A broad array of aging-related physiologic, psychological, and clinical benefits attributable to aerobic and strength activities has been discussed thus far. The following sections discuss relevant considerations and proposed strategies and recommendations for how to incorporate these exercise modalities into daily regimens to optimize health throughout the aging process.

Physical Activity Guidelines

Physical activity guidelines in the United States have evolved over the past several decades to reflect accumulated knowledge regarding the preventive and therapeutic health benefits of physical activity and in response to population trends in activity levels. In 1998, American College of Sports Medicine guidelines, specifically targeting older adults, called for a combination of aerobic (endurance) exercise and strength training and balance/posture and flexibility training to optimize health.[161] More recent physical activity guidelines aimed at improving and maintaining health among older adults, jointly released by the American College of Sports Medicine and the American Heart Association, recommend moderate-intensity aerobic physical activity for a minimum of 30 minutes on 5 days each week or vigorous-intensity aerobic activity for a minimum of 20 minutes on 3 days per week; large muscle group strength training at least 2 days per week; flexibility training at least 2 days per week (10 minutes each day); and, for those at risk of falls, balance exercises.[162]

Current US federal physical activity guidelines recommend 2.5 hours per week of moderate-intensity aerobic physical activity regardless of age or shorter durations of more vigorous physical activity.[162] In addition, strength training activities are recommended as part of a comprehensive regimen that includes at least two sessions a week. Older adults are advised to follow adult guidelines when it is within their physical capacity. When frailty or a chronic condition prohibits following the guidelines, however, activities are recommended as the capacity allows. Furthermore, exercise modalities should be more tailored among older adults who are frail, starting with exercises to build strength, stability, and balance, and progressing to aerobic modalities that relate to relevant functional goals (eg, walking, then adding hills, then adding stairs, then pushing a wheelchair). Among many infirm adults, it is recognized that exercises may become restricted to arm movements, seated machines, or water activities because disabilities preclude other options (see **Table 1**).

An Optimal Regimen

In concept, the combination of strength training and aerobic activities provides comprehensive health benefits. Strength or resistance training (eg, weight machines and free weights, lifting, carrying, and tai chi) helps increase muscle mass, bone density, physical strength, functional abilities, anabolic peptides IGF-I, and basal metabolic rate. Aerobic activity (eg, large muscle rhythmic activity, such as walking, swimming, and bicycling) provides complementary cardiovascular, autonomic,

Table 1
Physical activity recommendations for older adults

Activity Domain	Recommendations Based on this Review
Physical activity	Daily living should be as active as possible, in many cases including a designated exercise regimen. Ideally, 150 or more minutes per week of cumulative activity at light-moderate intensity is advised, which may involve time for "exercise" (detailed below). Total physical activity should include aerobic activities (eg, walking, grocery shopping, house chores) and strength activities (eg, carrying loads, yard work). It is important to avoid a sedentary lifestyle.
Aerobic exercise	Exercise intensity should ideally be at least moderate to achieve greater physiologic benefits in a regimen that accumulates 75 or more minutes per week, exercising on most days. Aerobic exercises are important for those who are deconditioned or frail and those who are more vigorous. • Frail: eg, walking, light chores, and yard work • Robust: eg, brisk walking, jogging, swimming, cycling, aerobics, and heavy yard work
Strength exercise	Strength training is particularly important in moderating the effects of sarcopenia with age, even for adults who maintain active daily aerobic activities. Ideally, adults should engage in 2–3 sessions per week of 2–3 sets, 8–12 repetitions of at least moderate intensity, involving large muscle groups. Intensity should be similar for frail and robust elderly, though this translates into very different training regimens. • Frail: eg, lifting body weight and light loads • Robust: eg, weight machines, free weights, and lifting heavy loads
Flexibility exercise	Two or more days per week, 10 minutes per day • Range-of-motion exercises for the neck, shoulder, elbow, wrist, hip, knee, and ankle
Balance exercise	For those at risk of falls • Backward, sideways, heel, and toe walking; standing from a sitting position
Warm up/cool down	For more vigorous exercises, a gradual increase (warm up) and decrease (cool down) in exercise intensity is advised, using the same exercise or an exercise that engages similar muscle groups.

metabolic, and cognitive benefits. Activities that incorporate strength and aerobic components thus produce a combination of benefits; in addition, they promote improved posture and reduced risks of falls. Balance training complements these postural benefits, with activities that include backward walking, sideways walking, heel walking, toe walking, and standing from a sitting position. Flexibility training adds to potential gains (eg, specific range-of-motion exercises for the neck, shoulder, elbow, wrist, hip, knee, and ankle that improve movement, balance, and proprioception).

In general, muscle strengthening exercises are oriented to legs, hips, chest, back, abdomen, shoulders, and arms as these all correspond to activities of daily living. Strength training sets usually entail 8 to 12 repetitions of moderate to heavy intensity. At least one set twice a week is beneficial, but 2 to 3 sets per session are recommended. Strength training sessions should usually be separated by at least 1 day, but frequency can increase as participants become stronger. Aerobic, balance, and flexibility exercises should also start slowly for many deconditioned or frail adults but can increase to daily routines as stamina increases.

Warm-up and cool-down activities are particularly important for elderly individuals. A warm-up before moderate- or high-intensity activity allows gradual increase in heart rate and breathing. Warm-up for strength training commonly involves doing exercises with less weight than during the strengthening activity. A cool-down allows a gradual decrease at the end of the activity.

It must be emphasized that the most successful regimens correspond to individual specific needs and preferences. Exercise adherence often ultimately relates to an individual's affinity for the activities themselves. Therefore, it is sometimes helpful to identify a specific activity that a patient prefers and to then initiate a regimen that involves strength or aerobic performance-enhancing exercises that complement this preference.

For those who are capable, engaging in exercises of higher intensity (eg, moderate to high intensity) elicits favorable cardiovascular adaptations not achieved with lower-intensity activity. Although the physiologic rationale for such higher intensity regimens is compelling, the associated gains must be balanced against the corresponding potential musculoskeletal, cardiovascular, or behavioral risks for individuals. In the case that an individual is unable to engage in higher-intensity activity, light to moderate activity can still help to lower blood pressure and reduce age-associated deterioration. Depending on an individual's functional capacity, participants may be advised to exercise at a level that feels "somewhat hard" for aerobic and strength training (ie, a level that usually corresponds to moderate exercise intensity and, therefore, leads to many key physiologic and clinical benefits). Such patients should, therefore, be counseled to exercise below a threshold at which they become short of breath as a means to maximize safety and comfort. Light- to moderate-intensity protocols can be recommended for patients who are exercising on their own (ie, greater safety concerns) or who are primarily trying to maintain their current capacity. Exercise progression, however, is particularly important for older adults who are initially frail and need to build muscle mass and capacity. In these cases, higher-intensity training goals with greater supervision may be most beneficial.

The benefits of pursuing higher intensity training goals pertain to multiple types of activities. High-intensity interval training is one form of high-intensity exercise that demonstrates compelling physiologic results and involves short bouts of vigorous exercise separated by periods of rest (or active recovery). The conceptual advantage is that the higher intensity maximizes physiologic benefit, and the rest interval aids in recovery and stabilization. In a 12-week-long trial involving elderly patients with HF, high-intensity aerobic interval training produced superior benefits in terms of aerobic capacity, left-ventricular remodeling, endothelial function, and mitochondrial function compared with moderate-intensity continuous aerobic training.[163] High-intensity interval training regimens have also been shown to induce favorable skeletal muscle adaptations,[164] work capacity, and aerobic power[165] and improvements to quality of life, cognitive function, and degree of independence.[166]

Strength training at higher intensities is similarly more likely to induce robust physiologic (eg, metabolic, bone strength, and muscle strength) adaptations. Benefits have been demonstrated with high-intensity strength training among frail nursing home residents, including improved muscle cross section area (3%–9%), strength (>100%), and functional performance measured as gait speed and stair climbing ability.[112] Relative improvements in skeletal muscle mass and function may be greatest among those who are the most deconditioned and frail at the onset.

Physical Activity for the Frail Elder

Exercise regimens for older adults must incorporate a range of strategies that respond to the corresponding range of health profiles that are associated with aging. In general, the specific types of activity and exercise do not differ between someone who is frail and someone who is robust; even the notion of exercising at moderate to heavy intensity is similar, but the specific volume and progression of activity must be adjusted to a patient's starting capacities (and limitations). Activity may need to be minimal at first (eg, less than 10 minutes of low-intensity walking) but then increasing in duration and frequency as fitness evolves. It should be noted, however, that it may take months to achieve guideline recommended exercise goals.

Training regimens must also emphasize safety and a foundation that fosters behaviors conducive to ongoing physical activity. Proper warm-up and stretching are particularly important with careful instruction on balance and breathing. A warm-up with aerobic activity usually consists of short intervals of low-intensity movement (eg, walking for 5 minutes). In persons who are too weak to sustain aerobic activities, strength training may be a critical first step toward increasing minimum strength and balance needed for aerobic capacity. In this case, goals may begin with using a patient's own bodyweight for resistance, then slowly progressing to strength training that uses resistance tubing and bands, ankle weights, and other weights over many weeks or months. Strength training sets are usually short with only one to two sessions per week. As strength increases, activity is best advanced by first increasing the number of repetitions before increasing the resistance. Such activity is progressively integrated with daily walking and other aerobic activities as they become tolerated. Supervision, monitoring, teaching, and encouragement are essential, recognizing that long adaptation periods may be needed as deconditioned elderly may develop aches and pains as they begin a more active lifestyle. Supervision is best when it comes from people familiar with the special needs of the elderly.

Barriers to Exercise

The far-reaching clinical and socioeconomic impacts of aging often translate into disproportionate fear, diminished self-efficacy, and reduced opportunities to exercise with surveillance and safety. Among the many common age-related concerns, many older adults fear precipitating a cardiac event, such as a myocardial infarction, musculoskeletal injury, or even embarrassment (eg, incontinence). Age-related hearing and visual impairments, cognitive slowing, and economic constraints add to apprehensiveness. Likewise, many older adults can no longer drive or afford alternate transportation (eg, taxis or shuttle services), and many are tethered by caregiver responsibilities to an infirmed spouse. Furthermore, many older adults also suffer from poor nutrition and poor sleep quality, which adds to their disinclination to exercise.

Overcoming these barriers requires a stepwise individual approach. Barriers specific to individuals should be identified and plans tailored accordingly. Fears can often be mitigated with supervision and education, especially by providing safeguards and insights to prevent injury and safely gauge exercise intensity. Likewise, physical activity can easily be structured as a seated exercise eliminating most of the fall-related apprehensions.

Muscle soreness is a common deterrent for physical activity among many older adults. Frequently, muscle soreness is innocuous and transient and can be modified with reduced training intensity, cold compresses, and sufficient time and patience to allow spontaneous healing to occur. With initiation of activity for someone who is sedentary, there is often a period of physiologic adaptation during which muscle soreness may occur. In most individuals this adaptation can take 2 to 3 weeks but may be longer in the elderly. Unfortunately, many older adults react to soreness with fear and apprehension and use this as rationale to abandon their fledgling exercise routines. If exercise is kept at a lower intensity and progresses modestly, however, soreness may be prevented or gradually resolve.

Barriers to age-related sensory impairment can be overcome or alleviated through the use of visual aids with large fonts and even color-coded hand weights. Emphasis on consistent room organization and proper lighting helps older adults with visual impairment to locate items they need for their routine. Sensory impairments, such as hearing loss, can make it difficult to instruct older adults. Therefore, speaking loudly and slowly, using visual aids, and demonstrating exercises are all techniques that help older adults become active.

Overcoming economic and transportation challenges can often be particularly difficult. There are many senior centers in cities throughout the country where exercise classes are offered daily, but they are of little value to those who lack essential transportation. Although many cities offer transportation assistance to get to medical appointments, such benefits rarely apply to exercise classes. Alternatively, it is usually not feasible to expect older adults, particularly those who are frail, to initiate exercise routines independently in their own homes. There remains a prominent need to develop physical activity training programs or low-cost transportation particularly suited for the needs of the growing older population.

Comprehensive behavioral strategies including social support and positive reinforcement are essential to help older adults initiate and maintain physical activity. Most adults know the importance of physical activity, but that alone is insufficient to motivate them to initiate and adhere to an exercise regimen. Hence, it is important to incorporate a comprehensive management strategy to maximize recruitment, increase teaching and safety, increase motivation, and minimize attrition.[167] Social support from family, friends, and physicians provides a key component to long-term adherence to physical activity.[167–169] The more involved older adults are with their physician, the more likely the physician will facilitate positive exercise behavior, set realistic goals and a course of action, and reinforce a commitment to the exercise routine.

Nonetheless, it remains a limitation that many patients rely exclusively on their primary physician to prescribe an exercise training protocol. Dauenhauer and colleagues demonstrated that 47% of primary care physicians do not prescribe exercise for older adults, and 85% reported having no formal training in exercise prescription.[170] Many physicians avoid giving their older patients written instructions due to feeling inadequately prepared to prescribe an exercise regimen in patients with complex medical conditions and medication regimens.[170,171]

Access

Home-based exercise takes place in an individual's residence, is not supervised, and is often conducted alone. Although convenient, home-based exercise presents many problems. Frail older adults tend to require personal instruction in how to perform the exercises to best insure the safety and efficacy of activity, but such guidance is difficult to acquire. Furthermore, lack of emergency care for home-based exercise compounds risk and apprehension.

Community-based exercise, alternatively, takes place in a setting such as a health or fitness center, is usually supervised, and allows several individuals to exercise together or at the same time. In addition to incorporating components of assessment, monitoring, and safety, community-based programs provide opportunities for social reinforcement and higher adherence. Community-based, supervised resistance training has more consistently achieved greater increases in lean mass and muscle strength than home-based programs.[172-175] Furthermore, community-based programs are better suited for older adults with baseline frailty or concomitant exercise risks, such as neurologic, cardiovascular, orthopedic, or pulmonary conditions.

Safety

Absolute contraindications for exercise testing or training include recent ECG changes or myocardial infarction, unstable angina, uncontrolled arrhythmias, acute HF, severe conduction disease, or other destabilizing cardiac conditions. Likewise, exercise is contraindicated in patients with acute noncardiac diseases that may be exacerbated by exercise (eg, infection, renal failure, or thyrotoxicosis). In contrast, although many other conditions may pose challenges (eg, arthritis, visual impairment, stroke, other neurologic conditions), they are not contraindications to participation in an exercise program.

Many caregivers recommend that an exercise stress test precede exercise activity, especially for sedentary older adults. Exercise testing helps rule out ischemia in a population that is inherently prone to coronary artery disease and to diabetes, hypertension, hypotension, renal disease, HF, arrhythmia, and other potentially destabilizing conditions. It is important to emphasize the value of functional exercise testing and resist the tendency of many stress labs to use chemical stress testing because this does not fully address the clinical parameters relevant for exercise training.

Not all clinicians feel stress testing is necessary, especially for patients they deem generally stable based on clinical examinations or who are fearful of exercise testing. In such cases, it is appropriate to initiate activity at modest duration and intensity with regimens that progress gradually over extended time intervals. Particularly in these circumstances, it is important to limit activity to what a patient feels is comfortable, progressing in small increments, and prioritizing longer duration over higher exercise intensity.

General recommendations for safety, particularly in the initial stages of exercise, include exercising with at least one other person, carrying a cell phone to facilitate calling for emergency help, and adhering to an activity level that is comfortable and in which breathing is normal (ie, without feeling breathless). Proper footwear and clothing, well-lit and ventilated rooms, good nutrition, sleep, and medication compliance are other features of successful activity. Likewise, resting as needed, avoiding rushing through an activity routine, and careful consideration of body position and breathing are important. If injury or illness interrupts an activity routine, resuming activity at a lower intensity level (usually a maximum of 50% of the previous intensity and duration) and with pain-free range-of-motion activities are priorities once sufficient healing has occurred.

Strength training using exercise machines has advantages for older adults, especially those who are frail, as the range of motion is easier to control, and the margin of safety is increased. Although free weights provide greater accessibility and cost advantages, teaching and monitoring are particularly important.

To the surprise of many patients, and even many clinicians, strength training is typically safer for cardiac patients compared with aerobic training from a cardiovascular perspective. Heart rates are usually slower, with less cardiac work demands and arrhythmia than aerobic training modalities.[176]

Comorbidities also may trigger patient and caregiver concerns and apprehensions about increasing physical activity. Benefits of exercise remain high, however, despite the inherent complexities associated with comorbid conditions.

Cardiac rehabilitation is particularly well-suited to guiding exercise training for older adults with cardiovascular disease, providing a standardized program of supervision and monitoring to improve exercise capacity for patients with prior heart disease, HF, valvular disease, arrhythmia, peripheral arterial disease or other cardiovascular problems. Such programs are well oriented to complexities of hemodynamic fluctuations, medication effects, glucose monitoring, and other relevant concerns. In most scenarios where there is significant comorbid disease (eg, arthritis, chronic obstructive pulmonary disease, diabetes, and depression), patients benefit from increased supervision and monitoring in terms of exercise efficacy and safety.

Healthful Lifestyle Recommendations

Although this review provides information about specific exercise modalities and their associated training benefits, it is important to emphasize the principles that some physical activity is generally better than no physical activity, and that physical activity does not need to be painful or cumbersome to provide health benefits. Even an accumulation of light-moderate activities throughout the day can have a significant effect on total energy expenditure and overall health outcomes. Useful goals include structuring activity into a normal daily routine. Self-transportation (eg, walking or bicycling), home and garden chores, grocery shopping, and other aspects of daily living are all potential opportunities to structure active, healthy lifestyles that deliver physiologic and clinical benefits. Engaging in a variety of activities is beneficial in terms of avoiding excessive strain, increasing pleasure, and achieving complementary benefits from different movements. Participation in activities that provide positive social and intellectual stimulation (eg, dancing) confers synergistic benefits on cognitive components of aging.[177]

The totality of evidence demonstrating the many physical and psychological benefits of physical activity supports the fundamental principle that in the absence of physical activity, it is difficult, if not impossible to age optimally. On the contrary, regular physical activity is a proved strategy to improve health and well-being at any age. The authors, therefore, strongly advocate that all older adults engage regularly in physical activity.

REFERENCES

1. Lunney JR, Lynn J, Foley DJ, et al. Patterns of functional decline at the end of life. JAMA 2003;289(18):2387–92.
2. Province MA, Hadley EC, Hornbrook MC, et al. The effects of exercise on falls in elderly patients. A preplanned meta-analysis of the FICSIT Trials. Frailty and injuries: cooperative studies of intervention techniques. JAMA 1995;273(17): 1341–7.

3. Rhodes RE, Martin AD, Taunton JE, et al. Factors associated with exercise adherence among older adults: an individual perspective. Sports Med 1999; 28(6):397–411.
4. DiPietro L. Physical activity in aging: changes in patterns and their relation to health and function. J Gerontol A Biol Sci Med Sci 2001;56A:13–22.
5. Lakatta EG, Levy D. Arterial and cardiac aging: major shareholders in cardiovascular disease enterprises: part I: aging arteries: a "Set Up" for vascular disease. Circulation 2003;107(1):139–46.
6. DeSouza CA, Shapiro LF, Clevenger CM, et al. Regular aerobic exercise prevents and restores age-related declines in endothelium-dependent vasodilation in healthy men. Circulation 2000;102(12):1351–7.
7. Kitzman DW. Diastolic heart failure in the elderly. Heart Fail Rev 2002;7(1):17–27.
8. Grewal J, McCully RB, Kane GC, et al. Left ventricular function and exercise capacity. JAMA 2009;301(3):286–94.
9. Xiao RP, Tomhave ED, Wang DJ, et al. Age-associated reductions in cardiac beta1- and beta2-adrenergic responses without changes in inhibitory G proteins or receptor kinases. J Clin Invest 1998;101(6):1273–82.
10. Kleiger RE, Stein PK, Bigger JT. Heart rate variability: measurement and clinical utility. Ann Noninvasive Electrocardiol 2005;10(1):1–14.
11. Grimby G, Saltin B. The ageing muscle. Clin Physiol 1983;3(3):209–18.
12. Visser M, Goodpaster BH, Kritchevsky SB, et al. Muscle mass, muscle strength, and muscle fat infiltration as predictors of incident mobility limitations in well-functioning older persons. J Gerontol A Biol Sci Med Sci 2005;60(3): 324–33.
13. Jette AM, Branch LG. The Framingham disability study: II. Physical disability among the aging. Am J Public Health 1981;71(11):1211–6.
14. Danneskiold-Samsøe B, Kofod V, Munter J, et al. Muscle strength and functional capacity in 78–81-year-old men and women. Eur J Appl Physiol Occup Physiol 1984;52(3):310–4.
15. Ji LL. Antioxidant signaling in skeletal muscle: a brief review. Exp Gerontol 2007; 42(7):582–93.
16. Vasan RS, Sullivan LM, Roubenoff R, et al. Inflammatory markers and risk of heart failure in elderly subjects without prior myocardial infarction: the Framingham heart study. Circulation 2003;107(11):1486–91.
17. Roubenoff R. Catabolism of aging: is it an inflammatory process? Curr Opin Clin Nutr Metab Care 2003;6(3):295–9.
18. Brinkley TE, Leng X, Miller ME, et al. Chronic inflammation is associated with low physical function in older adults across multiple comorbidities. J Gerontol A Biol Sci Med Sci 2009;64(4):455–61.
19. Reuben DB, Cheh AI, Harris TB, et al. Peripheral blood markers of inflammation predict mortality and functional decline in high-functioning community-dwelling older persons. J Am Geriatr Soc 2002;50(4):638–44.
20. Cappola AR, Xue Q-L, Ferrucci L, et al. Insulin-like growth factor I and Interleukin-6 contribute synergistically to disability and mortality in older women. J Clin Endocrinol Metab 2003;88(5):2019–25.
21. Demissie S, Levy D, Benjamin EJ, et al. Insulin resistance, oxidative stress, hypertension, and leukocyte telomere length in men from the Framingham heart study. Aging Cell 2006;5(4):325–30.
22. Festa A, D'Agostino R Jr, Williams K, et al. The relation of body fat mass and distribution to markers of chronic inflammation. Int J Obes Relat Metab Disord 2001;25(10):1407–15.

23. Cesari M, Kritchevsky SB, Baumgartner RN, et al. Sarcopenia, obesity, and inflammation—results from the trial of angiotensin converting enzyme inhibition and novel cardiovascular risk factors study. Am J Clin Nutr 2005;82(2):428–34.

24. Ettinger MP. Aging bone and osteoporosis: strategies for preventing fractures in the elderly. Arch Intern Med 2003;163(18):2237–46.

25. Looker AC, Orwoll ES, Johnston CCJ, et al. Prevalence of low femoral bone density in older U.S. adults from NHANES III. J Bone Miner Res 1997;12(11): 1761–8.

26. Wark JD. Osteoporosis: the emerging epidemic. Med J Aust 1996;164(6):327–8.

27. Fleg JL, Morrell CH, Bos AG, et al. Accelerated longitudinal decline of aerobic capacity in healthy older adults. Circulation 2005;112(5):674–82.

28. Koopman R, van Loon LJC. Aging, exercise and muscle protein metabolism. J Appl Physiol 2008, in press.

29. Physical Activity Guidelines Advisory Committee, Physical Activity Guidelines Advisory Committee Report, US Department of Health and Human Service. Washington, DC: 2008.

30. Gates PE, Seals DR. Decline in large elastic artery compliance with age: a therapeutic target for habitual exercise. Br J Sports Med 2006;40(11):897–9.

31. Seals DR, DeSouza CA, Donato AJ, et al. Habitual exercise and arterial aging. J Appl Physiol 2008;105(4):1323–32.

32. Tanabe T, Maeda S, Miyauchi T, et al. Exercise training improves ageing-induced decrease in eNOS expression of the aorta. Acta Physiol Scand 2003; 178(1):3–10.

33. Sugawara J, Otsuki T, Tanabe T, et al. Physical activity duration, intensity, and arterial stiffening in postmenopausal womenast. Am J Hypertens 2006;19(10): 1032–6.

34. Tanaka H, DeSouza CA, Seals DR. Absence of age-related increase in central arterial stiffness in physically active women. Arterioscler Thromb Vasc Biol 1998;18(1):127–32.

35. Taddei S, Galetta F, Virdis A, et al. Physical activity prevents age-related impairment in nitric oxide availability in elderly athletes. Circulation 2000;101(25): 2896–901.

36. Hambrecht R, Fiehn E, Weigl C, et al. Regular physical exercise corrects endothelial dysfunction and improves exercise capacity in patients with chronic heart failure. Circulation 1998;98(24):2709–15.

37. Stratton JR, Levy WC, Cerqueira MD, et al. Cardiovascular responses to exercise. Effects of aging and exercise training in healthy men. Circulation 1994; 89(4):1648–55.

38. Forman DE, Manning WJ, Hauser R, et al. Enhanced left ventricular diastolic filling associated with long-term endurance training. J Gerontol A Biol Sci Med Sci 1992;47(2):M56–8.

39. Leosco D, Rengo G, Iaccarino G, et al. Exercise training and beta-blocker treatment ameliorate age-dependent impairment of beta-adrenergic receptor signaling and enhance cardiac responsiveness to adrenergic stimulation. Am J Physiol Heart Circ Physiol 2007;293(3):H1596–603.

40. Lahiri MK, Kannankeril PJ, Goldberger JJ. Assessment of autonomic function in cardiovascular disease: physiological basis and prognostic implications. J Am Coll Cardiol 2008;51(18):1725–33.

41. Plisiene J, Blumberg A, Haager G, et al. Moderate physical exercise: a simplified approach for ventricular rate control in older patients with atrial fibrillation. Clin Res Cardiol 2008;97(11):820–6.

42. Earnest CP, Lavie CJ, Blair SN, et al. Heart rate variability characteristics in sedentary postmenopausal women following six months of exercise training: the DREW study. PLoS ONE 2008;3(6):e2288.
43. Melo RC, Santos MD, Silva E, et al. Effects of age and physical activity on the autonomic control of heart rate in healthy men. Braz J Med Biol Res 2005; 38(9):1331–8.
44. Buchheit MS, Simon C, Viola AU, et al. Heart rate variability in sportive elderly: relationship with daily physical activity. Med Sci Sports Exerc 2004;36(4): 601–5.
45. Dietrich DF, Ackermann-Liebrich U, Schindler C. Effect of physical activity on heart rate variability in normal weight, overweight and obese subjects: results from the SAPALDIA study. Eur J Appl Physiol 2008;104:557–65.
46. Adamo ML, Farrar RP. Resistance training, and IGF involvement in the maintenance of muscle mass during the aging process. Ageing Res Rev 2006;5(3):310–31.
47. Vale RG, de Oliveira RD, Pernambuco CS, et al. Effects of muscle strength and aerobic training on basal serum levels of IGF-1 and cortisol in elderly women. Arch Gerontol Geriatr 2009, Jan 6. [Epub ahead of print].
48. Abramson JL, Vaccarino V. Relationship between physical activity and inflammation among apparently healthy middle-aged and older US adults. Arch Intern Med 2002;162(11):1286–92.
49. Mora S, Lee IM, Buring JE, et al. Association of physical activity and body mass index with novel and traditional cardiovascular biomarkers in women. JAMA 2006;295(12):1412–9.
50. Pischon T, Hankinson SE, Hotamisligil GS, et al. Leisure-time physical activity and reduced plasma levels of obesity-related inflammatory markers. Obes Res 2003;11(9):1055–64.
51. Ford JL, Downes S. Cellularity of human annulus tissue: an investigation into the cellularity of tissue of different pathologies. Histopathology 2002;41(6):531–7.
52. Geffken DF, Cushman M, Burke GL, et al. Association between physical activity and markers of inflammation in a healthy elderly population. Am J Epidemiol 2001;153(3):242–50.
53. Reuben DB, Judd-Hamilton L, Harris TB, et al. The associations between physical activity and inflammatory markers in high-functioning older persons: macarthur studies of successful aging. J Am Geriatr Soc 2003;51(8): 1125–30.
54. Covas MI, Elosua R, Fito M, et al. Relationship between physical activity and oxidative stress biomarkers in women. Med Sci Sports Exerc 2002;34(5): 814–9.
55. Elosua R, Molina L, Fito M, et al. Response of oxidative stress biomarkers to a 16-week aerobic physical activity program, and to acute physical activity, in healthy young men and women. Atherosclerosis 2003;167(2):327–34.
56. Roberts CK, Won D, Pruthi S, et al. Effect of a short-term diet and exercise intervention on oxidative stress, inflammation, MMP-9, and monocyte chemotactic activity in men with metabolic syndrome factors. J Appl Physiol 2006;100(5): 1657–65.
57. Cherkas LF, Hunkin JL, Kato BS, et al. The association between physical activity in leisure time and leukocyte telomere length. Arch Intern Med 2008;168(2): 154–8.
58. Renehan AG, Tyson M, Egger M, et al. Body-mass index and incidence of cancer: a systematic review and meta-analysis of prospective observational studies. Lancet 2008;371(9612):569–78.

59. Field AE, Coakley EH, Must A, et al. Impact of overweight on the risk of developing common chronic diseases during a 10-year period. Arch Intern Med 2001;161(13):1581–6.

60. Klein S, Burke LE, Bray GA, et al. Clinical implications of obesity with specific focus on cardiovascular disease: a statement for professionals from the American Heart Association council on nutrition, physical activity, and metabolism: endorsed by the American College of Cardiology Foundation. Circulation 2004;110(18):2952–67.

61. Irwin ML, Yasui Y, Ulrich CM, et al. Effect of exercise on total and intra-abdominal body fat in postmenopausal women: a randomized controlled trial. JAMA 2003; 289(3):323–30.

62. Ross R, Janssen I, Dawson J, et al. Exercise-induced reduction in obesity and insulin resistance in women: a randomized controlled trial. Obesity Research 2004;12(5):789–98.

63. Olson TP, Dengel DR, Leon AS, et al. Changes in inflammatory biomarkers following one-year of moderate resistance training in overweight women. Int J Obes 2007;31(6):996–1003.

64. Iwamoto J, Takeda T, Ichimura S. Effect of exercise training and detraining on bone mineral density in postmenopausal women with osteoporosis. J Orthop Sci 2001;6(2):128–32.

65. Gass M, Dawson-Hughes B. Preventing osteoporosis-related fractures: an overview. Am J Med 2006;119(4 Suppl 1):S3–11.

66. Todd JA, Robinson RJ. Osteoporosis and exercise. Postgrad Med J 2003; 79(932):320–3.

67. Cussler EC, Going SB, Houtkooper LB, et al. Exercise frequency and calcium intake predict 4-year bone changes in postmenopausal women. Osteoporos Int 2005;16(12):2129–41.

68. Nelson ME, Fiatarone MA, Morganti CM, et al. Effects of high-intensity strength training on multiple risk factors for osteoporotic fractures. A randomized controlled trial. JAMA 1994;272(24):1909–14.

69. Goldspink DF, Burniston JG, Tan LB. Cardiomyocyte death and the ageing and failing heart. Exp Physiol 2003;88(3):447–58.

70. Pimentel AE, Gentile CL, Tanaka H, et al. Greater rate of decline in maximal aerobic capacity with age in endurance-trained than in sedentary men. J Appl Physiol 2003;94(6):2406–13.

71. Fleg JL, Pina IL, Balady GJ, et al. Assessment of functional capacity in clinical and research applications: an advisory from the committee on exercise, rehabilitation, and prevention, council on clinical cardiology, American Heart Association. Circulation 2000;102(13):1591–7.

72. Frontera WR, Meredith CN, O'Reilly KP, et al. Strength conditioning in older men: skeletal muscle hypertrophy and improved function. J Appl Physiol 1988;64(3): 1038–44.

73. Halverstadt A, Phares DA, Wilund KR, et al. Endurance exercise training raises high-density lipoprotein cholesterol and lowers small low-density lipoprotein and very low-density lipoprotein independent of body fat phenotypes in older men and women. Metabolism 2007;56(4):444–50.

74. Kelley GA, Kelley KS. Aerobic exercise and resting blood pressure in older adults: a meta-analytic review of randomized controlled trials. J Gerontol A Biol Sci Med Sci 2001;56(5):M298–303.

75. O'Rourke MF, Hashimoto J. Mechanical factors in arterial aging: a clinical perspective. J Am Coll Cardiol 2007;50(1):1–13.

76. Vaitkevicius PV, Fleg JL, Engel JH, et al. Effects of age and aerobic capacity on arterial stiffness in healthy adults. Circulation 1993;88(4):1456–62.
77. Jeon CY, Lokken RP, Hu FB, et al. Physical activity of moderate intensity and risk of type 2 diabetes: a systematic review. Diabetes Care 2007;30(3):744–52.
78. Helmrich SP, Ragland DR, Leung RW, et al. Physical activity and reduced occurrence of non-insulin-dependent diabetes mellitus. N Engl J Med 1991; 325(3):147–52.
79. Manson JE, Stampfer MJ, Colditz GA, et al. Physical activity and incidence of non-insulin-dependent diabetes mellitus in women. Lancet 1991;338(8770): 774–8.
80. Hu FB, Sigal RJ, Rich-Edwards JW, et al. Walking compared with vigorous physical activity and risk of type 2 diabetes in women: a prospective study. JAMA 1999;282(15):1433–9.
81. Hu G, Qiao Q, Silventoinen K, et al. Occupational, commuting, and leisure-time physical activity in relation to risk for type 2 diabetes in middle-aged Finnish men and women. Diabetologia 2003;46(3):322–9.
82. Lynch J, Helmrich SP, Lakka TA, et al. Moderately intense physical activities and high levels of cardiorespiratory fitness reduce the risk of non-insulin-dependent diabetes mellitus in middle-aged men. Arch Intern Med 1996; 156(12):1307–14.
83. Pan XR, Li GW, Hu YH, et al. Effects of diet and exercise in preventing NIDDM in people with impaired glucose tolerance. The Da Qing IGT and Diabetes Study. Diabetes Care 1997;20(4):537–44.
84. Eriksson J, Lindström J, Valle T, et al. Prevention of type II diabetes in subjects with impaired glucose tolerance: the diabetes prevention study (DPS) in Finland. Study design and 1-year interim report on the feasibility of the lifestyle intervention programme. Diabetologia 1999;42(7):793–801.
85. Tuomilehto J, Lindstrom J, Eriksson JG, et al. Prevention of type 2 diabetes mellitus by changes in lifestyle among subjects with impaired glucose tolerance. N Engl J Med 2001;344(18):1343–50.
86. Hsia J, Wu L, Allen C, et al. Physical activity and diabetes risk in postmenopausal women. Am J Prev Med 2005;28(1):19–25.
87. Folsom AR, Kushi LH, Ching-Ping H. Physical activity and mellitus in postmenopausal women. Am J Public Health 2000;90(1):134–8.
88. Schneider SH, Amorosa LF, Khachadurian AK, et al. Studies on the mechanism of improved glucose control during regular exercise in type 2 (non-insulin-dependent) diabetes. Diabetologia 1984;26(5):355–60.
89. Lanza IR, Short DK, Short KR, et al. Endurance exercise as a countermeasure for aging. Diabetes 2008;57(11):2933–42.
90. Snowling NJ, Hopkins WG. Effects of different modes of exercise training on glucose control and risk factors for complications in type 2 diabetic patients: a meta-analysis. Diabetes Care 2006;29(11):2518–27.
91. DiPietro L, Seeman TE, Stachenfeld NS, et al. Moderate-intensity aerobic training improves glucose tolerance in aging independent of abdominal adiposity. J Am Geriatr Soc 1998;46(7):875–9.
92. Van Dam RM, Schuit AJ, Feskens EJ, et al. Physical activity and glucose tolerance in elderly men: the Zutphen Elderly study. Med Sci Sports Exerc 2002; 34(7):1132–6.
93. Hu G, Eriksson J, Barengo NC, et al. Occupational, commuting, and leisure-time physical activity in relation to total and cardiovascular mortality among Finnish subjects with type 2 diabetes. Circulation 2004;110(6):666–73.

94. Tanasescu M, Leitzmann MF, Rimm EB, et al. Physical activity in relation to cardiovascular disease and total mortality among men with type 2 diabetes. Circulation 2003;107(19):2435–9.

95. Hu FB, Stampfer MJ, Solomon C, et al. Physical activity and risk for cardiovascular events in diabetic women. Ann Intern Med 2001;134(2):96–105.

96. Balducci S, Iacobellis G, Parisi L, et al. Exercise training can modify the natural history of diabetic peripheral neuropathy. J Diabetes Complications 2006;20(4): 216–23.

97. Sofi F, Capalbo A, Cesari F, et al. Physical activity during leisure time and primary prevention of coronary heart disease: an updated meta-analysis of cohort studies. Eur J Cardiovasc Prev Rehabil 2008;15(3):247–57.

98. Kohl HW 3rd. Physical activity and cardiovascular disease: evidence for a dose response. Med Sci Sports Exerc 2001;33(6):S472–83.

99. Tanasescu M, Leitzmann MF, Rimm EB, et al. Exercise type and intensity in relation to coronary heart disease in men. JAMA 2002;288(16):1994–2000.

100. Manson JE, Hu FB, Rich-Edwards JW, et al. A prospective study of walking as compared with vigorous exercise in the prevention of coronary heart disease in women. N Engl J Med 1999;341(9):650–8.

101. Donahue RP, Abbott RD, Reed DM, et al. Physical activity and coronary heart disease in middle-aged and elderly men: the Honolulu Heart Program. Am J Public Health 1988;78(6):683–5.

102. Hakim AA, Curb JD, Petrovitch H, et al. Effects of walking on coronary heart disease in elderly men: the Honolulu Heart Program. Circulation 1999;100(1):9–13.

103. Smith SC Jr, Allen J, Blair SN, et al. AHA/ACC guidelines for secondary prevention for patients with coronary and other atherosclerotic vascular disease: 2006 update: endorsed by the national heart, lung, and blood institute. J Am Coll Cardiol 2006;47(10):2130–9.

104. Suaya JA, Shepard DS, Normand S-LT, et al. Use of cardiac rehabilitation by medicare beneficiaries after myocardial infarction or coronary bypass surgery. Circulation 2007;116(15):1653–62.

105. Thomas S, Rich MW. Epidemiology, pathophysiology, and prognosis of heart failure in the elderly. Heart Fail Clin 2007;3(4):381–7.

106. Kitzman DW, Gardin JM, Gottdiener JS, et al. Importance of heart failure with preserved systolic function in patients ≥ 65 years of age. Am J Cardiol 2001; 87(4):413–9.

107. Kitzman DW, Daniel KR. Diastolic heart failure in the elderly. Heart Fail Clin 2007; 3(4):437–53.

108. Kenchaiah S, Sesso HD, Gaziano JM. Body mass index and vigorous physical activity and the risk of heart failure among men. Circulation 2009;119(1):44–52.

109. O'Connor CM, Whellan DJ, Lee KL, et al. Efficacy and safety of exercise training in patients with chronic heart failure: HF-ACTION randomized controlled trial. JAMA 2009;301(14):1439–50.

110. Duscha BD, Schulze PC, Robbins JL, et al. Implications of chronic heart failure on peripheral vasculature and skeletal muscle before and after exercise training. Heart Fail Rev 2008;13(1):21–37.

111. Witham MD, Struthers AD, McMurdo ME. Exercise training as a therapy for chronic heart failure: can older people benefit? J Am Geriatr Soc 2003;51(5): 699–709.

112. Fiatarone M, O'Neill E, Ryan N, et al. Exercise training and nutritional supplementation for physical frailty in very elderly people. N Engl J Med 1994; 330(25):1769–75.

113. Trappe S, Williamson D, Godard M. Maintenance of whole muscle strength and size following resistance training in older men. J Gerontol A Biol Sci Med Sci 2002;57(4):B138–43.
114. Binder EF, Yarasheski KE, Steger-May K, et al. Effects of progressive resistance training on body composition in frail older adults: results of a randomized, controlled trial. J Gerontol A Biol Sci Med Sci 2005;60(11):1425–31.
115. Nordström A, Karlsson C, Nyquist F, et al. Bone loss and fracture risk after reduced physical activity. J Bone Miner Res 2005;20(2):202–7.
116. Ringsberg KA, Gärdsell P, Johnell O, et al. The impact of long-term moderate physical activity on functional performance, bone mineral density and fracture incidence in elderly women. Gerontology 2001;47(1):15–20.
117. Vogel T, Brechat PH, Lepretre PM, et al. Health benefits of physical activity in older patients: a review. Int J Clin Pract 2009;63(2):303–20.
118. Kohrt WM, Bloomfield SA, Little KD, et al. American College of Sports Medicine Position Stand: physical activity and bone health. Med Sci Sports Exerc 2004; 36(11):1985–96.
119. Campbell AJ, Borrie MJ, Spears GF. Risk factors for falls in a community-based prospective study of people 70 years and older. J Gerontol A Biol Sci Med Sci 1989;44(4):M112–7.
120. Nevitt MC, Cummings SR, Hudes ES. Risk factors for injurious falls: a prospective study. J Gerontol A Biol Sci Med Sci 1991;46(5):M164–70.
121. Tinetti ME. Preventing falls in elderly persons. N Engl J Med 2003;348(1):42–9.
122. Chang JT, Morton SC, Rubenstein LZ, et al. Interventions for the prevention of falls in older adults: systematic review and meta-analysis of randomised clinical trials. BMJ 2004;328(7441):680.
123. Sherrington C, Lord SR, Finch CF. Physical activity interventions to prevent falls among older people: update of the evidence. J Sci Med Sport 2004;7(1 Suppl):43–51.
124. Baker MK, Atlantis E, Fiatarone Singh MA. Multi-modal exercise programs for older adults. Age Ageing 2007;36(4):375–81.
125. Robertson MC, Campbell AJ, Gardner MM, et al. Preventing injuries in older people by preventing falls: a meta-analysis of individual-level data. J Am Geriatr Soc 2002;50(5):905–11.
126. Li F, Harmer P, Fisher KJ, et al. Tai Chi and fall reductions in older adults: a randomized controlled trial. J Gerontol A Biol Sci Med Sci 2005;60(2):187–94.
127. Klein PJ, Adams WD. Comprehensive therapeutic benefits of Taiji: a critical review. Am J Phys Med Rehabil 2004;83(9):735–45.
128. Voukelatos A, Cumming RG, Lord SR, et al. A randomized, controlled trial of tai chi for the prevention of falls: the Central Sydney tai chi trial. J Am Geriatr Soc 2007;55(8):1185–91.
129. Kramer AF, Erickson KI, Colcombe SJ. Exercise, cognition, and the aging brain. J Appl Physiol 2006;101(4):1237–42.
130. Yaffe K, Barnes D, Nevitt M, et al. A prospective study of physical activity and cognitive decline in elderly women: women who walk. Arch Intern Med 2001; 161(14):1703–8.
131. Weuve J, Kang JH, Manson JE, et al. Physical activity, including walking, and cognitive function in older women. JAMA 2004;292(12):1454–61.
132. Hamer M, Chida Y. Physical activity and risk of neurodegenerative disease: a systematic review of prospective evidence. Psychol Med 2009;39(01):3–11.
133. Rovio S, Kåreholt I, Helkala E-L, et al. Leisure-time physical activity at midlife and the risk of dementia and Alzheimer's disease. Lancet Neurol 2005;4(11): 705–11.

134. Abbott RD, White LR, Ross GW, et al. Walking and dementia in physically capable elderly men. JAMA 2004;292(12):1447–53.
135. Lautenschlager NT, Cox KL, Flicker L, et al. Effect of physical activity on cognitive function in older adults at risk for Alzheimer disease: a randomized trial. JAMA 2008;300(9):1027–37.
136. Heckman GA, McKelvie RS. Cardiovascular aging and exercise in healthy older adults. Clin J Sport Med 2008;18(6):479–85.
137. Churchill JD, Galvez R, Colcombe S, et al. Exercise, experience and the aging brain. Neurobiol Aging 2002;23(5):941–55.
138. Cotman CW, Berchtold NC. Exercise: a behavioral intervention to enhance brain health and plasticity. Trends Neurosci 2002;25(6):295–301.
139. van Praag H, Shubert T, Zhao C, et al. Exercise enhances learning and hippocampal neurogenesis in aged mice. J Neurosci 2005;25(38):8680–5.
140. Lopez-Lopez C, LeRoith D, Torres-Aleman I. Insulin-like growth factor I is required for vessel remodeling in the adult brain. Proc Natl Acad Sci USA 2004;101(26):9833–8.
141. Jonker JT, De Laet C, Franco OH, et al. Physical activity and life expectancy with and without diabetes: life table analysis of the Framingham heart study. Diabetes Care 2006;29(1):38–43.
142. Wannamethee SG, Shaper AG, Walker M. Physical activity and mortality in older men with diagnosed coronary heart disease. Circulation 2000;102(12):1358–63.
143. Landi F, Cesari M, Onder G, et al. Physical activity and mortality in frail, community-living elderly patients. J Gerontol A Biol Sci Med Sci 2004;59(8):833–7.
144. Fried LP, Kronmal RA, Newman AB, et al. Risk factors for 5-year mortality in older adults: the cardiovascular health study. JAMA 1998;279(8):585–92.
145. Sundquist K, Qvist J, Sundquist J, et al. Frequent and occasional physical activity in the elderly: a 12-year follow-up study of mortality. Am J Prev Med 2004;27(1):22–7.
146. Hakim AA, Petrovitch H, Burchfiel CM, et al. Effects of walking on mortality among nonsmoking retired men. N Engl J Med 1998;338(2):94–9.
147. Knoops KT, de Groot LC, Kromhout D, et al. Mediterranean diet, lifestyle factors, and 10-year mortality in elderly european men and women: the HALE project. JAMA 2004;292(12):1433–9.
148. Pressman SD, Cohen S. Does positive affect influence health? Psychol Bull 2005;131(6):925–71.
149. Wolin KY, Glynn RJ, Colditz GA, et al. Long-term physical activity patterns and health-related quality of life in U.S. women. Am J Prev Med 2007;32(6):490–9.
150. Kruger J, Bowles HR, Jones DA, et al. Health-related quality of life, BMI and physical activity among US adults (ges18 years): national physical activity and weight loss survey, 2002. Int J Obes 2006;31(2):321–7.
151. Shih M, Hootman JM, Kruger J, et al. Physical activity in men and women with arthritis: national health interview survey, 2002. Am J Prev Med 2006;30(5):385–93.
152. Rejeski WJ, Mihalko SL. Physical activity and quality of life in older adults. J Gerontol A Biol Sci Med Sci 2001;56(2):23–35.
153. Drewnowski A, Evans WJ. Nutrition, physical activity, and quality of life in older adults: summary. J Gerontol A Biol Sci Med Sci 2001;56(2):89–94.
154. Brown DW, Balluz LS, Heath GW, et al. Associations between recommended levels of physical activity and health-related quality of life Findings from the 2001 Behavioral Risk Factor Surveillance System (BRFSS) survey. Prev Med 2003;37(5):520–8.

155. Penedo FJ, Dahn JR. Exercise and well-being: a review of mental and physical health benefits associated with physical activity. Curr Opin Psychiatry 2005; 18(2):189–93.
156. Bazargan M. Self-reported sleep disturbance among African-American elderly: the effects of depression, health status, exercise, and social support. Int J Aging Hum Dev 1996;42(2):143–60.
157. Morgan K. Daytime activity and risk factors for late-life insomnia. J Sleep Res 2003;12(3):231–8.
158. Ohayon MM. Interactions between sleep normative data and sociocultural characteristics in the elderly. J Psychosom Res 2004;56(5):479–86.
159. King AC, Oman RF, Brassington GS, et al. Moderate-intensity exercise and self-rated quality of sleep in older adults. A randomized controlled trial. JAMA 1997; 277(1):32–7.
160. Singh NA, Clements KM, Fiatarone MA. A randomized controlled trial of the effect of exercise on sleep. Sleep 1997;20(2):95–101.
161. Mazzeo RS, Cavanagh P, Evans WJ, et al. Exercise and physical activity for older adults: ACSM position statement. Med Sci Sports Exerc 1998;30(6): 992–1008.
162. Nelson ME, Rejeski WJ, Blair SN, et al. Physical activity and public health in older adults: recommendation from the American College of Sports Medicine and the American Heart Association. Med Sci Sports Exerc 2007;39(8):1435–45.
163. Wisloff U, Stoylen A, Loennechen JP, et al. Superior cardiovascular effect of aerobic interval training versus moderate continuous training in heart failure patients: a randomized study. Circulation 2007;115(24):3086–94.
164. Vogiatzis I, Terzis G, Nanas S, et al. Skeletal muscle adaptations to interval training in patients with advanced COPD*. Chest 2005;128(6):3838–45.
165. Broman G, Quintana M, Lindberg T, et al. High intensity deep water training can improve aerobic power in elderly women. Eur J Appl Physiol 2006;98(2):117–23.
166. Cancela Carral JM, Ayán Pérez C. Effects of high-intensity combined training on women over 65. Gerontology 2007;53(6):340–6.
167. Cress EM, Buchner DM, Prohaska T, et al. Physical activity programs and behavior counseling in older adult populations. Med Sci Sports Exerc 2004; 36(11):1997–2003.
168. Oka R, King A. Sources of social support as predictors of exercise adherence in women and men age 50 to 65 years. Womens Health 1995;1:161–75.
169. Petrella PJ, Koval JJ, Cunningham DA, et al. Can primary care doctors prescribe exercise to improve fitness? Am J Prev Med 2003;24(4):316–22.
170. Dauenhauer JA, Podgorski CA, Karuza J. Prescribing exercise for older adults: a needs assessment comparing primary care physician, nurse practitioners, and physician assistants. Gerontol Geriatr Educ 2006;26(3):81–99.
171. Andersen RE, Blair SN, Cheskin LJ, et al. Encouraging patients to become more physically active: the physician's role. Ann Intern Med 1997;127:395–400.
172. Dunstan DW, Daly RM, Owen N, et al. Home-based resistance training in not sufficient to maintain improved glycemic control following supervised training in older individuals with type 2 diabetes. Diabetes Care 2005;28(1):3–9.
173. Nelson M, Layne J, Bernstein M, et al. The effects of multidimensional home-based exercise on functional performance in elderly people. J Gerontol A Biol Sci Med Sci 2004;59(2):154–60.
174. Ransdell L, Taylor A, Oakland D, et al. Daughters and mothers exercising together: effects of home- and community-based programs. Med Sci Sports Exerc 2003;35(2):286–96.

175. Ravaud P, Giraudeau B, Logeart I, et al. Management of osteoarthritis (OA) with an unsupervised home based exercise programme and/or patient administered assessment tools. A cluster randomised controlled trial with a 2x2 factorial design. Ann Rheum Dis 2004;63(6):703–8.

176. Daub WD, Knapik GP, Black WR. Strength training early after myocardial infarction. J Cardiopulm Rehabil 1996;16(2):100–9.

177. Belardinelli R, Lacalaprice F, Ventrella C, et al. Waltz dancing in patients with chronic heart failure: new form of exercise training. Circ Heart Fail 2008;1(2): 107–14.

Impact of Strength and Resistance Training on Cardiovascular Disease Risk Factors and Outcomes in Older Adults

Mark A. Williams, PhD, FACSM, FAACVPR,[a,b,*],
Kerry J. Stewart, EdD, FAHA, FAACVPR, FACSM, FSGC[c,d]

KEYWORDS

- Strength • Cardiovascular disease risk factors • Older adults
- Resistance training • Resistance exercise prescription

In older persons with and without cardiovascular disease, muscular strength and endurance significantly contribute to improved functional independence and quality of life,[1,2] while reducing disability. Unfortunately, muscle atrophy results from aging and inactivity, leading to a loss of strength and power,[3,4] the latter being a function of both force and the speed of the movement. This article reviews the physiologic response to resistance training in older adults and discusses the impact of resistance exercise training on cardiovascular disease risk factors, particularly obesity and diabetes.

RESISTANCE EXERCISE TRAINING RESPONSES IN OLDER ADULTS

Regardless of age, skeletal muscle responds to progressive overload through resistance training. Strength improves through neuromuscular adaptation, muscle fiber hypertrophy, and muscle strength. In older adults, muscle strength and the ability to move quickly appear to have an inverse relationship with risk for falls.[5] In particular,

---

[a] Division of Cardiology, Department of Medicine, Creighton University School of Medicine, Omaha, NE, USA
[b] Cardiovascular Disease Prevention and Rehabilitation, Cardiac Center of Creighton University, 3006 Webster Street, Omaha, NE 68131, USA
[c] Department of Medicine, Johns Hopkins University School of Medicine, Baltimore, MD, USA
[d] Clinical and Research Exercise Physiology, Johns Hopkins Bayview Medical Center, 4940 Eastern Avenue, Baltimore, MD 21224, USA
* Corresponding author. Cardiovascular Disease Prevention and Rehabilitation, Cardiac Center of Creighton University, 3006 Webster Street, Omaha, NE 68131.
E-mail address: mawilli@creighton.edu (M.A. Williams).

Clin Geriatr Med 25 (2009) 703–714
doi:10.1016/j.cger.2009.07.003
0749-0690/09/$ – see front matter © 2009 Elsevier Inc. All rights reserved.
geriatric.theclinics.com

low- to moderate-intensity resistance training incorporating increased movement velocity (ie, power) has been shown to improve performance of activities of daily living and balance.[6–10]

Resistance training appears to increase muscle oxidative capacity and the capacity for aerobic endurance exercise.[11] The most likely reason for this is that resistance training programs in older adults are usually a mix of strength development and aerobic exercise resulting from the circuit training format using moderate-intensity resistance (**Fig. 1**).[12] This approach has been demonstrated to maintain or increase capillary density, mitochondrial content, and oxidative capacity.

Benefits of Resistance Exercise Training in Older Persons

Improved physical function results from substantial increases in upper- and lower-body muscle strength and endurance.[9,13,14] In both older men and women, resistance training improves several components of function, including walking endurance, walking speed, and dynamic balance.[9,13–19] Even in the oldest persons (nursing home residents; mean age, 87 years), Fiatarone and colleagues[17] demonstrated that 10 weeks of resistance training significantly improved strength, gait velocity, and stair-climbing power in association with an increase in thigh muscle cross-sectional area. Nakamura and colleagues[20] showed that training frequencies ranging from 1 to 3 days per week, which included both aerobic and resistance types of exercise, produced similar increases in strength, but that 3 days per week was superior for muscle endurance, coordination, balance, and cardiovascular endurance. With regard to increasing strength, modest- to high-intensity resistance programs have demonstrated similar improvements in strength in some studies,[11,21,22] while other studies found that high-intensity effort produced the greatest benefit in strength in older adults.[23–26]

In older women with cardiovascular disease and at least moderate mobility limitation, Brochu and colleagues[27] and Ades and colleagues[28] showed that, compared

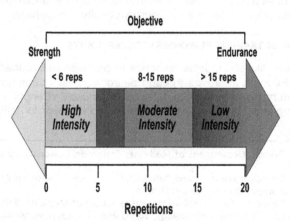

Fig. 1. Classification of weight training intensity (resistance). A lower repetition range with a heavier weight may better optimize strength and power, whereas a higher repetition range with a lighter weight may better enhance muscular endurance. Using weight loads that permit 8 to 15 repetitions (reps) will generally facilitate improvements in muscular strength and endurance. (*Reprinted from* Williams MA, Haskell WL, Ades PA, et al. Resistance exercise in individuals with and without cardiovascular disease: 2007 update. Circulation 2007;116:579; with permission.)

with controls, resistance training improved upper- and lower-body strength (increased 18% and 23%, respectively), balance and coordination (improved 29%), walking endurance (increased 15%), and the overall physical activity summary score (improved 24%). Total energy expenditure was estimated to have increased by 150 to 175 kcal/d resulting from increased total physical activity and resting metabolic rate.[11,27,29]

CARDIOVASCULAR DISEASE RISK MODIFICATION

Skeletal muscle is the primary tissue for glucose and triglyceride metabolism, and muscle mass is thus a determinant of resting metabolic rate. Loss of muscle mass with aging slows the metabolic rate and reduces caloric expenditure. This effect is exacerbated with decreased physical activity, which also contributes to the risk of developing obesity, insulin resistance, type 2 diabetes, dyslipidemia, and hypertension.[30–35] Muscular strength is inversely associated with the prevalence of metabolic syndrome, independent of aerobic fitness levels.[36–38] Nonetheless, as yet there remains little evidence to demonstrate that resistance training decreases cardiovascular disease risk, particularly in older adults.

Hypertension

It is well established that regular aerobic training can reduce blood pressure. Several health organizations, including the American Heart Association[12] and the American College of Sports Medicine,[39] have recommended moderate-intensity resistance training as an adjunct to aerobic exercise programs for preventing and treating hypertension. These recommendations are supported by studies of resistance training alone and combined aerobic and resistance training.

The effect of resistance training on blood pressure was examined in two meta-analyses. Kelley and colleagues[40] found decreases of approximately 3 mm Hg for both systolic blood pressure (SBP) and diastolic blood pressure (DBP) in a review of 11 studies, including 182 resistance training subjects and 138 controls. Overall, these changes represented 2% and 4% reductions in resting SBP and DBP, respectively. There were no differences for changes in resting blood pressure between studies that used resistance training alone compared with a circuit resistance training protocol. Resistance training alone generally consisted of lifting heavier weights with longer rest periods, while circuit protocols usually involve lifting weights at a moderate intensity, generally 50% of the one-repetition maximum (ie, the maximal amount of weight that can be moved one time [eg, lifted, pushed, or pulled]) with short rest periods between exercises. Circuit weight training, which uses lighter weights with higher repetitions, improves aerobic capacity as well as strength.[41] The meta-analysis of resistance training alone and resting blood pressure by Cornelissen and Fagard[42] (12 studies, 341 patients) showed reductions of 6 and 3 mm Hg for SBP and DBP, respectively. Less than 20% of subjects in these studies had both initial resting SBP equal to or greater than 140 mm Hg and initial resting DBP equal to or greater than 90 mm Hg.

In a 10-week study, men (mean age 54 years old) with mild hypertension performed combined resistance training and aerobic training and were randomly assigned to beta-blockers, calcium channel blockers, or placebo.[43,44] The key finding was that all three groups decreased SBP and DBP by 13 mm Hg each. The investigators concluded that drug therapy provided no additive benefit to the antihypertensive effects of exercise. Stewart and colleagues,[45] using a similar combined resistance training and aerobic training program in 104 older adults (55–75 years) with undertreated hypertension, found that exercisers significantly improved aerobic and strength fitness, increased lean mass, and reduced general and abdominal obesity. Mean decreases in SBP and DBP were 5.3 and 3.7 mm Hg, respectively, among exercisers and 4.5 and 1.5 mm Hg among controls (P<.001 for all). There were no significant group differences in mean SBP change from baseline (−0.8 mm Hg, P = .67) although the mean DBP reduction was greater among exercisers (−2.2 mm Hg, P = .02). Aortic stiffness was unchanged in both groups. Body composition improvements explained 8% of the SBP reduction (P = .006) and 17% of the DBP reduction (P<.001). Thus, relative to controls, this program of combined resistance training and aerobic training significantly lowered DBP but not SBP in older adults with mild hypertension. The lack of improvement in aortic stiffness in exercisers suggests that older persons may be resistant to exercise-induced reductions in SBP. Body composition improvements were associated with blood pressure reductions and may be a pathway by which exercise training improves cardiovascular health in older men and women.

Overall, the evidence for resistance training alone as a mode of exercise to reduce blood pressure is mixed. This is reflected in existing guidelines that endorse combined resistance training and aerobic training as the best opportunity for reducing blood pressure with exercise. However, the magnitude of benefit of exercise for reducing blood pressure may be attenuated with aging, suggesting a need to combine exercise with other interventions, including improved diet, weight loss, and antihypertensive drug therapy.

Dyslipidemia

The effect of resistance training on the lipid profile is equivocal, and few studies have investigated the effects of resistance training on lipid metabolism in individuals, especially older individually, who actually have lipid disorders. Most studies of resistance training have involved younger individuals with normal lipid profiles at baseline. In a study of 8499 men (mean age 40.5 ± 10.7 years), Tucker and Sylvester[46] showed a decreased risk of hypercholesterolemia in individuals participating in resistance training, but after adjusting for other factors, including age, only those participating 4 h/w or more maintained a decrease in risk. In contrast, Kohl and colleagues,[47] in a study of 1193 women and 5460 men, found no relationship between muscle strength and levels of either total cholesterol or low-density lipoprotein cholesterol. However, among men, increased upper- and lower-body strength was associated with lower triglyceride levels. In a randomized trial of 33 patients with type 2 diabetes, mean age 57 years, Cauza and colleagues[48] found that those randomized to resistance training had significantly greater decreases in total cholesterol, low-density lipoprotein cholesterol, and triglycerides compared with an aerobic exercise group. For patients with components of the metabolic syndrome, combining resistance training with aerobic exercise may be more beneficial in older adults.[45,49] In these studies, exercisers significantly increased aerobic capacity, muscular endurance, lean body mass, and high-density lipoprotein cholesterol, while reducing total and abdominal fat and blood pressure, thereby resulting in a lower prevalence of metabolic syndrome compared with nonexercisers.

Body Composition

Randomized studies of resistance training consistently show increases in muscle mass and quality (ie, increased strength for same muscle mass), especially in older men.[15] This increase in muscle mass and quality should assist in weight control and improve muscle metabolism. In theory, increased muscle mass increases resting energy expenditure and may prevent or reverse age-associated increases in body fat.[50,51] In addition, data suggest that even without a change in resting energy expenditure, maintaining muscle mass with aging is valuable in preventing age-associated fat gains.[52–55] Resistance training is also associated with decreased abdominal visceral adipose tissue, a significant component of the metabolic syndrome.[45,49,55–58] Hunter and colleagues[29] and McCarthy and colleagues[59] have reported increased lean body mass and decreased adipose tissue in older adults participating in resistance training, when weight is controlled. Resistance training can also increase muscle mass in older persons with sarcopenia.[60,61]

The value of resistance training for total body weight loss without concomitant dietary changes appears limited. Total body weight does not usually change significantly because loss of fat mass is offset by the gain in muscle mass.[62] In one study, for example, 6 months of combined resistance training and aerobic training in persons 55 to 75 years old resulted in significant reductions in waist circumference and total body and abdominal obesity, as well as an increase in lean mass, yet total body weight decreased by only 2.2 kg.[45,49]

Glycemic Control

The risk of developing type 2 diabetes, insulin resistance, and impaired glucose tolerance increases with age, especially in individuals who are overweight, obese, and physically inactive. Maintaining normal body weight and being physically active can help to prevent these conditions, which are also major risk factors for developing cardiovascular disease. Maintaining glycemic control relies on improving insulin availability or secretion and increasing insulin sensitivity. In persons who have established diabetes, even when glycemia is under good control with diet and medication, reducing insulin resistance by resistance training should be considered to avoid disease progression and to reverse some of its adverse consequences.

Miller and colleagues,[33] Smutok and colleagues,[63] and Ishii and colleagues[64] have demonstrated that muscle contraction with resistance training increases both glucose uptake and insulin sensitivity in skeletal muscle, thereby providing a rationale for resistance training in individuals with glucose intolerance. The greatest impact of resistance training on glycemic control appears to occur when baseline glucose tolerance is more severely impaired rather than when there is no or only mild impairment.[32,33,65–70] Resistance training increases insulin sensitivity and glucose clearance in healthy and diabetic individuals and decreases hemoglobin A1c levels in persons with diabetes.[32,33,65–71]

Improved glycemic control is related to increased muscle mass as well as local adaptation in the muscle tissue. Cauza and colleagues[48,72] found that, in contrast to endurance training, only resistance training was associated with improvement in acute and chronic blood glucose and hemoglobin A1c levels. In another study of 251 adults age 39 to 70 years with type 2 diabetes, 6 months of either aerobic or resistance training lowered HbA1c, but improvements were greater with combined aerobic and resistance training.[73] The absolute change in hemoglobin A1c in the combined exercise training group was −0.97% versus −0.51% in the aerobic training group ($P = .014$) and −0.38% in the resistance training group ($P = .001$). The additional benefit of combined training may be attributable to total duration of exercise being longer than in the aerobic training and resistance training groups. Differences in results among studies are likely due to differences in study populations, length of training, types of equipment used, and intensity of exercise. Nevertheless, resistance training clearly plays an important role in the management of impaired glucose tolerance and diabetes. However, data showing that resistance training prevents type 2 diabetes or reduces clinical event rates are lacking.

Resistance Training: The Exercise Prescription

At the initiation of a resistance training program or when significant increases in muscular work or frequency of training are made to an existing program, emphasis must be placed on allowing adequate time for musculoskeletal adaptation and practicing good technique, thereby limiting the potential for excessive muscle soreness and injury.[12] This is particularly important in older individuals, especially those with cardiovascular disease. The initial workload intensity and frequency of training should be at a modest level to permit the participant to use proper body mechanics, to avoid straining during training sessions, and to prevent injuries associated with overuse, either acutely or over a period of time. The initial exercise prescription and subsequent progression of resistance training should be undertaken with caution, particularly in persons with hypertension, arthritis, cardiovascular disease, or other debilitating illnesses.[74] Alternatives to traditional resistance training may be considered. Alternatives include, for example, aquatic resistance exercise and modification of the exercise components, such as variation of activities, more gradual progression, and rest periods within each session.[74] **Box 1** describes considerations and methodology for the prescription of resistance training. In general, the methods for prescribing resistance training in older adults are not different from those for younger persons, although adjustments may need to be made to accommodate health conditions and other individual limitations.[12] Although most studies have involved facility-based resistance training, favorable results also have been obtained with elders exercising at home.[16,18]

Because the effect of physical conditioning is specific to the muscle group being trained, resistance training regimens should include exercises involving all major muscle groups.[75] To approximate the appropriate limb-specific weight loads (intensity) for resistance training, one can determine the maximum weight that can be lifted or pushed one time (one repetition maximum [1 RM]) during a given exercise (eg, bench press, leg press, or biceps curl) and then lift a defined percentage of that amount during each set of the exercise. An initial intensity that corresponds to 30% to 40% of 1 RM for the upper body and 50% to 60% of 1 RM for the hips and legs is recommended (see Box 1).[12] Although there are few data to determine the appropriate time to initiate resistance training after a cardiac event, conventional guidelines frequently suggest a somewhat restrictive maximal weight limit (of 10–20 lb) for up 3 months, particularly in unsupervised activities. However, Stewart and colleagues[76] initiated resistance training as part of a combined aerobic and resistance training program as early as 6 weeks after myocardial infarction. Maximal oxygen uptake increased 14% ($P<.01$) and cycle time increased 10% ($P<.01$) in the combined training group; by comparison, 8% increases in maximal oxygen uptake and cycle time in a cycling-only group were not significant. Arm and leg strength increased ($P<.01$) in each group although the change was greater for the combined training group, 31% versus 16% ($P<.03$) for leg strength and 20% versus 10% ($P<.001$) for arm strength. There were no changes for either group in resting hemodynamics, body weight and composition, left ventricular wall motion, left ventricular fractional shortening, or early diastolic function, and there were no adverse clinical or exercise-related events.

As resistance training progresses, the exercise workload (intensity) can be increased to facilitate further improvement. In older persons, this increased "overload" should be achieved by increasing the resistance or weight or by adding a second set per exercise. Increasing the number of repetitions within a set or decreasing the rest period between sets or exercises is generally not recommended for this age group.[12] When the participant can comfortably achieve the "upper limit" of the repetition range for a specific exercise (eg, 12–15 repetitions) an increase in training

Box 1.
Prescription of resistance training in older adults (age >50 years)

Select six to eight different resistance training exercises that involve major muscle groups

Upper body

Chest press

Shoulder press

Triceps extension

Biceps curl

Lateral pull-down (upper back)

Midsection of the body

Lower-back extension

Abdominal crunch/curl-up

Lower body

Quadriceps extension or leg press

Leg curls (hamstrings)

Calf raise

Resistance training exercise prescription components

Initially, use single sets of six to eight varied exercises, 2 days per week

Each set should include 10 to 15 repetitions at less than 40% of one repetition maximum (1 RM). One repetition maximum (1 RM) is the greatest amount of resistance (ie, weight) that can be lifted or pushed with a single effort. As an alternative to the method of resistance training prescription using 1 RM, trial and error can be used to determine a level of resistance for which the participant can appropriately accomplish 10 repetitions. The participant can then work toward comfortably accomplishing up to 15 repetitions at this level before increasing resistance.

Provide 1 to 2 minutes rest between exercises

Alternate between upper- and lower-body work

Resistance training exercise technique

Perform each exercise through a full range of motion, in a controlled rhythmic manner, and at a slow to moderate speed

Avoid breath-holding and straining (Valsalva maneuver) by exhaling during the contraction or exertion phase of the exercise and inhaling during the relaxation or rest phase of the exercise

Emphasize proper body mechanics throughout each exercise

Updating the resistance training exercise prescription

As resistance training exercise repetitions (12–15 repetitions) become easily accomplished, consider updating the resistance training prescription in the following order:

Varying the type of resistance training exercises

Increasing the level of resistance; increasing by 5% of 1 RM, up to 40% of 1 RM for arm exercises and up to 60% of 1 RM for leg exercises

Adding a second set of exercises without increasing level of resistance

Adding a third day of resistance training during the week

workload can be considered for that particular exercise. An increase in load of approximately 5% may be implemented, which in general is about 2 to 5 lb for arm exercises and 5 to 10 lb for leg exercises.[12]

Measures of cardiovascular responses to resistance training in older persons should include heart rate, blood pressure, and perceived exertion. Although the heart rate response is generally lower during resistance training compared with response during aerobic exercise, blood pressure response may be higher; thus, heart rate alone may not accurately reflect the overall work of the heart.[77] In older persons, many of whom are hypertensive, it is useful to evaluate the blood pressure response to resistance training, particularly in those who have known heart disease.[78] However, blood pressure measured immediately after rather than during actual resistance exercise is likely to underestimate the pressure response.[79] During resistance training, participants can work to a perceived exertion rating of 11 to 14 ("fairly light" to "somewhat hard") on the Borg category scale,[80] assessed during the last couple of repetitions.[12] Participants should be frequently reminded that if adverse signs and symptoms occur, such as dizziness, excessive shortness of breath, chest discomfort, heart rhythm irregularities, or acute pain in the muscles or joints, resistance training should be immediately discontinued.[12,78,80]

Equipment

The types of resistance exercise equipment vary greatly in cost, complexity, requirements for neuromusculoskeletal coordination, and time commitment. Within these considerations, the essential element is to select a modality that the participant enjoys, as well as one that is safe, effective, and accessible. Often, good first choices are low-cost approaches to resistance training that have been shown to be effective while allowing for gradual progression, such as resistance bands, hand or wrist weights, and body-support calisthenics (eg, modified push-ups or sit-ups). If more expensive and complex resistance equipment or machines are of interest, participants should be encouraged to experiment with various devices at gyms or health clubs and seek advice from exercise professionals before initiating a resistance training program.

SUMMARY

In older adults, resistance training is associated with increased physical function and quality of life. Resistance training should be used to complement aerobic exercise training for reducing risk of cardiovascular disease. Available data indicate that resistance training is associated with modest improvements in blood pressure in hypertensive adults, equivocal effects on lipids, and significant mild to moderate improvements in glycemic control. The role of resistance training in glycemic control is intriguing and is an important area for future research; specifically, the value of high-intensity resistance training in various population subgroups, including the elderly, warrants further investigation.

REFERENCES

1. Beniamini Y, Rubinstein JJ, Faigenbaum AD, et al. High-intensity strength training of patients enrolled in an outpatient cardiac rehabilitation program. J Cardiopulm Rehabil 1999;19:8–17.
2. McCartney N, McKelvie RS, Haslam DR, et al. Usefulness of weightlifting training in improving strength and maximal power output in coronary artery disease. Am J Cardiol 1991;67:939–45.

3. Frontera WR, Hughes VA, Lutz KJ, et al. A cross-sectional study of muscle strength and mass in 45- to 78-year old men and women. J Appl Physiol 1991; 71:644–50.

4. Hakkinen K, Hakkinen A. Neuromuscular adaptations during intensive strength training in middle-aged and elderly males and females. Electromyogr Clin Neurophysiol 1995;35:137–47.

5. Pijnappels M, van der Burg JCE, Reeves ND, et al. Identification of elderly fallers by muscle strength measures. Eur J Appl Physiol 2008;102:585–92.

6. Bottaro M, Machado SN, Nogueira W, et al. Effect of high versus low-velocity resistance training on muscular fitness and functional performance in older men. Eur J Appl Physiol 2007;99:257–64.

7. De Vos NJ, Singh NA, Ross DA, et al. Optimal load for increasing muscle power during explosive resistance training in older adults. J Gerontol A Biol Sci Med Sci 2005;60:638–47.

8. Henwood TR, Taaffe DR. Improved physical performance in older adults undertaking a short-term programme of high velocity resistance training. Gerontology 2005;51:108–15.

9. Orr R, de Vos NJ, Singh NA, et al. Power training improves balance in healthy older adults. J Gerontol A Biol Sci Med Sci 2006;61:78–85.

10. Signorile JF, Carmel MP, Lai S, et al. Early plateau of power and torque gains during high- and low-speed resistance training in older women. J Appl Physiol 2005;98:1213–20.

11. Ades PA, Savage PD, Brochu M, et al. Resistance training increases total daily energy expenditure in disabled older women with coronary heart disease. J Appl Physiol 2005;98:1280–5.

12. Williams MA, Haskell WL, Ades PA, et al. Resistance exercise in individuals with and without cardiovascular disease: 2007 update. Circulation 2007;116:572–84.

13. Campbell AJ, Robertson MC, Gardner MM, et al. Randomised controlled trial of a general practice programme of home based exercise to prevent falls in elderly women. BMJ 1997;315:1065–9.

14. Ades PA, Ballor DL, Ashikaga T, et al. Weight training improves walking endurance in healthy elderly persons. Ann Intern Med 1996;124:568–72.

15. Hunter GR, McCarthy JP, Bamman MM, et al. Effects of resistance exercise training on older adults. Sports Med 2004;34:329–48.

16. Seguin R, Nelson ME. The benefits of strength training for older adults. Am J Prev Med 2003;25(Suppl 2):141–9.

17. Fiatarone MA, O'Neill EF, Ryan ND, et al. Exercise training and nutritional supplementation for physical frailty in very elderly people. N Engl J Med 1994;330: 1769–75.

18. Jette AM, Lachman M, Giorgetti MM, et al. Exercise: It's never too late: the Strong-for-Life Program. Am J Public Health 1999;89:66–72.

19. Vincent KR, Braith RW, Feldman RA, et al. Improved cardiorespiratory endurance following 6 months of resistance exercise in elderly men and women. Arch Intern Med 2002;162:673–8.

20. Nakamura Y, Tanaka K, Yabushita N, et al. Effects of exercise frequency on functional status in older adult women. Arch Gerontol Geriatr 2007;44:163–73.

21. Harris C, Debeliso MA, Spitzer-Gibson TA, et al. The effect of resistance-training on strength-gain response in the older adult. J Strength Cond Res 2004;18: 833–8.

22. Hunter GR, Wetzstein CJ, McLafferty CL, et al. High-resistance versus variable-resistance training in older adults. Med Sci Sports Exerc 2001;33:1759–64.

23. Fatouros IG, Tournis S, Leontsini D, et al. Liptin and adiponectin responses in overweight and inactive elderly following resistance training and detraining are intensity related. J Clin Endocrinol Metab 2005;90:5970–7.

24. Fatouros IG, Kambas A, Katrabasas I, et al. Resistance training and detraining effects on flexibility performance in the elderly are intensity-dependent. J Strength Cond Res 2006;20:634–42.

25. Kalapotharakos V, Mechalopoulos M, Godolia G, et al. The effect of high- and moderate-resistance training on muscle function in the elderly. J Aging Phys Act 2004;11:131–43.

26. Kalapotharakos V, Mechalopoulos M, Tokmakidis SP, et al. Effects of a heavy and a moderate resistance training on functional performance in older adults. J Strength Cond Res 2005;19:652–7.

27. Brochu M, Savage P, Lee M, et al. Effects of resistance training on physical function in older disabled women with coronary heart disease. J Appl Physiol 2002; 92:672–8.

28. Ades PA, Savage PD, Cress ME, et al. Resistance training on physical performance in disabled older female cardiac patients. Med Sci Sports Exerc 2003; 35:1265–70.

29. Hunter GR, Wetstein CJ, Fields DA, et al. Resistance training increases total energy expenditure and free-living physical activity in older adults. J Appl Physiol 2000;89:977–84.

30. Fletcher GF, Balady G, Blair SN, et al. Statement on exercise: benefits and recommendations for physical activity programs for all Americans. Circulation 1996;94: 857–62.

31. Klein S, Burke LE, Bray GA, et al. Clinical implications of obesity with specific focus on cardiovascular disease. Circulation 2004;110:2952–67.

32. Hurley BF, Hagberg JM, Goldberg AP, et al. Resistive training can reduce coronary risk factors without altering VO2max or percent body fat. Med Sci Sports Exerc 1988;20:150–4.

33. Miller JP, Pratley RE, Goldberg AP, et al. Strength training increases insulin action in healthy 50- to 65-yr-old men. J Appl Physiol 1994;77:1122–7.

34. Poehlman ET, Denino WF, Beckett T, et al. Effects of endurance and resistance training on total daily energy expenditure in young women: a controlled randomized trial. J Clin Endocrinol Metab 2002;87:1004–9.

35. Braith RW, Stewart KJ. Resistance exercise training: its role in the prevention of cardiovascular disease. Circulation 2006;113:2642–50.

36. Fitzgerald SJ, Barlowe CE, Kampert JB, et al. Muscular fitness and all-cause mortality: prospective observations. J Phys Act Health 2004;1:7–18.

37. Jurca R, Lamonte MJ, Barlowe CE, et al. Association of muscular strength with incidence of metabolic syndrome in men. Med Sci Sports Exerc 2005;37: 1849–55.

38. Jurca R, Lamonte MJ, Church TS, et al. Associations of muscle strength and fitness with metabolic syndrome in men. Med Sci Sports Exerc 2004;36:1301–7.

39. Pescatello LS, Franklin BA, Fagard R, et al. American College of Sports Medicine position stand. Exercise and hypertension. Med Sci Sports Exerc 2004;36: 533–53.

40. Kelley GA, Kelley KS. Progressive resistance exercise and resting blood pressure: a meta-analysis of randomized controlled trials. Hypertension 2000;35: 838–43.

41. Stewart KJ. Weight training in coronary artery disease and hypertension. Prog Cardiovasc Dis 1992;35:159–68.

42. Cornelissen VA, Fagard RH. Effect of resistance training on resting blood pressure: a meta-analysis of randomized controlled trials. J Hypertens 2005;23: 251–9.
43. Kelemen MH, Effron MB, Valenti SA, et al. Exercise training combined with antihypertensive drug therapy: effects on lipids, blood pressure, and left ventricular mass. JAMA 1990;263:2766–71.
44. Stewart KJ, Effron MB, Valenti SA, et al. Effects of diltiazem or propranolol during exercise training of hypertensive men. Med Sci Sports Exerc 1990;22:171–7.
45. Stewart KJ, Bacher AC, Turner KL, et al. Effect of exercise on blood pressure in older persons: a randomized controlled trial. Arch Intern Med 2005;165: 756–62.
46. Tucker LA, Sylvester LJ. Strength training and hypercholesterolemia: an epidemiologic study of 8499 employed men. Am J Health Promot 1996;11:35–41.
47. Kohl HW 3rd, Gordon NF, Scott CB, et al. Musculoskeletal strength and serum lipid levels in men and women. Med Sci Sports Exerc 1992;24:1080–7.
48. Cauza E, Hanusch-Enserer U, Strasser B, et al. The relative benefits of endurance and strength training on the metabolic factors and muscle function of people with type 2 diabetes mellitus. Arch Phys Med Rehabil 2005;86:1527–33.
49. Stewart KJ, Bachner AC, Turner K, et al. Exercise and risk factors associated with metabolic syndrome in older adults. Am J Prev Med 2005;28:9–18.
50. Weinsier RL, Shulzt Y, Bracco D. Reexamination of the relationship of resting metabolic rate to fat-free mass and to the metabolically active components of fat-free mass in humans. Am J Clin Nutr 1992;55:790–4.
51. Pratley R, Nicklas B, Rubin M, et al. Strength training increases resting metabolic rate and norepinephrine levels in healthy 50- to 65-yr old men. J Appl Physiol 1994;76:133–7.
52. Ryan AS, Pratley RE, Elahi D, et al. Resistive training increases fat-free mass and maintains RMR despite weight loss in postmenopausal women. J Applied Physiol 1995;79:818–23.
53. Campbell WW, Crim MC, Young VR, et al. Increased energy requirements and changes in body composition with resistance training in older adults. Am J Clin Nutr 1994;60:167–75.
54. Schmitz KH, Jensen MD, Kugler KC, et al. Strength training for obesity prevention in midlife women. Int J Obes Relat Metab Disord 2003;27:326–33.
55. Treuth MS, Ryan AS, Pratley RE, et al. Effects of strength training on total and regional body composition in older men. J Appl Physiol 1994;77:614–20.
56. Treuth MS, Hunter GR, Kekes-Szabo T, et al. Reduction in intra-abdominal adipose tissue after strength training in older women. J Appl Physiol 1995;78: 1425–31.
57. Ross R, Rissanen J. Mobilization of visceral and subcutaneous adipose tissue in response to energy restriction and exercise. Am J Clin Nutr 1994;60:695–703.
58. Ross R, Rissanen J, Pedwell H, et al. Influence of diet and exercise on skeletal muscle and visceral adipose tissue in men. J Appl Physiol 1996;81:2445–55.
59. McCarthy JP, Agre JC, Graf BK, et al. Compatibility of adaptive responses with combining strength and endurance training. Med Sci Sports Exerc 1995;27: 429–36.
60. Kim JS, Cross JM, Bamman MM. Impact of resistance loading on myostatin expression and cell cycle regulation in young and older men and women. Am J Physiol Endrocrinol Metab 2005;288:e1110–9.
61. Lemmer JT, Hurlburt GE, Martel DF, et al. Age and gender responses to strength training and detraining. Med Sci Sports Exerc 2000;32:1505–12.

62. Donnelly JE, Smith B, Jacobsen DJ, et al. The role of exercise for weight loss and maintenance. Best Pract Res Clin Gastroenterol 2004;18:1009–29.

63. Smutok MA, Reece C, Kokkinos PF, et al. Effects of exercise training modality on glucose tolerance in men with abnormal glucose regulation. Int J Sports Med 1994;15:283–9.

64. Ishii T, Yamakita T, Sato T, et al. Resistance training improves insulin sensitivity in NIDDM subjects without altering maximal oxygen uptake. Diabetes Care 1998; 21:1353–5.

65. Castaneda C, Layne JE, Munoz-Orians, et al. A randomized controlled trial of resistance exercise training to improve glycemic control in older adults with type 2 diabetes. Diabetes Care 2002;25:2335–41.

66. Fenicchia LM, Kanaly JA, Azevedo JL, et al. Influence of resistance exercise training on glucose control in women with type 2 diabetes. Metabolism 2004; 53:284–9.

67. Reynolds TH, Supiano JA, Dengel JL, et al. Resistance training enhances insulin-mediated glucose disposal with minimal effect on the tumor necrosis factor-alpha system in older hypertensives. Metabolism 2004;53:397–402.

68. Ibanez J, Izquierdo M, Arguelles I, et al. Twice-weekly progressive resistance training decreases abdominal fat and improves insulin sensitivity in older men with type 2 diabetes. Diabetes Care 2005;28:662–7.

69. Dunstan DW, Daly RM, Owen N, et al. High-intensity resistance training improves glycemic control in older patients with type 2 diabetes. Diabetes Care 2002;25: 1729–36.

70. Honkola A, Forsen T, Ericksson J. Resistance training improves the metabolic profile in individuals with type 2 diabetes. Acta Diabetol 1997;34:245–8.

71. Durak EP, Janovic-Peterson L, Peterson CM. Randomized crossover study of effect of resistance training on glycemic control, muscular strength, and cholesterol in type 1 diabetic men. Diabetes Care 1990;13:1039–43.

72. Cauza E, Hanusch-Enserer U, Strasser B, et al. Strength and endurance training lead to different postexercise glucose profiles in diabetic participants using a continuous subcutaneous glucose monitoring system. Eur J Clin Invest 2005; 35:745–51.

73. Sigal RJ, Kenny GP, Boule NG, et al. Effects of aerobic training, resistance training, or both on glycemic control in type 2 diabetes: a randomized trial. Ann Intern Med 2007;147:357–69.

74. Ratamess NA, Alvar BA, Evetoch TK, et al. Progression models in resistance training for healthy adults. Med Sci Sports Exerc 2009;41:687–708.

75. Anderson K, Behm DG. Trunk muscle activity increases with unstable squat movements. Can J Appl Physiol 2005;30:33–45.

76. Stewart KJ, McFarland LD, Weinhofer JJ, et al. Safety and efficacy of weight training soon after acute myocardial infarction. J Cardiopulm Rehabil 1988;18:37–44.

77. Hunter GR. Changes in body composition, body build and performance associated with different weight training frequencies in males and females. NSCA J 1985;7:26–8.

78. Hass C, Garzarella L, Dehoyos D, et al. Single versus multiple sets and long-term recreational weightlifters. Med Sci Sports Exerc 2000;32:235–42.

79. Hurley BF, Kokkinos PF. Effects of weight training on risk factors for coronary heart disease. Sports Med 1987;4:231–8.

80. Hatfield DL, Kraemer WJ, Spiering BA, et al. The impact of velocity of movement on performance factors in resistance training. J Strength Cond Res 2006;20: 760–6.

Cellular Mechanisms of Cardioprotection by Calorie Restriction: State of the Science and Future Perspectives

Emanuele Marzetti, MD, PhD[a,d,*], Stephanie E. Wohlgemuth, PhD[b],
Stephen D. Anton, PhD[c], Roberto Bernabei, MD[e], Christy S. Carter, PhD[f],
Christiaan Leeuwenburgh, PhD[f,**]

KEYWORDS

- Cardiovascular disease • Oxidative stress • Inflammation
- Apoptosis • Autophagy • Calorie restriction mimetics

Cardiovascular disease (CVD) is the leading cause of morbidity and mortality in Western countries,[1] and it is estimated that by 2020 up to 40% of all deaths will be due to CVD.[2] The impact of CVD is especially pronounced in older populations, in whom remarkably high prevalence of CVD and incident events are observed, resulting

This research was supported by grants to C.L. (NIA R01-AG17994 and AG21042) and C.S.C, (NIH R01-AG024526-02), and the University of Florida Institute on Aging and Claude D. Pepper Older Americans Independence Center (1 P30AG028740).

[a] Department of Aging and Geriatric Research, Institute on Aging, Division of Biology of Aging, University of Florida, 1600 SW Archer Road, Room P1-09, PO Box 100143, Gainesville, FL 32610-0143, USA

[b] Department of Aging and Geriatric Research, Institute on Aging, Division of Biology of Aging, University of Florida, 1600 SW Archer Road, Room P1-08, PO Box 100143, Gainesville, FL 32610-0143, USA

[c] Department of Aging and Geriatric Research, Institute on Aging, University of Florida, PO Box 112610, Gainesville, FL 32610-0143, USA

[d] Department of Orthopaedics and Traumatology, Catholic University of the Sacred Heart, Largo F. Vito, 1, 00168, Rome 00168, Italy

[e] Department of Gerontology, Geriatrics and Physiatrics, Catholic University of the Sacred Heart, Large F. Vito, 1, 00168, Rome, Italy

[f] Department of Aging and Geriatric Research, Institute on Aging, Division of Biology of Aging, University of Florida, 210 East Mowry Drive, PO Box 112610, Gainesville, FL 32611, USA

* Corresponding author. Department of Aging and Geriatric Research, Institute on Aging, Division of Biology of Aging, University of Florida, 1600 SW Archer Road, Room P1-09, PO Box 100143, Gainesville, FL 32610.

E-mail address: emarzetti@aging.ufl.edu (E. Marzetti).

** Corresponding author.

E-mail address: cleeuwen@aging.ufl.edu (C. Leeuwenburgh).

in high levels of disability and mortality.[3] Numerous modifiable risk factors for CVD have been identified, including smoking, hypertension, dyslipidemia, abdominal obesity, impaired insulin sensitivity, and sedentary lifestyle.[4] In addition, advances in cardiovascular biology have unveiled several biomarkers associated with increased CVD risk. Examples include alterations in the redox state favoring a pro-oxidant milieu, enhanced production of inflammatory cytokines, and high levels of proinflammatory enzymes, hemostatic factors, and adhesion molecules.[3,5]

Despite great progress in the diagnosis and management of CVD, the prevalence of heart failure (HF), the final common pathway of many heart diseases, has reached epidemic proportions among older persons.[6] This condition represents a major determinant of chronic disability in the elderly.[7] Furthermore, HF is characterized by extremely poor prognosis, with 1-year mortality rate exceeding 50% in those aged 85 years or older.[8] Hence, there is an urgent need for effective strategies to reduce the incidence and improve the prognosis of CVD, especially in geriatric populations.

Calorie restriction (CR) without malnutrition is to date the most effective intervention for improving health, maintaining function, and increasing mean and maximum lifespan in a variety of species.[9] The antiaging properties of CR reside in the prevention or retardation of several degenerative diseases, including CVD, cancer, neurodegenerative disorders, diabetes, and autoimmune diseases.[10] As a result, experimental rodents subjected to lifelong CR display up to 60% maximum lifespan extension compared with ad libitum (AL)-fed controls.[11] The magnitude of this effect suggests that dietary restriction affects global and fundamental biologic processes underlying aging. In support of this, CR has been shown to delay the onset of age-related cardiac alterations and ameliorate virtually all known CVD risk factors both in experimental animals and humans.[12–14] This protection stems from a multitude of adaptations, such as blood pressure reduction, alterations of the lipoprotein profile, improved glucoregulation, reduction in sympathetic nervous system drive, and hormonal changes.[10]

CELLULAR MECHANISMS OF CARDIOPROTECTION BY CALORIE RESTRICTION

At the cellular level, cardioprotection by CR is mediated by various mechanisms, among which attenuation of oxidative stress, mitochondrial dysfunction and inflammation, and a favorable modulation of apoptosis and autophagy are prominent contributors (**Table 1**). The role that each of these adaptations plays in cardioprotection is discussed in this brief review.

Oxidative Stress and Mitochondrial Dysfunction

The free radical theory of aging, first proposed by Haman in the 1950s[15] and subsequently refined,[16–19] is currently the most widely accepted theory of aging. The main tenet of this theory is that the accumulation of oxidative damage to cellular constituents over the lifespan causes age-related tissue deterioration and ultimately disease conditions. Free radicals and other reactive species are continuously generated by numerous biologic processes, with mitochondrial respiration considered the main source. To protect itself against oxidative damage, the cell is equipped with enzymatic (eg, superoxide dismutase [SOD], glutathione peroxidase [GPx], catalase, thioredoxins) as well as nonenzymatic (eg, glutathione, vitamin E, vitamin C, β-carotene, uric acid) antioxidant defenses. Redox imbalance, resulting from increased oxidant generation and/or reduced antioxidant capacity, causes structural and functional cellular alterations, eventually leading to aging and disease.

Table 1
CR-induced cellular and molecular changes in aging and CVD

	Effects of CR	
	Aging	CVD
Oxidative stress		
Cardiac DNA damage	↓	—
Heart mitochondrial DNA damage	↓	—
Cardiac protein oxidation	↓	—
Heart mitochondrial protein oxidation	↓	—
Heart mitochondrial oxidant generation	↓	—
Heart antioxidant defenses	↑	↑
Cardiac nitrosative damage	↓	—
Cardiac lipid peroxidation	↓	↓
Endothelium mitochondrial oxidant generation	—	↓
Vascular oxidative damage	↓	↓
Endothelial NO availability	—	↑
Inflammation		
Myocardial TNF-α expression	—	↓
Myocardial IL-1β expression	—	↓
Systemic TNF-α levels	↓	↓
Systemic soluble TNF-α receptor 1 levels	↓	—
Systemic IL-6 levels	↓	↓
Systemic CRP levels	↓	—
Systemic CAM levels	↓	—
Vascular CAM expression	↓	—
Vascular TGF-β₁ levels	—	↓
Apoptosis		
Cardiomyocyte apoptosis	↓	↓
Heart mitochondrial apoptotic signaling	↓	—
Autophagy		
Cardiac autophagy	↑	—
Vascular autophagy	—	—

Abbreviations: CAM, cellular adhesion molecule; CR, calorie restriction; CRP, C-reactive protein; CVD, cardiovascular disease; IL, interleukin; NO, nitric oxide; TGF, transforming growth factor; TNF, tumor necrosis factor.
↑ = increase; ↓ = decrease; — = not investigated.

Analyses of heart tissues of old rodents[20–25] and humans[26] have shown evidence of elevated levels of oxidative damage to proteins, lipids, and DNA. Oxidative stress is involved in the pathogenesis of myocardial ischemia-reperfusion injury,[27] cardiac remodeling after myocardial infarction,[28] left ventricular hypertrophy (LVH), and HF.[29] Furthermore, oxidative damage plays a central role in endothelial dysfunction both during aging[30] and in the setting of CVD.[31]

Studies have shown that CR can prevent or even reverse the cardiovascular accrual of oxidative damage in a variety of experimental settings. Sohal and colleagues[21] found that cardiac DNA oxidative damage, as determined by 8-hydroxydeoxyguanosine content, was increased in old mice compared with younger controls. Of note, mice subjected to 40% CR displayed a significant reduction in DNA oxidation relative to AL-fed rodents. Similar findings were reported in rats kept on an alternate-day fasting regimen.[23] In addition, protein carbonyl content (a marker of protein oxidation) increased in the heart of AL-fed rats over the course of aging, which was attenuated by lifelong 40% food intake reduction.[20] Mitigation of protein oxidative damage was sustained by reduced mitochondrial generation of superoxide anion (O_2^-) and hydrogen peroxide (H_2O_2).[20] In addition, catalase activity was reduced during aging in AL-fed mice, whereas an opposite pattern was evident in CR animals. Furthermore, Leeuwenburgh and colleagues[22] demonstrated that lifelong 40% CR prevented the age-related accumulation of o-tyrosine and o,o'-dityrosine in the mouse heart. It has also been reported that 12-month 40% CR decreases mitochondrial H_2O_2 generation, free radical leak and oxidative damage to mitochondrial DNA (mtDNA) in the heart of aged rats.[32] A similar dietary regimen also counteracted the age-dependent increase in glycoxidative and lipoxidative damage to rat heart mitochondrial proteins.[33] A later study from the same group demonstrated that even 4-month 40% CR was sufficient to elicit a significant reduction in mitochondrial protein glycoxidation and lipoxidation in the heart of young rats.[34] The efficacy of short-term CR in attenuating heart oxidative stress was further demonstrated by Diniz and colleagues,[35] who reported decreased myocardial levels of lipoperoxidation in young rats subjected to 50% CR for 35 days. In addition, CR rats displayed increased activity of the antioxidant enzymes GPx and catalase relative to AL-fed controls. Finally, 40% CR for 3 months reduced cardiac mitochondrial H_2O_2 generation and protein carbonyl content in middle-aged rats.[36]

Although most studies have shown attenuation of cardiac oxidative damage or mitochondrial oxidant generation with CR, a few reports did not detect such adaptations.[37,38] This discrepancy may be ascribed to differences in the dietary regimens employed or species-specific differential susceptibility to CR. However, it should also be considered that the heart, similar to skeletal muscle, contains two bioenergetically[39] and structurally[40] distinct mitochondrial subpopulations: subsarcolemmal mitochondria (SSM), located beneath the sarcolemma, and intermyofibrillar mitochondria (IFM), arranged in parallel rows between the myofibrils. Of note, these two populations are differentially affected by aging and display different susceptibility to CR.[25] However, most studies have analyzed either SSM only or a mixed population of SSM and IFM. Our laboratory has recently investigated the effect of lifelong mild CR (ie, 8% calorie intake reduction), alone or in combination with voluntary wheel running, on mitochondrial H_2O_2 generation and markers of oxidative stress in cardiac SSM and IFM of old rats.[41] CR combined with exercise reduced H_2O_2 generation in both mitochondrial populations. In addition, activity of the mitochondrial SOD isoenzyme (MnSOD) was significantly decreased in SSM and IFM from wheel runners, likely as a result of reduced $O_2^{\bullet-}$ production. However, despite the attenuation of mitochondrial oxidant generation, levels of protein and lipid oxidative damage were not affected by either intervention. In another study, Kalani and colleagues,[42] employing an analogous experimental model, found increased plasma total antioxidant capacity in 8% CR rats either sedentary or exercised.

Besides cardiac aging, oxidative stress is also involved in the pathogenesis of several cardiovascular conditions. Mitochondria of the failing heart produce large amounts of reactive oxygen species (ROS).[43] Moreover, other sources of oxidants (eg, xanthine oxidase and nonphagocytic nicotinamide adenine dinucleotide phosphate [NADPH] oxidase) can contribute to the development of HF, cardiac remodeling, and LVH.[44–46] Furthermore, xanthine oxidase and NADPH oxidase-derived free radicals play a role in the pathogenesis of endothelial dysfunction via scavenging of nitric oxide (NO) by $O_2^{\bullet-}$.[47,48] Increased ROS generation and oxidative damage are also responsible for cardiac contractile dysfunction following ischemia-reperfusion.[27] Seymour and colleagues[49] demonstrated that 15% CR reduced cardiac lipid peroxidation in Dahl salt-sensitive rats fed a high-salt diet. Mitigation of oxidative stress ameliorated left ventricular remodeling, improved diastolic function and cardiac index, and delayed the onset of cardiac cachexia. It was also reported that lifelong 40% CR attenuated cardiac oxidative damage in middle-aged rats following myocardial ischemia-reperfusion.[50]

Regarding the effects of CR on endothelial function, short-term (ie, 3 months) 30% food restriction abolished the increases in mitochondrial ROS generation and NADPH-dependent $O_2^{\bullet-}$ production in the coronary endothelium and aortic wall of spontaneously diabetic rats.[51] Furthermore, CR prevented the decrease in total SOD activity in the thoracic aorta. These changes resulted in reduced levels of lipid peroxidation and increased NO availability. Moreover, CR combined with low-intensity physical activity reduced oxidative stress and improved acetylcholine-dependent vasodilatation in healthy, middle-aged obese subjects.[52]

In summary, although the magnitude of the antioxidant effect is influenced by several factors, including the degree of dietary restriction, the age at which CR is initiated, and the duration of the intervention, a wealth of evidence supports a protective effect of CR against oxidative stress in the cardiovascular system.

Inflammation

Chronic low-grade inflammation is acknowledged as a powerful, independent risk factor for CVD.[53] Moreover, chronic inflammation may be a converging process linking normal aging with age-related diseases.[54] According to this proposition, the age-dependent increase in oxidative stress activates redox-sensitive transcription factors (eg, nuclear factor-κB), which in turn enhance the expression of inflammatory cytokines, cellular adhesion molecules (CAMs), and proinflammatory enzymes.[54] Among the inflammatory biomarkers predictive of cardiovascular events, C-reactive protein (CRP), interleukin-6 (IL-6), and tumor necrosis factor-α (TNF-α) have been the most extensively investigated. In addition, myeloperoxidase (MPO) has recently emerged as a novel biomarker of inflammation and oxidative stress in CVD.[55] Of note, it has become clear that these molecules are not mere risk markers, but they indeed play an active role in the pathogenesis of CVD.[55–58] Besides cytokines, CAMs have also been identified as important mediators in the inflammatory process involved in atherosclerosis.[59] Notably, TNF-α and IL-1β are potent inducers of CAM expression.[60]

Convincing evidence indicates that CR attenuates the age-related increase in systemic inflammation. Old rodents kept on lifelong 40% CR displayed reduced levels of various inflammatory biomarkers, including TNF-α, IL-6, CRP and several CAMs.[42,61–63] Furthermore, Kalani and colleagues[42] found that lifelong 8% CR either alone or combined with voluntary wheel running prevented the increase in plasma CRP levels in old rats. In addition, CR attenuated the age-related increase in MPO activity in the rat kidney.[64] Mitigation of systemic inflammation by CR has also been reported in nonhuman primates.[65] Moreover, similar anti-inflammatory effects can be obtained with CR in human subjects,[14,66,67] even when dietary restriction is initiated late in life.[68]

Regarding the effects of CR on inflammation in the presence of CVD, lifelong 40% food intake reduction attenuated the myocardial inflammatory response to ischemia-reperfusion in rats.[50] Furthermore, 15% CR reduced the plasma levels of IL-6 and TNF-α in salt-sensitive rats fed a high-salt diet.[49] Three-month 30% CR also prevented the increase in transforming growth factor-β₁ (TGF-β₁) levels in the aorta of spontaneously diabetic rats.[51]

In summary, available evidence indicates that CR protects against elevation in systemic inflammation. Moreover, this effect may be obtained even with mild restrictions in food intake, which is likely to be more feasible for humans to maintain over the long term.

Apoptosis

Apoptosis is a highly conserved and tightly regulated process of programmed cell death, resulting in cellular self-destruction without the induction of inflammation or damage to the surrounding tissue. Apoptosis is essential for numerous biologic processes, including embryogenesis and development, cellular turnover, tissue homeostasis, and several immunologic functions.[69] However, it is postulated that accelerated elimination of irreplaceable postmitotic cells, such as cardiomyocytes, may contribute to age-associated loss of function and diseases.[70] Cardiomyocyte removal through apoptosis increases with advancing age.[71] It is hypothesized that enhanced cardiomyocyte apoptosis combined with insufficient replenishment by cardiac stem cells may play a central role in age-related heart remodeling.[72,73] Apart from aging, cardiomyocyte apoptosis occurs as a consequence of ischemia-reperfusion insult.[74] In addition, myocyte loss due to apoptosis is increased in patients with end-stage HF.[75] Elevated levels of cardiomyocyte apoptosis have also been detected in diabetic patients,[76] suggesting a role for programmed cell death in diabetic cardiomyopathy. Moreover, apoptosis of smooth muscle cells and macrophages within atherosclerotic plaques contributes to disease progression and plaque instability.[77]

Recent evidence indicates that CR mitigates age-related apoptosis in the heart. Analysis of high-density oligonucleotide microarrays revealed that 40% CR started at middle age reduced the expression of proapoptotic genes and upregulated antiapoptotic transcripts in aged mouse heart.[78] In addition, short-term mild CR may protect the aging myocardium from apoptosis by promoting a splicing shift of the apoptosis regulator Bcl-X, favoring the antiapoptotic variant Bcl-X$_L$.[79] A recent study from our laboratory has also shown that lifelong 40% CR counteracts the age-related increase in mitochondrial permeability transition pore (mPTP) opening susceptibility in rat cardiac IFM.[80] Opening of the mPTP is considered an important mechanism for the initiation of mitochondria-mediated apoptosis.[81] Six-month 35% CR reduced the extent of cardiac apoptotic DNA fragmentation in rats subjected to ischemia-reperfusion injury.[82] This effect translated into improved recovery of left ventricular function and limitation of infarct size.

These findings collectively indicate that CR attenuates age-associated cardiomyocyte apoptosis. The effectiveness of dietary restriction in mitigating cell death in CVD has not yet been thoroughly investigated. However, given the major role of inflammation[83] and oxidative stress[84] in both age- and disease-related apoptosis, it is conceivable that CR may also counteract cardiomyocyte loss associated with CVD progression.

Autophagy

Autophagy is an evolutionary conserved process that allows eukaryotic cells to degrade and recycle long-lived proteins and organelles.[85] Besides this housekeeping function, the autophagic program is also involved in regulating cell growth and the cellular response to starvation, hypoxia, and invading pathogens.[86] As a cellular quality control mechanism, autophagy is essential for degradation of defective intracellular components, thus preventing the accumulation of cellular "garbage" and its detrimental consequences.[19] Three types of autophagy have been described: macroautophagy, microautophagy, and chaperone-mediated autophagy.[87] Of note, macroautophagy is the only mechanism so far attributed to the degradation of dysfunctional and damaged mitochondria. During macroautophagy (subsequently referred to as autophagy), cells typically sequester portions of cytoplasm, which can include organelles, into double membrane-bound vacuoles (autophagosomes) that are then delivered to lysosomes for degradation.[88] Imperfect autophagy results in altered turnover of cellular constituents, including mitochondria. Furthermore, insufficient digestion of oxidatively damaged macromolecules and organelles leads to the accumulation of undegradable material (eg, lipofuscin) within the lysosomal compartment.[89] In turn, lipofuscin accumulation may act as a sink for lysosomal enzymes, further impairing the degradation of damaged mitochondria.[19]

The importance of autophagy for cardiomyocyte health and survival has been demonstrated in autophagy-deficient animals and cell models. For example, in adult mice, cardiac-specific, temporarily controlled deficiency of Atg5, a protein required for autophagy, led to cardiac hypertrophy, left ventricular dilatation, and contractile dysfunction, accompanied by increased levels of ubiquitination (a process targeting proteins for degradation).[90] In the same study, Atg7, a protein essential for autophagosome formation, was silenced in rat neonatal cardiomyocytes, resulting in reduction of cell viability as well as morphologic and biochemical features of cardiomyocyte hypertrophy.[90] Furthermore, lysosome-associated membrane protein 2 (LAMP2)-deficient mice showed excessive accumulation of autophagic vacuoles and impaired autophagic degradation of long-lived proteins, resulting in cardiomyopathy.[91] These findings collectively indicate that constitutive cardiomyocyte autophagy is required for protein quality control, and normal cellular structure and function under the basal state.

The role of autophagy in cardiac disease is still controversial. Increased numbers of autophagosomes have been observed in cardiac tissues of patients with cardiovascular disorders such as LVH,[92] aortic valve stenosis,[93] hibernating myocardium,[94] and HF.[95] However, it is unclear whether autophagy contributed to cell death in these conditions or was upregulated in an attempt to prevent it. On the other hand, Yan and colleagues[96] proposed that in chronically ischemic myocardium, autophagy might function cardioprotectively. This hypothesis was supported by a significant increase in the expression of autophagic proteins and the occurrence of autophagic vacuoles in viable but unlysed cells. In contrast, autophagic markers were downregulated in the infarcted myocardium. In addition, the autophagic degradation of damaged organelles, misfolded proteins and protein aggregates, and the importance of autophagy in nutrient supply and maintenance of energy homeostasis in times of limitation (eg, during ischemia) suggest a cardioprotective role.

Preservation of well-functioning autophagy may be particularly important during aging. In fact, the increase in oxidative damage and the concomitant increased frequency of misfolded and damaged proteins, protein aggregates, and damaged cell organelles impose a higher demand for functional autophagic cellular quality control in old age. However, it seems that the efficiency of autophagy decreases with age.[97–99] CR has been shown to attenuate the age-related decline of autophagy in the rat liver.[100] Although starvation has often been utilized to stimulate autophagy, there are limited data on the effect of lifelong CR on age-related changes in autophagy in the heart. The authors have recently reported that lifelong 40% CR increased the expression of autophagic markers in the heart from adult and old rats compared with AL controls.[101] Although further research is warranted, it is conceivable that upregulation of autophagy by CR may play a cardioprotective role by attenuating oxidative damage accrual during aging and CVD.

EVIDENCE FOR CARDIOPROTECTION BY CALORIE RESTRICTION IN HUMANS

Adaptations elicited by long-term CR in human subjects appear to resemble those observed in animal models. Inhabitants of Okinawa Island, whose traditional diet contains approximately 20% and 40% fewer calories compared with inland Japan and the United States, respectively, have the longest life expectancy and the greatest percentage of centenarians in the world. The extraordinary longevity and disability-free lifespan of Okinawans result from decreased incidence of conditions such as CVD, stroke, and cancer. Although Okinawan centenarians seem to possess a genetic "survival advantage,"[102] it is likely that a significant part of their longevity secret resides in their nutrient-rich, low-calorie diet.[103]

Apart from this case of naturally occurring CR, accumulating evidence indicates that dietary restriction results in significant improvements in traditional cardiovascular risk factors (eg, blood pressure, blood glucose, lipids, body composition) among overweight and obese subjects[104–109] as well as in lean individuals.[14,66,110] In contrast, the effect of CR on emerging CVD risk factors (eg, biomarkers of oxidative stress and inflammation) is less established. However, recent studies suggest that CR may have significant effects on these biologic processes as well. Lower levels of CRP, TNF-α, and TGF-β_1 have been detected in middle-aged healthy persons on long-term CR (ie, 3–15 years) compared with age- and gender-matched healthy controls consuming typical Western diets.[14,66] Diastolic heart function, as assessed by Doppler echocardiography, displayed a more youthful pattern in CR individuals relative to controls.[14] Furthermore, in a 6-month randomized controlled trial examining the effect of CR (25% of baseline energy requirements) on biomarkers of longevity and oxidative stress in healthy, nonobese adults, dietary restriction was found to reduce DNA damage in white blood cells (WBC),[111] improve whole body insulin sensitivity,[111] enhance skeletal muscle mitochondrial biogenesis,[112] and produce favorable changes in systemic inflammation, coagulation, lipid, and blood pressure.[113,114] In a recent study, 12-month CR (20% of baseline energy requirements) improved glucose tolerance and reduced DNA and RNA oxidative damage in WBC of healthy normal and overweight persons 50 to 60 years old.[115,116] Furthermore, Bosutti and colleagues[67] reported that 20% CR for 2 weeks prevented the increase in circulating levels of CRP and IL-6 in normal-weight, healthy men subjected to experimental bed rest. In addition, an 8-day very low calorie diet[117] (600 kcal/d) increased plasma levels of antioxidants and erythrocyte SOD activity, while decreasing levels of lipid peroxidation, in middle-aged obese subjects.

The biologic effects of CR in older persons have not yet been thoroughly investigated. However, in a large-scale trial conducted in obese, older adults (≥ 60 years, n = 316), 18-month diet-induced weight loss reduced markers of systemic inflammation (ie, CRP, IL-6, and soluble TNF-α receptor 1).[68] Weight loss induced by combining diet and exercise did not modify any of the inflammatory biomarkers to a greater extent than diet alone. However, the magnitude of weight loss was lower in the combined program, suggesting that the degree of weight loss or CR may be the key factor contributing to these changes.

In summary, based on studies conducted to date, moderate CR seems to be an effective means for reducing CVD risk in both younger and older persons, including normal-weight and overweight individuals. As observed in experimental animals, cardioprotection by CR in humans seems to be mediated by improvement in mitochondrial function, and reduction in systemic levels of oxidative stress and inflammation.

APPLICABILITY OF CALORIE RESTRICTION: CALORIE RESTRICTION MIMETICS AS AN ALTERNATIVE STRATEGY

Findings from the obesity literature indicate that most persons are reluctant to engage in long-term CR. In addition, many individuals are unable to sustain CR-induced weight loss, possibly due to internal feedback systems that signal the body to increase food intake or decrease energy expenditure in response to weight loss. Moreover, weight loss may not be advisable in older persons, as it can accelerate age-related muscle loss.[118] Of note, low body mass index has been associated with increased risk of disability and mortality in older populations.[119,120] Furthermore, people practicing long-term severe CR may experience several adverse events, including undesired changes in physical appearance, loss of strength and stamina, menstrual irregularities,

Table 2
Candidate primary CR mimetics listed in alphabetical order

Compound	CR Mimicking Properties
2-Deoxyglucose	Glycolytic inhibitor
4-Phenylbutyrate	Antioxidant
Acarbose	Glucose absorption inhibitor
3,5-Dimethylpyrazole	Insulin secretion inhibitor, autophagy enhancer
Adiponectin	IGF-1 signaling inhibitor
All-*trans* retinoic acid	IGF-1 signaling inhibitor
α-Lipoic acid	Antioxidant
α-Phenyl-*tert*-butyl nitrone	Anti-inflammatory, antioxidant
Aminoguanidine	Antiglycator
Brain-derived neurotrophic factor	Neuroprotector
Buformin	Gluconeogenesis inhibitor, insulin sensitizer
Butein	Sirtuin activator
Carnitine	Mitochondrial function preserver
Carnosine	Antiglycator
Coenzyme Q10	Antioxidant
Daidzein	IGF-1 signaling inhibitor, glucagon inhibitor
Fenretinide	IGF-1 signaling inhibitor
Fisetin	Sirtuin activator
Genistein	IGF-1 signaling inhibitor
Glyburide	Insulin sensitizer
Gymnemoside	Glucose absorption inhibitor
Iodoacetate	Glycolytic inhibitor
Kaempferol	IGF-1 signaling inhibitor, antioxidant
Metformin	Gluconeogenesis inhibitor, insulin sensitizer
ω-3 polyunsaturated fatty acids	Anti-inflammatory
Octreotide	IGF-1 signaling inhibitor
Phlorizin	Urinary glucose excretion promoter
Piceatannol	Sirtuin activator
Pioglitazone	PPAR-γ agonist and insulin sensitizer
Quercetin	IGF-1 signaling inhibitor, antioxidant
Rapamycin	IGF-1 signaling inhibitor
Resveratrol	Sirtuin activator, anti-inflammatory, antioxidant
Rosiglitazone	PPAR-γ agonist, insulin sensitizer
SC-ααδ9	IGF-1 signaling inhibitor
Tamoxifen	IGF-1 signaling inhibitor

IGF-1, insulin-like growth factor 1; PPAR-γ, peroxisome proliferator-activated receptor γ.

infertility, loss of libido, osteoporosis, cold sensitivity, slower wound healing, and psychological conditions such as food obsession, depression, and irritability.[10]

Thus, a critical research question is: what degree of CR is tolerable in humans to obtain beneficial physiologic changes without incurring adverse events? Animal studies have shown that even mild CR (ie, 8% calorie intake reduction) may elicit cardioprotective effects,[41,42] thus obviating the need for substantial food intake reductions. If findings from animal studies can be translated to humans, then the amount of CR required for cardioprotection may be more achievable than previously thought. Nevertheless, it will likely be decades before this issue is resolved.

Given the questionable feasibility of long-term dietary restriction, CR mimetics has become a topic of increasing scientific focus. As a general definition, CR mimetics are agents or interventions that are capable of reproducing the effects of CR without requiring food intake reduction.[121] Since the identification of the first agent (2-deoxy-D-glucose) by Lane and colleagues[122] in 1998, the list of putative CR mimetics has increasingly grown (**Table 2**). For many of these agents, however, there is little, if any, scientific evidence supporting their efficacy or safety.

Among CR mimetics, resveratrol has received the greatest attention. Resveratrol is a naturally occurring polyphenol found in red wine, the notorious cardioprotective effects of which are invoked to explain the so-called French paradox.[123] One salient feature of resveratrol resides in its ability to activate sirtuins, which in turn are prominent mediators of lifespan extension by CR.[124] In fact, resveratrol was found to extend the lifespan and delay the onset of aging phenotypes in short-lived organisms by modulating sirtuin signaling.[125–127] With respect to the cardiovascular system, resveratrol has been shown to inhibit cardiomyocyte apoptosis,[128] protect the myocardium against ischemia-reperfusion injury,[129] prevent LVH,[130] improve endothelial function,[131] inhibit platelet aggregation,[132] and reduce inflammation.[133] In a recent study, resveratrol improved survival and reduced the prevalence of cardiac pathology in mice fed a high-calorie diet.[134] Moreover, resveratrol-supplemented mice displayed better insulin sensitivity and enhanced liver mitochondrial biogenesis compared with animals fed either a standard or high-calorie diet. Of note, short-term supplementation with a nutraceutical mixture containing resveratrol induced a transcriptional shift in murine heart resembling that detected with long-term CR.[135] Lekakis and colleagues[136] reported that consumption of a red grape polyphenol extract containing resveratrol improved endothelial function in patients with coronary heart disease. Furthermore, 4-week supplementation with a lyophilized grape powder reduced blood lipids, plasma TNF-α, and urinary F(2)-isoprostane levels in both pre- and postmenopausal women.[137]

In summary, preclinical studies, as well as small clinical trials, seem to support a cardioprotective effect of resveratrol. Results from the numerous ongoing clinical trials testing this CR mimetic will likely provide insightful information concerning the efficacy and long-term safety of resveratrol supplementation in human populations.

SUMMARY

Despite the indisputable evidence supporting a wide range of beneficial effects of CR, excessive consumption of calorie-dense, nutrient-poor foods, combined with a sedentary lifestyle, has provoked an obesity epidemic in industrialized countries. Adoption of healthier eating habits is feasible by virtually anybody; however, most people are unwilling or unable to engage in substantial food intake restrictions, such as those employed in experimental settings. Furthermore, older persons may be especially prone to experience detrimental effects from dietary restriction if it is excessive or implemented too rapidly. Hence, the optimal level of CR, tailored to specific age groups, is currently unknown and needs to be explored in future studies. Mild CR regimens may provide a valid alternative, as they produce, at least in animal models, significant cardioprotective effects. An intriguing option is represented by CR mimetics, among which resveratrol has emerged as the leading candidate. Results from ongoing clinical trials will reveal whether resveratrol supplementation may provide an effective and safe strategy to improve cardiovascular health in human subjects. Until then, when indulging ourselves with a glass of wine, we can entertain the hope that it does not just warm our heart: it might actually protect it!

ACKNOWLEDGMENTS

The authors recognize that not all of the excellent scientific work in this area could be included or cited due to the vast literature on the subject and space limitations. The authors wish to thank Ms Hazel Lees for her assistance in the preparation of this article.

REFERENCES

1. Murray CJ, Lopez AD. Global mortality, disability, and the contribution of risk factors: Global Burden of Disease Study. Lancet 1997;349:1436–42.
2. Braunwald E. Shattuck lecture—cardiovascular medicine at the turn of the millennium: triumphs, concerns, and opportunities. N Engl J Med 1997;337: 1360–9.
3. Carbonin P, Zuccala G, Marzetti E, et al. Coronary risk factors in the elderly: their interactions and treatment. Curr Pharm Des 2003;9:2465–78.
4. Kannel WB. Cardiovascular risk factors in the elderly. Coron Artery Dis 1997;8: 565–75.
5. Chung HY, Cesari M, Anton S, et al. Molecular inflammation: underpinnings of aging and age-related diseases. Ageing Res Rev 2009;8:18–30.
6. McCullough PA, Philbin EF, Spertus JA, et al. Confirmation of a heart failure epidemic: findings from the Resource Utilization Among Congestive Heart Failure (REACH) study. J Am Coll Cardiol 2002;39:60–9.
7. Rich MW. Epidemiology, pathophysiology, and etiology of congestive heart failure in older adults. J Am Geriatr Soc 1997;45:968–74.
8. MacIntyre K, Capewell S, Stewart S, et al. Evidence of improving prognosis in heart failure: trends in case fatality in 66547 patients hospitalized between 1986 and 1995. Circulation 2000;102:1126–31.
9. Weindruch R, Walford RL. The retardation of aging and disease by dietary restriction. Springfield (IL): Charles C Thomas Publisher; 1988.
10. Dirks AJ, Leeuwenburgh C. Caloric restriction in humans: potential pitfalls and health concerns. Mech Ageing Dev 2006;127:1–7.
11. Weindruch R, Walford RL, Fligiel S, et al. The retardation of aging in mice by dietary restriction: longevity, cancer, immunity and lifetime energy intake. J Nutr 1986;116:641–54.
12. Kemi M, Keenan KP, McCoy C, et al. The relative protective effects of moderate dietary restriction versus dietary modification on spontaneous cardiomyopathy in male Sprague-Dawley rats. Toxicol Pathol 2000;28:285–96.
13. Fontana L, Meyer TE, Klein S, et al. Long-term calorie restriction is highly effective in reducing the risk for atherosclerosis in humans. Proc Natl Acad Sci U S A 2004;101:6659–63.

14. Meyer TE, Kovacs SJ, Ehsani AA, et al. Long-term caloric restriction ameliorates the decline in diastolic function in humans. J Am Coll Cardiol 2006;47:398–402.
15. Harman D. Aging: a theory based on free radical and radiation chemistry. J Gerontol 1956;11:298–300.
16. Harman D. The biologic clock: the mitochondria? J Am Geriatr Soc 1972;20: 145–7.
17. Yu BP, Yang R. Critical evaluation of the free radical theory of aging. A proposal for the oxidative stress hypothesis. Ann N Y Acad Sci 1996;786:1–11.
18. de Grey AD. A proposed refinement of the mitochondrial free radical theory of aging. Bioessays 1997;19:161–6.
19. Brunk UT, Terman A. The mitochondrial-lysosomal axis theory of aging: accumulation of damaged mitochondria as a result of imperfect autophagocytosis. Eur J Biochem 2002;269:1996–2002.
20. Sohal RS, Ku HH, Agarwal S, et al. Oxidative damage, mitochondrial oxidant generation and antioxidant defenses during aging and in response to food restriction in the mouse. Mech Ageing Dev 1994;74:121–33.
21. Sohal RS, Agarwal S, Candas M, et al. Effect of age and caloric restriction on DNA oxidative damage in different tissues of C57BL/6 mice. Mech Ageing Dev 1994;76:215–24.
22. Leeuwenburgh C, Wagner P, Holloszy JO, et al. Caloric restriction attenuates dityrosine cross-linking of cardiac and skeletal muscle proteins in aging mice. Arch Biochem Biophys 1997;346:74–80.
23. Kaneko T, Tahara S, Matsuo M. Retarding effect of dietary restriction on the accumulation of 8-hydroxy-2'-deoxyguanosine in organs of Fischer 344 rats during aging. Free Radic Biol Med 1997;23:76–81.
24. Barja G, Herrero A. Oxidative damage to mitochondrial DNA is inversely related to maximum life span in the heart and brain of mammals. FASEB J 2000;14:312–8.
25. Judge S, Jang YM, Smith A, et al. Age-associated increases in oxidative stress and antioxidant enzyme activities in cardiac interfibrillar mitochondria: implications for the mitochondrial theory of aging. FASEB J 2005;19:419–21.
26. Hayakawa M, Hattori K, Sugiyama S, et al. Age-associated oxygen damage and mutations in mitochondrial DNA in human hearts. Biochem Biophys Res Commun 1992;189:979–85.
27. Dhalla NS, Golfman L, Takeda S, et al. Evidence for the role of oxidative stress in acute ischemic heart disease: a brief review. Can J Cardiol 1999;15:587–93.
28. Grieve DJ, Byrne JA, Cave AC, et al. Role of oxidative stress in cardiac remodelling after myocardial infarction. Heart Lung Circ 2004;13:132–8.
29. Seddon M, Looi YH, Shah AM. Oxidative stress and redox signalling in cardiac hypertrophy and heart failure. Heart 2007;93:903–7.
30. Rodriguez-Manas L, El-Assar M, Vallejo S, et al. Endothelial dysfunction in aged humans is related with oxidative stress and vascular inflammation. Aging Cell 2009;8: 226–38.
31. Ogita H, Liao J. Endothelial function and oxidative stress. Endothelium 2004;11: 123–32.
32. Gredilla R, Sanz A, Lopez-Torres M, et al. Caloric restriction decreases mitochondrial free radical generation at complex I and lowers oxidative damage to mitochondrial DNA in the rat heart. FASEB J 2001;15:1589–91.
33. Pamplona R, Portero-Otin M, Bellmun MJ, et al. Aging increases Nepsilon-(carboxymethyl)lysine and caloric restriction decreases Nepsilon-(carboxyethyl) lysine and Nepsilon-(malondialdehyde)lysine in rat heart mitochondrial proteins. Free Radic Res 2002;36:47–54.

34. Pamplona R, Portero-Otin M, Requena J, et al. Oxidative, glycoxidative and lipoxidative damage to rat heart mitochondrial proteins is lower after 4 months of caloric restriction than in age-matched controls. Mech Ageing Dev 2002;123:1437–46.

35. Diniz YS, Cicogna AC, Padovani CR, et al. Dietary restriction and fibre supplementation: oxidative stress and metabolic shifting for cardiac health. Can J Physiol Pharmacol 2003;81:1042–8.

36. Colom B, Oliver J, Roca P, et al. Caloric restriction and gender modulate cardiac muscle mitochondrial H_2O_2 production and oxidative damage. Cardiovasc Res 2007;74:456–65.

37. Drew B, Phaneuf S, Dirks A, et al. Effects of aging and caloric restriction on mitochondrial energy production in gastrocnemius muscle and heart. Am J Physiol Regul Integr Comp Physiol 2003;284:R474–80.

38. Colotti C, Cavallini G, Vitale RL, et al. Effects of aging and anti-aging caloric restrictions on carbonyl and heat shock protein levels and expression. Biogerontology 2005;6:397–406.

39. Palmer JW, Tandler B, Hoppel CL. Biochemical properties of subsarcolemmal and interfibrillar mitochondria isolated from rat cardiac muscle. J Biol Chem 1977;252:8731–9.

40. Riva A, Tandler B, Lesnefsky EJ, et al. Structure of cristae in cardiac mitochondria of aged rat. Mech Ageing Dev 2006;127:917–21.

41. Judge S, Jang YM, Smith A, et al. Exercise by lifelong voluntary wheel running reduces subsarcolemmal and interfibrillar mitochondrial hydrogen peroxide production in the heart. Am J Physiol Regul Integr Comp Physiol 2005;289:R1564–72.

42. Kalani R, Judge S, Carter C, et al. Effects of caloric restriction and exercise on age-related, chronic inflammation assessed by C-reactive protein and interleukin-6. J Gerontol A Biol Sci Med Sci 2006;61:211–7.

43. Ide T, Tsutsui H, Kinugawa S, et al. Mitochondrial electron transport complex I is a potential source of oxygen free radicals in the failing myocardium. Circ Res 1999;85:357–63.

44. Li JM, Gall NP, Grieve DJ, et al. Activation of NADPH oxidase during progression of cardiac hypertrophy to failure. Hypertension 2002;40:477–84.

45. Minhas KM, Saraiva RM, Schuleri KH, et al. Xanthine oxidoreductase inhibition causes reverse remodeling in rats with dilated cardiomyopathy. Circ Res 2006;98:271–9.

46. Xu X, Hu X, Lu Z, et al. Xanthine oxidase inhibition with febuxostat attenuates systolic overload-induced left ventricular hypertrophy and dysfunction in mice. J Card Fail 2008;14:746–53.

47. Guthikonda S, Sinkey C, Barenz T, et al. Xanthine oxidase inhibition reverses endothelial dysfunction in heavy smokers. Circulation 2003;107:416–21.

48. Edirimanne VE, Woo CW, Siow YL, et al. Homocysteine stimulates NADPH oxidase-mediated superoxide production leading to endothelial dysfunction in rats. Can J Physiol Pharmacol 2007;85:1236–47.

49. Seymour EM, Parikh RV, Singer AA, et al. Moderate calorie restriction improves cardiac remodeling and diastolic dysfunction in the Dahl-SS rat. J Mol Cell Cardiol 2006;41:661–8.

50. Chandrasekar B, Nelson JF, Colston JT, et al. Calorie restriction attenuates inflammatory responses to myocardial ischemia-reperfusion injury. Am J Physiol Heart Circ Physiol 2001;280:H2094–102.

51. Minamiyama Y, Bito Y, Takemura S, et al. Calorie restriction improves cardiovascular risk factors via reduction of mitochondrial reactive oxygen species in type II diabetic rats. J Pharmacol Exp Ther 2007;320:535–43.

52. Sciacqua A, Candigliota M, Ceravolo R, et al. Weight loss in combination with physical activity improves endothelial dysfunction in human obesity. Diabetes Care 2003;26:1673–8.

53. Ross R. Atherosclerosis—an inflammatory disease. N Engl J Med 1999;340: 115–26.

54. Chung HY, Sung B, Jung KJ, et al. The molecular inflammatory process in aging. Antioxid Redox Signal 2006;8:572–81.

55. Sinning C, Schnabel R, Peacock WF, et al. Up-and-coming markers: myeloperoxidase, a novel biomarker test for heart failure and acute coronary syndrome application? Congest Heart Fail 2008;14:46–8.

56. Venugopal SK, Devaraj S, Yuhanna I, et al. Demonstration that C-reactive protein decreases eNOS expression and bioactivity in human aortic endothelial cells. Circulation 2002;106:1439–41.

57. Retter AS, Frishman WH. The role of tumor necrosis factor in cardiac disease. Heart Dis 2001;3:319–25.

58. Kanda T, Takahashi T. Interleukin-6 and cardiovascular diseases. Jpn Heart J 2004;45:183–93.

59. Blankenberg S, Barbaux S, Tiret L. Adhesion molecules and atherosclerosis. Atherosclerosis 2003;170:191–203.

60. Meager A. Cytokine regulation of cellular adhesion molecule expression in inflammation. Cytokine Growth Factor Rev 1999;10:27–39.

61. Zou Y, Jung KJ, Kim JW, et al. Alteration of soluble adhesion molecules during aging and their modulation by calorie restriction. FASEB J 2004;18: 320–2.

62. Phillips T, Leeuwenburgh C. Muscle fiber specific apoptosis and TNF-alpha signaling in sarcopenia are attenuated by life-long calorie restriction. FASEB J 2005;19:668–70.

63. You T, Sonntag WE, Leng X, et al. Lifelong caloric restriction and interleukin-6 secretion from adipose tissue: effects on physical performance decline in aged rats. J Gerontol A Biol Sci Med Sci 2007;62:1082–7.

64. Son TG, Zou Y, Yu BP, et al. Aging effect on myeloperoxidase in rat kidney and its modulation by calorie restriction. Free Radic Res 2005;39:283–9.

65. Lane MA, Reznick AZ, Tilmont EM, et al. Aging and food restriction alter some indices of bone metabolism in male rhesus monkeys (Macaca mulatta). J Nutr 1995;125:1600–10.

66. Fontana L, Klein S, Holloszy JO, et al. Effect of long-term calorie restriction with adequate protein and micronutrients on thyroid hormones. J Clin Endocrinol Metab 2006;91:3232–5.

67. Bosutti A, Malaponte G, Zanetti M, et al. Calorie restriction modulates inactivity-induced changes in the inflammatory markers C-reactive protein and pentraxin-3. J Clin Endocrinol Metab 2008;93:3226–9.

68. Nicklas BJ, Ambrosius W, Messier SP, et al. Diet-induced weight loss, exercise, and chronic inflammation in older, obese adults: a randomized controlled clinical trial. Am J Clin Nutr 2004;79:544–51.

69. Kerr JF, Wyllie AH, Currie AR. Apoptosis: a basic biological phenomenon with wide-ranging implications in tissue kinetics. Br J Cancer 1972;26:239–57.

70. Pollack M, Phaneuf S, Dirks A, et al. The role of apoptosis in the normal aging brain, skeletal muscle, and heart. Ann N Y Acad Sci 2002;959:93–107.

71. Centurione L, Antonucci A, Miscia S, et al. Age-related death-survival balance in myocardium: an immunohistochemical and biochemical study. Mech Ageing Dev 2002;123:341–50.

72. Kwak HB, Song W, Lawler JM. Exercise training attenuates age-induced elevation in Bax/Bcl-2 ratio, apoptosis, and remodeling in the rat heart. FASEB J 2006; 20:791–3.
73. Sussman MA, Anversa P. Myocardial aging and senescence: where have the stem cells gone? Annu Rev Physiol 2004;66:29–48.
74. Gottlieb RA, Burleson KO, Kloner RA, et al. Reperfusion injury induces apoptosis in rabbit cardiomyocytes. J Clin Invest 1994;94:1621–8.
75. Narula J, Haider N, Virmani R, et al. Apoptosis in myocytes in end-stage heart failure. N Engl J Med 1996;335:1182–9.
76. Frustaci A, Kajstura J, Chimenti C, et al. Myocardial cell death in human diabetes. Circ Res 2000;87:1123–32.
77. Kockx MM, De Meyer GR, Muhring J, et al. Apoptosis and related proteins in different stages of human atherosclerotic plaques. Circulation 1998;97: 2307–15.
78. Lee CK, Allison DB, Brand J, et al. Transcriptional profiles associated with aging and middle age-onset caloric restriction in mouse hearts. Proc Natl Acad Sci U S A 2002;99:14988–93.
79. Rohrbach S, Niemann B, Abushouk AM, et al. Caloric restriction and mitochondrial function in the ageing myocardium. Exp Gerontol 2006;41:525–31.
80. Hofer T, Servais S, Seo AY, et al. Bioenergetics and permeability transition pore opening in heart subsarcolemmal and interfibrillar mitochondria: Effects of aging and lifelong calorie restriction. Mech Ageing Dev 2009;130:297–307.
81. Crompton M. The mitochondrial permeability transition pore and its role in cell death. Biochem J 1999;341(Pt 2):233–49.
82. Shinmura K, Tamaki K, Bolli R. Impact of 6-mo caloric restriction on myocardial ischemic tolerance: possible involvement of nitric oxide-dependent increase in nuclear Sirt1. Am J Physiol Heart Circ Physiol 2008;295:H2348–55.
83. Pulkki KJ. Cytokines and cardiomyocyte death. Ann Med 1997;29:339–43.
84. Kumar D, Lou H, Singal PK. Oxidative stress and apoptosis in heart dysfunction. Herz 2002;27:662–8.
85. Levine B, Klionsky DJ. Development by self-digestion: molecular mechanisms and biological functions of autophagy. Dev Cell 2004;6:463–77.
86. Shintani T, Klionsky DJ. Autophagy in health and disease: a double-edged sword. Science 2004;306:990–5.
87. Cuervo AM. Autophagy: many paths to the same end. Mol Cell Biochem 2004; 263:55–72.
88. Wang CW, Klionsky DJ. The molecular mechanism of autophagy. Mol Med 2003; 9:65–76.
89. Terman A, Brunk UT. Oxidative stress, accumulation of biological 'garbage', and aging. Antioxid Redox Signal 2006;8:197–204.
90. Nakai A, Yamaguchi O, Takeda T, et al. The role of autophagy in cardiomyocytes in the basal state and in response to hemodynamic stress. Nat Med 2007;13: 619–24.
91. Tanaka Y, Guhde G, Suter A, et al. Accumulation of autophagic vacuoles and cardiomyopathy in LAMP-2-deficient mice. Nature 2000;406:902–6.
92. Yamamoto S, Sawada K, Shimomura H, et al. On the nature of cell death during remodeling of hypertrophied human myocardium. J Mol Cell Cardiol 2000;32: 161–75.
93. Hein S, Arnon E, Kostin S, et al. Progression from compensated hypertrophy to failure in the pressure-overloaded human heart: structural deterioration and compensatory mechanisms. Circulation 2003;107:984–91.

94. Elsasser A, Vogt AM, Nef H, et al. Human hibernating myocardium is jeopardized by apoptotic and autophagic cell death. J Am Coll Cardiol 2004;43:2191–9.
95. Kostin S, Pool L, Elsasser A, et al. Myocytes die by multiple mechanisms in failing human hearts. Circ Res 2003;92:715–24.
96. Yan L, Vatner DE, Kim SJ, et al. Autophagy in chronically ischemic myocardium. Proc Natl Acad Sci U S A 2005;102:13807–12.
97. Cuervo AM, Dice JF. When lysosomes get old. Exp Gerontol 2000;35:119–31.
98. Bergamini E, Cavallini G, Donati A, et al. The role of macroautophagy in the ageing process, anti-ageing intervention and age-associated diseases. Int J Biochem Cell Biol 2004;36:2392–404.
99. Terman A, Brunk UT. Autophagy in cardiac myocyte homeostasis, aging, and pathology. Cardiovasc Res 2005;68:355–65.
100. Donati A, Cavallini G, Paradiso C, et al. Age-related changes in the autophagic proteolysis of rat isolated liver cells: effects of antiaging dietary restrictions. J Gerontol A Biol Sci Med Sci 2001;56:B375–83.
101. Wohlgemuth SE, Julian D, Akin DE, et al. Autophagy in the heart and liver during normal aging and calorie restriction. Rejuvenation Res 2007;10:281–92.
102. Willcox BJ, Willcox DC, He Q, et al. Siblings of Okinawan centenarians share lifelong mortality advantages. J Gerontol A Biol Sci Med Sci 2006;61:345–54.
103. Kagawa Y. Impact of Westernization on the nutrition of Japanese: changes in physique, cancer, longevity and centenarians. Prev Med 1978;7:205–17.
104. Wing RR, Jeffery RW. Effect of modest weight loss on changes in cardiovascular risk factors: are there differences between men and women or between weight loss and maintenance? Int J Obes Relat Metab Disord 1995;19:67–73.
105. McTigue KM, Harris R, Hemphill B, et al. Screening and interventions for obesity in adults: summary of the evidence for the U.S. Preventive Services Task Force. Ann Intern Med 2003;139:933–49.
106. Racette SB, Weiss EP, Villareal DT, et al. One year of caloric restriction in humans: feasibility and effects on body composition and abdominal adipose tissue. J Gerontol A Biol Sci Med Sci 2006;61:943–50.
107. Fontana L, Villareal DT, Weiss EP, et al. Calorie restriction or exercise: effects on coronary heart disease risk factors. A randomized, controlled trial. Am J Physiol Endocrinol Metab 2007;293:E197–202.
108. Ashida T, Ono C, Sugiyama T. Effects of short-term hypocaloric diet on sympatho-vagal interaction assessed by spectral analysis of heart rate and blood pressure variability during stress tests in obese hypertensive patients. Hypertens Res 2007;30:1199–203.
109. Hammer S, Snel M, Lamb HJ, et al. Prolonged caloric restriction in obese patients with type 2 diabetes mellitus decreases myocardial triglyceride content and improves myocardial function. J Am Coll Cardiol 2008;52:1006–12.
110. Fontana L, Weiss EP, Villareal DT, et al. Long-term effects of calorie or protein restriction on serum IGF-1 and IGFBP-3 concentration in humans. Aging Cell 2008;7:681–7.
111. Heilbronn LK, de JL, Frisard MI, et al. Effect of 6-month calorie restriction on biomarkers of longevity, metabolic adaptation, and oxidative stress in overweight individuals: a randomized controlled trial. JAMA 2006;295:1539–48.
112. Civitarese AE, Carling S, Heilbronn LK, et al. Calorie restriction increases muscle mitochondrial biogenesis in healthy humans. PLoS Med 2007;4:e76.
113. Lefevre M, Redman LM, Heilbronn LK, et al. Caloric restriction alone and with exercise improves CVD risk in healthy non-obese individuals. Atherosclerosis 2009;203:206–13.

114. Larson-Meyer DE, Newcomer BR, Heilbronn LK, et al. Effect of 6-month calorie restriction and exercise on serum and liver lipids and markers of liver function. Obesity (Silver Spring) 2008;16:1355–62.
115. Weiss EP, Racette SB, Villareal DT, et al. Improvements in glucose tolerance and insulin action induced by increasing energy expenditure or decreasing energy intake: a randomized controlled trial. Am J Clin Nutr 2006;84: 1033–42.
116. Hofer T, Fontana L, Anton SD, et al. Long-term effects of caloric restriction or exercise on DNA and RNA oxidation levels in white blood cells and urine in humans. Rejuvenation Res 2008;11:793–9.
117. Skrha J, Kunesová M, Hilgertová J, et al. Short-term very low calorie diet reduces oxidative stress in obese type 2 diabetic patients. Physiol Res 2005; 54:33–9.
118. Miller SL, Wolfe RR. The danger of weight loss in the elderly. J Nutr Health Aging 2008;12:487–91.
119. Landi F, Zuccala G, Gambassi G, et al. Body mass index and mortality among older people living in the community. J Am Geriatr Soc 1999;47:1072–6.
120. Landi F, Onder G, Gambassi G, et al. Body mass index and mortality among hospitalized patients. Arch Intern Med 2000;160:2641–4.
121. Roth GS, Lane MA, Ingram DK. Caloric restriction mimetics: the next phase. Ann N Y Acad Sci 2005;1057:365–71.
122. Lane MA, Ingram DK, Roth DG. 2-Deoxy-D-glucose feeding in rats mimics physiological effects of calorie restriction. J Anti Aging Med 1998;1:327–37.
123. Kopp P. Resveratrol, a phytoestrogen found in red wine. A possible explanation for the conundrum of the 'French paradox'? Eur J Endocrinol 1998;138:619–20.
124. Guarente L, Picard F. Calorie restriction—the SIR2 connection. Cell 2005;120: 473–82.
125. Howitz KT, Bitterman KJ, Cohen HY, et al. Small molecule activators of sirtuins extend *Saccharomyces cerevisiae* lifespan. Nature 2003;425:191–6.
126. Viswanathan M, Kim SK, Berdichevsky A, et al. A role for SIR-2.1 regulation of ER stress response genes in determining *C. elegans* life span. Dev Cell 2005; 9:605–15.
127. Valenzano DR, Terzibasi E, Genade T, et al. Resveratrol prolongs lifespan and retards the onset of age-related markers in a short-lived vertebrate. Curr Biol 2006;16:296–300.
128. Seya K, Kanemaru K, Sugimoto C, et al. Opposite effects of two resveratrol (trans-3,5,4'-trihydroxystilbene) tetramers, vitisin A and hopeaphenol, on apoptosis of myocytes isolated from adult rat heart. J Pharmacol Exp Ther 2009;328:90–8.
129. Ray PS, Maulik G, Cordis GA, et al. The red wine antioxidant resveratrol protects isolated rat hearts from ischemia reperfusion injury. Free Radic Biol Med 1999; 27:160–9.
130. Juric D, Wojciechowski P, Das DK, et al. Prevention of concentric hypertrophy and diastolic impairment in aortic-banded rats treated with resveratrol. Am J Physiol Heart Circ Physiol 2007;292:H2138–43.
131. Chen CK, Pace-Asciak CR. Vasorelaxing activity of resveratrol and quercetin in isolated rat aorta. Gen Pharmacol 1996;27:363–6.
132. Bertelli AA, Giovannini L, Giannessi D, et al. Antiplatelet activity of synthetic and natural resveratrol in red wine. Int J Tissue React 1995;17:1–3.
133. Csiszar A, Labinskyy N, Podlutsky A, et al. Vasoprotective effects of resveratrol and SIRT1: attenuation of cigarette smoke-induced oxidative stress and

proinflammatory phenotypic alterations. Am J Physiol Heart Circ Physiol 2008; 294:H2721–35.

134. Baur JA, Pearson KJ, Price NL, et al. Resveratrol improves health and survival of mice on a high-calorie diet. Nature 2006;444:337–42.

135. Barger JL, Kayo T, Pugh TD, et al. Short-term consumption of a resveratrol-containing nutraceutical mixture mimics gene expression of long-term caloric restriction in mouse heart. Exp Gerontol 2008;43:859–66.

136. Lekakis J, Rallidis LS, Andreadou I, et al. Polyphenolic compounds from red grapes acutely improve endothelial function in patients with coronary heart disease. Eur J Cardiovasc Prev Rehabil 2005;12:596–600.

137. Zern TL, Wood RJ, Greene C, et al. Grape polyphenols exert a cardioprotective effect in pre- and postmenopausal women by lowering plasma lipids and reducing oxidative stress. J Nutr 2005;135:1911–7.

Effects of Caloric Restriction on Cardiovascular Aging in Non-human Primates and Humans

Christina Cruzen, DVM, Ricki J. Colman, PhD*

KEYWORDS

• Calorie restriction • Rhesus monkey • Cardiovascular disease
• Metabolic syndrome • Aging

Heart disease is the leading cause of death in the United States,[1] and has been for nearly a century,[2] while stroke is the number three cause of death.[3] Approximately 80 million, or one in three American adults have some form of cardiovascular disease (CVD). In 2004, one of every 2.8 deaths in the United States was attributable to CVD.[1] CVD claims more lives each year than cancer, chronic lower respiratory diseases, accidents, and diabetes mellitus combined.[4] As the population ages and the epidemic of obesity continues, the number of people living with heart disease also continues to rise, and an increasing number of younger individuals are being diagnosed with CVD.[5,6]

HEART DISEASE AND AGING

Due in large part to a 20-year increase in average life span during the second half of the 20th century, the median age of the world's population is increasing, and this trend is expected to continue worldwide, with the average life span rising another 10 years by 2050.[7] In the United States, the proportion of the population over 65 years of age is projected to increase from 12.4% in 2000 to 19.6% in 2030.[8] The number of persons over 65 years of age is expected to increase from approximately 35 million in 2000 to an estimated 71 million in 2030,[8] and the number of persons over 80 years of age is

This work was supported by grants P01 AG-11915 (National Institute on Aging) and P51 RR000167 (National Center for Research Resources [NCRR]). This research was conducted in part at a facility constructed with support from Research Facilities Improvement Program grant numbers RR15459-01 and RR020141-01 from NCRR.

Wisconsin National Primate Research Center, University of Wisconsin, Madison, 1220 Capitol Court, Madison, WI 53715, USA

* Corresponding author.

E-mail address: rcolman@primate.wisc.edu (R.J. Colman).

Clin Geriatr Med 25 (2009) 733–743

doi:10.1016/j.cger.2009.07.001

expected to increase from 9.3 million in 2000 to 19.5 million in 2030.[8] Because age is the major risk factor for CVD,[1] deaths caused by CVD are expected to increase substantially. In addition to the actual increase in prevalence of heart diseases with aging, several major risk factors for CVD (ie, blood lipids, blood pressure, hemostatic factors, inflammatory markers, and endothelial function) increase with age.[9] Given the substantial morbidity and mortality associated with CVD, in addition to its economic impact on the individual, the family, the nation, and the world, identification of interventions that can decrease the incidence or severity of CVD successfully would be expected to have a major impact on global health and related health care costs.

CARDIOVASCULAR DISEASE AND OBESITY

The link between obesity and CVD has been established clearly. Left ventricular hypertrophy, hypertension, diastolic dysfunction, poor cardiac contractility, and dyslipidemia are recognized cardiovascular complications of obesity.[10,11] In the past. it was believed that poor cardiovascular health in adults was a long-term effect of increased body mass. Recent studies, however, show that even obese children are developing signs of heart disease.[12,13] Currently, nearly 20% of US children are obese, and the percentage is even higher among certain minority groups (as high as 50% in some groups, ie, African Americans and Hispanics).[2,5,6,14] If the current trends continue, 45% of children in the United States will be obese within the next 10 years.[5] Unfortunately, 80% of these obese children will remain obese as adults.[15] This is due in part to the persistence of early-established lifestyle habits into adulthood, but also because of physiologic changes that make it more difficult to achieve and maintain an ideal body weight.[2,5,6] Early diagnosis and intervention for CVD prevention, therefore, has become a critical component of pediatric health.

As body mass increases, overall heart size increases because of increased cardiac workload.[16] In people, morbid obesity leads to concentric hypertrophy (ie, thickening of the walls with impingement of the chamber) and increased left ventricular mass, clearly established independent risk factors for CVD.[17,18] Although some hypertrophy of the left ventricle may be a normal physiologic response to increased body mass, the degree of hypertrophy that is considered normal is controversial.[16,19] Cardiac health is compromised when hypertrophy adversely affects cardiac function (diastolic dysfunction). Lean body mass appears to have a linear relationship with cardiac size.[20] The effects of fat mass, however, are less clear. In the past 20 years, body mass index (BMI) and waist circumference measurements have been used to categorize obesity and to assess CVD risk. Recent studies have found these methods to be unreliable and suggest that CVD is linked more closely to percent fat mass.[20–22] Additionally, the distribution of fat may play a role in its effect on cardiovascular risk.[23] Central fat appears to have a more detrimental effect on heart health than peripheral fat.[23] In monkeys, the effect of increased body fat on overall cardiac health is unknown, but obese and lean animals of the same weight would not be expected to have equivalent cardiac wall and chamber dimensions.

CARDIOVASCULAR DISEASE AND METABOLIC SYNDROME

Metabolic syndrome, an increasingly common human age-related disorder driven mainly by the rising prevalence of obesity,[24] originally was recognized in 1988 as a multiplex risk for CVD. It includes components of insulin resistance, hyperinsulinemia, glucose intolerance, increased triglycerides, decreased high-density lipoprotein (HDL) cholesterol, and hypertension.[25] More recent definitions include obesity, or specifically abdominal obesity, in the diagnostic criteria.[26–31] Although there is ongoing debate regarding the existence of and diagnostic criteria for metabolic syndrome,[32] it is known to be a clustering of risk factors associated with increased risk of cardiovascular morbidity and mortality. A recent meta-analysis has shown that metabolic syndrome almost doubles the risk of developing CVD, and that an excess risk for cardiovascular events and death remains even after adjusting for traditional cardiovascular risk factors in people with metabolic syndrome.[33]

Debate regarding the primary etiology of metabolic syndrome centers on theories starting with either insulin resistance or obesity.[34] It seems likely, however, that insulin resistance is a result of increasing adiposity, with inflammation being the key mediating factor.[35,36] Systemic inflammation can cause impaired insulin action, and it is associated strongly with adipose tissue deposition. Adipocytes and monocyte-derived macrophages resident in the expanded adipose depot lead to increased generation of proinflammatory cytokines.[37-39] It is unclear, however, if inflammation is the cause or a consequence in metabolic syndrome. Circulating markers of systemic inflammation such as C-reactive protein (CRP), tumor necrosis factor-α, and interleukin-6 clearly are associated with metabolic syndrome,[40-45] but there is also evidence that CRP levels can predict the development of metabolic syndrome in healthy people.[46,47] In addition, several components of the metabolic syndrome may lead to chronic low levels of inflammation. It is also possible that resistance to the anti-inflammatory actions of insulin contributes to the increased levels of inflammatory cytokines, thereby maintaining low-grade inflammation.[42] Furthermore, the increased morbidity and mortality associated with metabolic syndrome may in part be a consequence of exaggerated acute postprandial responses. For example, there is recent evidence that postprandial vascular dysfunction is more pronounced in individuals with metabolic syndrome.[48]

CALORIC RESTRICTION

Caloric restriction (CR) offers a powerful way to explore the aging process, because it is the only environmental or lifestyle intervention that has repeatedly and strongly been shown to increase maximum life span and retard aging in laboratory rodents.[49-52] The ability of CR to increase life span extends to fish, spiders, and other animals. Dogs on CR show an increased healthy life span and average life span.[53,54] In most rodent CR studies, mice or rats are fed 50% to 70% as many calories as controls, while avoiding deficiencies in essential nutrients. The beneficial actions of CR described here depend on chronic restriction of calorie intake without malnutrition.

Currently, most CR research can be divided into three general areas. First, studies are being conducted to understand the mechanism(s) by which CR is able to extend median and maximal lifespan. Most of this work is being undertaken in model organisms such as *Saccharomyces cerevisiae* (yeast), *Caenorhabditis elegans* (worms), *Drosophila melanogaster* (fruit flies), mice, and rats. Second, there are explorations underway to determine if the positive effects of CR that have been documented in rodents extend to primates, both nonhuman and human. Finally, efforts are underway to identify or develop potential CR mimetics that would allow the positive effects of CR to be realized without the need for dietary manipulation. The remainder of this article focuses mainly on studies in nonhuman primates, specifically rhesus monkeys, and people.

THE RHESUS MONKEY MODEL OF CALORIC RESTRICTION

The rhesus monkey (*Macaca mulatta*), an Old World primate of either Indian or Asian origin, is a commonly used and extensively characterized biomedical model. Because of their evolutionary proximity to people, data from this model are easily translatable to human medicine.[55–58] Similarities between rhesus monkeys and people extend to almost all aspects of anatomy, physiology, neurology, endocrinology, immunology, behavior, and aging processes.[59,60] Of particular importance, rhesus monkeys develop spontaneous obesity, metabolic syndrome, and CVD.[61–63] As in people, they form advanced atherosclerotic lesions, demonstrate plaque mineralization, and are subject to complications[64–66] including myocardial infarction.[65]

Two studies designed to test the long-term effects of CR in nonhuman primates are ongoing, one at the National Institute on Aging (NIA)[67,68] and at the Wisconsin National Primate Research Center (WNPRC).[69,70] Both trials have shown that long-term CR can be carried out safely and is associated with indications of improved health. Additional support for the beneficial effects of CR in nonhuman primates derives from a long-term study at the University of Maryland that focuses specifically on obesity and diabetes,[71] and from a 4-year study in cynomolgus macaques (Macaca fascicularis) designed to evaluate the effects of CR on the development of atherosclerosis.[72] Among the many improvements in health, monkeys on long-term, moderate CR show improvements in many factors related to the metabolic syndrome, including decreased body weight and fat mass, and improved glucoregulatory function and lipid profile compared with ad libitum fed controls (**Table 1**).

It is not surprising that nonhuman primates on long-term CR have lower body weight when compared with ad libitum fed animals. By design, animals assigned to the CR group in the NIA and WNPRC studies receive approximately 70% of their ad libitum food allotment.[67,69] Correspondingly, the CR animals weigh approximately 30% less than their age- and sex-matched control counterparts. It is also not surprising that most of this weight difference is accounted for by a decrease in fat mass. As fat distribution is known to play a role in relative risk for CVD, it is important to note that CR animals had reductions not only in total body fat, but also in fat located specifically in the abdominal region as measured by dual-energy x-ray absorptiometry (DXA),[73] and in the abdomen and intra-abdominal compartment as measured by computed tomogrpahy.[74]

Glucoregulatory function is impaired by advancing age and obesity. With the aging of the human population and the growing obesity epidemic, diabetes has become an international health concern. Notably, the benefits of CR on glucoregulatory function are among the most consistent findings in the nonhuman primate studies. Specifically,

Table 1
Effects of caloric restriction on factors of the metabolic syndrome in nonhuman primates and people

Measurement	Nonhuman Primates	People
Body weight	↓ 69,70,73,74,81,99,100	↓ 92–94
Body fat	↓ 69,73,74,81,99–101	↓ 92–94
Basal glucose/insulin	↓ 75–78	↓ 90–92,95,96
Insulin sensitivity	↑ 74–78,81	↑ 90,91
Blood pressure	↓ 68,82	↓ 89,92,102
Triglycerides	↓ 83,85,103	↓ 95,98
HDL cholesterol	↑ 84,85,103	↑ 95,98

↑ Indicates an increase in the measured parameter with CR.
↓ Indicates a decrease in the measured parameter with CR.
Abbreviations: CR, caloric restriction; HDL, high-density lipoprotein.

both short- and long-term CR potently lowers fasting insulin and improves fasting glucose and glycosylated hemoglobin measures.[70,75–78] Furthermore, insulin sensitivity, as measured by the minimal model assessment or the hyperinsulinemic euglycemic clamp method, consistently is increased by CR.[70,75–81]

Aging and obesity also are associated with a rise in systolic blood pressure, another well-recognized risk factor for CVD. There is evidence that 3 years of CR lowers blood pressure in female rhesus monkeys.[82] With regard to lipids, both the NIA and WNPRC studies have shown that CR favorably alters lipid profiles.[83–85] In particular, triglyceride levels were significantly lower in CR animals compared with controls. In addition, adult CR animals had increased levels of HDL2b, the HDL fraction associated with cardioprotection. Furthermore, CR induced compositional changes in low-density lipoprotein (LDL) cholesterol particles that reduced their participation in a potentially atherogenic interaction. LDL particles from CR animals were lower in molecular weight and were depleted in triglycerides and phospholipids. In addition, LDL binding with arterial proteoglycan was reduced.

CR IN PEOPLE

The efficacy of CR in nonhuman primates[86] suggests that CR might be beneficial in people also. Epidemiological data additionally suggest an inverse relationship between caloric intake and aging in people.[51,87,88] Further evidence in support of benefits from moderate CR in people derives from an unplanned observation from the Biosphere 2 experiment. In this project, eight individuals, four men and four women, lived in a completely enclosed environment that was meant to contain all necessary supplies. Unfortunately, food supplies ran short, and the individuals in the Biosphere effectively were subjected to a 2-year period of moderate CR. As in the nonhuman primate studies, participants lost weight and fat mass, and these changes were accompanied by improvements in basal glucose, basal insulin, insulin sensitivity, and blood pressure (**Table 1**).[89–91]

More recently, a controlled trial in people was initiated to study the effects of CR in healthy adults. Sponsored by the NIA, CALERIE (Comprehensive Assessment of the Long-term Effect of Reducing Intake of Energy) is a multicenter (Washington University in St. Louis, MO, Tufts University in Boston, MA, and the Pennington Biomedical Research Center in Baton Rouge, LA) study of moderate (25%) CR in approximately 150 nonobese healthy men and women between the ages of 25 and 45 years. Data from independent phase 1 trials performed at each site prior to the multicenter trial indicate that CR in people results in some of the same changes described in the nonhuman primate studies and in the Biosphere 2 experiment. Specifically, CR led to decreased body weight and fat mass,[92–94] decreased basal insulin and glucose levels,[92,95,96] increased insulin sensitivity,[97] decreased blood pressure,[92] decreased triglycerides,[92,95,98] and increased HDL levels (**Table 1**).[92,98]

Because of the myriad factors that affect life span in people, the ability of CR to extend median and maximal lifespan in people may never be known. Nonetheless, evidence from animal models and recent human experiments suggests that CR may be able to extend the healthy period of life, regardless of its ability to ultimately extend lifespan.

SUMMARY

CVD is a major public health concern in the United States, affecting approximately one in three adults and accounting for one of every 2.8 deaths. With the aging of the population and the increasing obesity epidemic, incidence and prevalence rates of CVD will continue to increase. CR is the only intervention shown to increase maximum life-span and retard aging in laboratory rodents and nonhuman primates. There is also strong evidence that CR improves several components of the metabolic syndrome in nonhuman primates, thereby reducing the risk of CVD and related complications. Recent data from human studies indicate that CR is likely to have similar positive effects in people.

ACKNOWLEDGMENTS

The authors gratefully acknowledge the excellent technical assistance provided by S. Baum, J. Christensen, J. A. Adriansjach, C. E. Armstrong, and the Animal Care, Veterinary, and Pathology Staff of the WNPRC.

REFERENCES

1. Rosamond W, Flegal K, Friday G, et al. Heart disease and stroke statistics—2007 update: a report from the American Heart Association Statistics Committee and Stroke Statistics Subcommittee. Circulation 2007;115:e69–e171.
2. Odgen CL, Carroll MD, Curtin LR, et al. Prevalence of overweight and obesity in the United States, 1999–2004. JAMA 2006;295:1549–55.
3. Rosamond W, Flegal K, Furie K, et al. Heart disease and stroke statistics—2008 update: a report from the American Heart Association Statistics Committee and Stroke Statistics Subcommittee. Circulation 2008;117:e25–e146.
4. Minino AM, Heron MP, Smith BL. Deaths: preliminary data for 2004. Natl Vital Stat Rep 2006;54:1–49.
5. Ludwig DS. Childhood obesity—the shape of things to come. N Engl J Med 2007;357:2325–7.
6. von Haehling S, Doehner W, Anker SD. Obesity and the heart: a weighty issue. J Am Coll Cardiol 2006;47:2274–6.
7. United Nations. Report of the second world assembly on aging. Madrid (Spain): United Nations; 2002.
8. US Census Bureau. International database. Table 094. Midyear population, by age and sex. Available at: http://www.census.gov/population/www/projections/natdet-D1A.html. Accessed June 24, 2009.
9. Chobanian AV, Bakris GL, Black HR, et al. The Seventh Report of the Joint National Committee on Prevention, Detection, Evaluation, and Treatment of High Blood Pressure: the JNC 7 report. JAMA 2003;289:2560–72.
10. Daniels SR. Obesity in the pediatric patient: cardiovascular complications. Prog Pediatr Cardiol 2001;12:161–7.
11. Rabbia F, Silke B, Conterno A, et al. Assessment of cardiac autonomic modulation during adolescent obesity. Obes Res 2003;11:541–8.
12. Gidding SS. Clinical and epidemiological significance of left ventricular mass assessed in children and adolescents. Circulation 1998;97:1893–4.
13. Lorch SM, Sharkey A. Myocardial velocity, strain, and strain rate abnormalities in healthy obese children. J Cardiometab Syndr 2007;2:30–4.
14. Barrett J. The price of childhood obesity: why the costs could catastrophic if we don't stop the epidemic now. Newsweek. Accessed December 5, 2007.
15. Schonfeld-Warden N, Warden C. Pediatric obesity: an overview of etiology and treatment. Pediatr Clin North Am 1997;44:339–61.
16. Chinalli M, De Simone G, Roman M, et al. Impact of obesity on cardiac geometry and function in a population of adolescents: the strong heart study. J Am Col Cardiol 2006;47:2267–76 [commentary].

17. Friberg P, Allansdotter-Johnsson A, Ambring A, et al. Increased left ventricular mass in obese adolescents. Eur Heart J 2004;25:987–92.
18. Shub C, Klein AL, Zachariah PK, et al. Determination of left ventricular mass by echocardiography in a normal population: effect of age and sex in addition to body size. Mayo Clin Proc 1994;69:205–11.
19. Foppa M, Duncan BB, Rohde LE. Echocardiography-based left ventricular mass estimation. How should we define hypertrophy? Cardiovasc Ultrasound 2005;3:17.
20. Bosy-Westphal A, Geisler C, Onur S, et al. Value of body fat mass vs anthropometric obesity indices in the assessment of metabolic risk factors. Int J Obes (Lond) 2006;30:475–83.
21. Iacobellis G, Sharma AM. Obesity and the heart: redefinition of the relationship. Obes Rev 2007;8:35–9.
22. Wong C, Moore-Sullivan T, Leano R, et al. Alterations of left ventricular myocardial characteristics associated with obesity. Circulation 2004;110:3081–7.
23. Ferreira I, Snijder MB, Twisk JW, et al. Central fat mass versus peripheral fat and lean mass: opposite (adverse versus favorable) associations with arterial stiffness? The Amsterdam Growth and Health Longitudinal Study. J Clin Endocrinol Metab 2004;89:2632–9.
24. Eckel RH, Grundy SM, Zimmet PZ. The metabolic syndrome. Lancet 2005;365:1415–28.
25. Reaven GM. Banting lecture 1988. Role of insulin resistance in human disease; 1988. Nutrition 1997;13:65 [discussion: 64, 66].
26. The IDF consensus worldwide definition of the metabolic syndrome. Available at: http://www.idf.org/webdata/docs/MetS_def_update2006.pdf. Accessed June 24, 2009.
27. Alberti KG, Zimmet PZ. Definition, diagnosis, and classification of diabetes mellitus and its complications. Part 1: diagnosis and classification of diabetes mellitus, provisional report of a WHO consultation. Diabet Med 1998;15:539–53.
28. Balkau B, Charles MA. Comment on the provisional report from the WHO consultation. European Group for the Study of Insulin Resistance (EGIR). Diabet Med 1999;16:442–3.
29. Einhorn D, Reaven GM, Cobin RH, et al. American College of Endocrinology position statement on the insulin resistance syndrome. Endocr Pract 2003;9:237–52.
30. Grundy SM, Brewer HB Jr, Cleeman JI, et al. Definition of metabolic syndrome: report of the National Heart, Lung, and Blood Institute/American Heart Association conference on scientific issues related to definition. Arterioscler Thromb Vasc Biol 2004;24:e13–8.
31. Grundy SM, Cleeman JI, Daniels SR, et al. Diagnosis and management of the metabolic syndrome: an American Heart Association/National Heart, Lung, and Blood Institute Scientific Statement. Circulation 2005;112:2735–52.
32. Day C. Metabolic syndrome, or what you will: definitions and epidemiology. Diab Vasc Dis Res 2007;4:32–8.
33. Gami AS, Witt BJ, Howard DE, et al. Metabolic syndrome and risk of incident cardiovascular events and death: a systematic review and meta-analysis of longitudinal studies. J Am Coll Cardiol 2007;49:403–14.
34. Penno G, Miccoli R, Pucci L, et al. The metabolic syndrome: beyond the insulin resistance syndrome. Pharmacol Res 2006;53:457–68.
35. Sutherland JP, McKinley B, Eckel RH. The metabolic syndrome and inflammation. Metab Syndr Relat Disord 2004;2:82–104.

36. Tataranni PA, Ortega E. A burning question: does an adipokine-induced activation of the immune system mediate the effect of overnutrition on type 2 diabetes? Diabetes 2005;54:917–27.
37. Di Gregorio GB, Yao-Borengasser A, Rasouli N, et al. Expression of CD68 and macrophage chemoattractant protein-1 genes in human adipose and muscle tissues: association with cytokine expression, insulin resistance, and reduction by pioglitazone. Diabetes 2005;54:2305–13.
38. Weisberg SP, McCann D, Desai M, et al. Obesity is associated with macrophage accumulation in adipose tissue. J Clin Invest 2003;112:1796–808.
39. Xu H, Barnes GT, Yang Q, et al. Chronic inflammation in fat plays a crucial role in the development of obesity-related insulin resistance. J Clin Invest 2003;112: 1821–30.
40. Chapidze G, Dolidze N, Enquobahrie DA, et al. Metabolic syndrome and C-reactive protein among cardiology patients. Arch Med Res 2007;38:783–8.
41. Festa A, D'Agostino R Jr, Howard G, et al. Chronic subclinical inflammation as part of the insulin resistance syndrome: the Insulin Resistance Atherosclerosis Study (IRAS). Circulation 2000;102:42–7.
42. Gustafson B, Hammarstedt A, Andersson CX, et al. Inflamed adipose tissue: a culprit underlying the metabolic syndrome and atherosclerosis. Arterioscler Thromb Vasc Biol 2007;27:2276–83.
43. Ridker PM, Buring JE, Cook NR, et al. C-reactive protein, the metabolic syndrome, and risk of incident cardiovascular events: an 8-year follow-up of 14,719 initially healthy American women. Circulation 2003;107:391–7.
44. Rutter MK, Meigs JB, Sullivan LM, et al. C-reactive protein, the metabolic syndrome, and prediction of cardiovascular events in the Framingham Offspring Study. Circulation 2004;110:380–5.
45. Ye X, Yu Z, Li H, et al. Distributions of C-reactive protein and its association with metabolic syndrome in middle-aged and older Chinese people. J Am Coll Cardiol 2007;49:1798–805.
46. Han TS, Sattar N, Williams K, et al. Prospective study of C-reactive protein in relation to the development of diabetes and metabolic syndrome in the Mexico City Diabetes Study. Diabet Care 2002;25:2016–21.
47. Laaksonen DE, Niskanen L, Nyyssonen K, et al. C-reactive protein and the development of the metabolic syndrome and diabetes in middle-aged men. Diabetologia 2004;47:1403–10.
48. Esposito K, Ciotola M, Sasso FC, et al. Effect of a single high-fat meal on endothelial function in patients with the metabolic syndrome: role of tumor necrosis factor-alpha. Nutr Metab Cardiovasc Dis 2007;17:274–9.
49. Masoro EJ. Dietary restriction: current status. Aging 2001;13:261–2.
50. Masoro EJ. Overview of caloric restriction and ageing. Mech Ageing Dev 2005; 126:913–22.
51. Weindruch R, Walford RL. The retardation of aging and disease by dietary restriction. Springfield (IL): Charles C. Thomas; 1988.
52. Yu BP. How diet influences the aging process of the rat. Proc Soc Exp Biol Med 2004;205:97–105.
53. Kealy RD, Lawler DF, Ballam JM, et al. Effects of diet restriction on life span and age-related changes in dogs. J Am Vet Med Assoc 2002;220:1315–20.
54. Lawler DF, Larson BT, Ballam JM, et al. Diet restriction and ageing in the dog: major observations over two decades. Br J Nutr 2008;99:793–805.
55. Bontrop RE. Nonhuman primates: essential partners in biomedical research. Immunol Rev 2001;183:5–9.

56. King FA, Yarbrough CJ, Anderson DC, et al. Primates. Science 1988;240: 1475–82.

57. Sibley CG, Ahlquist JE. DNA hybridization evidence of hominoid phylogeny: results from an expanded data set. J Mol Evol 1987;26:99–121.

58. Sibley CG, Comstock JA, Ahlquist JE. DNA hybridization evidence of hominoid phylogeny: a reanalysis of the data. J Mol Evol 1990;30:202–36.

59. Colman RJ, Binkley N. Skeletal aging in macaque monkeys. In: Erwin JM, Hof PR, editors, Aging in nonhuman primates. Interdisciplinary topics in gerontology. Basel (Switzerland): Karger; 2002. p. 32–47.

60. Colman RJ, Kemnitz JW. Aging experiments in nonhuman primates. In: Yu BP, editor. Methods in aging research. Boca Raton (FL): CRC Press; 1998. p. 249–67.

61. Bodkin NL, Pill J, Meyer K, et al. The effects of K-111, a new insulin-sensitizer, on metabolic syndrome in obese prediabetic rhesus monkeys. Horm Metab Res 2003;35:617–24.

62. Hannah JS, Verdery RB, Bodkin NL, et al. Changes in lipoprotein concentrations during the development of noninsulin-dependent diabetes mellitus in obese rhesus monkeys (Macaca mulatta). J Clin Endocrinol Metab 1991;72: 1067–72.

63. Hansen BC, Bodkin NL. Heterogeneity of insulin responses: phases leading to type 2 (noninsulin-dependent) diabetes mellitus in the rhesus monkey. Diabetologia 1986;29:713–9.

64. Hamm TE Jr, Kaplan JR, Clarkson TB, et al. Effects of gender and social behavior on the development of coronary artery atherosclerosis in cynomolgus macaques. Atherosclerosis 1983;48:221–33.

65. Pick R, Johnson PJ, Glick G. Deleterious effects of hypertension on the development of aortic and coronary atherosclerosis in stumptail macaques (Macaca speciosa) on an atherogenic diet. Circ Res 1974;35:472–82.

66. Taylor CB, Cox GE, Manalo-Estrella P, et al. Atherosclerosis in rhesus monkeys. II. Arterial lesions associated with hypercholesteremia induced by dietary fat and cholesterol. Arch Pathol 1962;74:16–34.

67. Lane MA, Black A, Handy A, et al. Caloric restriction in primates. Ann N Y Acad Sci 2001;928:287–95.

68. Mattison JA, Roth GS, Lane MA, et al. Dietary restriction in aging nonhuman primates. Interdiscip Top Gerontol 2007;35:137–58.

69. Kemnitz JW, Weindruch R, Roecker EB, et al. Dietary restriction of adult male rhesus monkeys: design, methodology, and preliminary findings from the first year of study. J Gerontol 1993;48:B17–26.

70. Ramsey JJ, Colman RJ, Binkley NC, et al. Dietary restriction and aging in rhesus monkeys: the University of Wisconsin study. Exp Gerontol 2000;35:1131–49.

71. Bodkin NL, Alexander TM, Ortmeyer HK, et al. Mortality and morbidity in laboratory-maintained rhesus monkeys and effects of long-term dietary restriction. J Gerontol 2003;58:212–9.

72. Cefalu WT, Wagner JD, Wang ZQ, et al. A study of caloric restriction and cardiovascular aging in cynomolgus monkeys (Macaca fascicularis): a potential model for aging research. J Gerontol A Biol Sci Med Sci 1997;52:B10–9.

73. Colman RJ, Ramsey JJ, Roecker EB, et al. Body fat distribution with long-term dietary restriction in adult male rhesus macaques. J Gerontol Biol Sci 1999; 54A:B283–90.

74. Cefalu WT, Wang ZQ, Bell-Farrow AD, et al. Caloric restriction and cardiovascular aging in cynomolgus monkeys (Macaca fascicularis): metabolic,

physiologic, and atherosclerotic measures from a 4-year intervention trial. J Gerontol A Biol Sci Med Sci 2004;59:1007–14.

75. Gresl TA, Colman RJ, Havighurst TC, et al. Dietary restriction and beta-cell sensitivity to glucose in adult male rhesus monkeys. J Gerontol A Biol Sci Med Sci 2003;58:598–610.

76. Gresl TA, Colman RJ, Roecker EB, et al. Dietary restriction and glucose regulation in aging rhesus monkeys: a follow-up report at 8.5 yr. Am J Physiol Endocrinol Metab 2001;281:E757–65.

77. Kemnitz JW, Roecker EB, Weindruch R, et al. Dietary restriction increases insulin sensitivity and lowers blood glucose in rhesus monkeys. Am J Physiol 1994;266: E540–7.

78. Lane MA, Ball SS, Ingram DK, et al. Diet restriction in rhesus monkeys lowers fasting and glucose-stimulated glucoregulatory end points. Am J Physiol 1995;268:E941–8.

79. Bodkin NL, Ortmeyer HK, Hansen BC. Long-term dietary restriction in older-aged rhesus monkeys: effects on insulin resistance. J Gerontol A Biol Sci Med Sci 1995;50:B142–7.

80. Cefalu WT, Wagner JD, Bell-Farrow AD, et al. Influence of caloric restriction on the development of atherosclerosis in nonhuman primates: progress to date. Toxicol Sci 1999;52:49–55.

81. Hansen BC, Bodkin NL. Primary prevention of diabetes mellitus by prevention of obesity in monkeys. Diabetes 1993;42:1809–14.

82. Lane MA, Black A, Ingram DK, et al. Calorie restriction in nonhuman primates: implications for age-related disease risk. J Antiaging Med 1998;1: 315–26.

83. Edwards IJ, Rudel LL, Terry JG, et al. Caloric restriction in rhesus monkeys reduces low-density lipoprotein interaction with arterial proteoglycans. J Gerontol A Biol Sci Med Sci 1998;53:B443–8.

84. Edwards IJ, Rudel LL, Terry JG, et al. Caloric restriction lowers plasma lipoprotein (a) in male but not female rhesus monkeys. Exp Gerontol 2001;36: 1413–8.

85. Verdery RB, Ingram DK, Roth GS, et al. Caloric restriction increases HDL2 levels in rhesus monkeys (Macaca mulatta). Am J Physiol 1997;273:E714–9.

86. Colman RJ, Anderson RM, Johnson SC, et al. Caloric restriction delays disease onset and mortality in rhesus monkeys. Science 2009;325:201–4.

87. Lee IM, Blair SN, Allison DB, et al. Epidemiologic data on the relationships of caloric intake, energy balance, and weight gain over the life span with longevity and morbidity. J Gerontol 2001;56:7–19.

88. Weindruch R, Sohal RS. Seminars in medicine of the Beth Israel Deaconess Medical Center. Caloric intake and aging. N Engl J Med 1997;337:986–94.

89. Walford RL, Harris SB, Gunion MW. The calorically restricted low-fat nutrient-dense diet in Biosphere 2 significantly lowers blood glucose, total leukocyte count, cholesterol, and blood pressure in humans. Proc Natl Acad Sci U S A 1992;89:11533–7.

90. Walford RL, Mock D, MacCallum T, et al. Physiologic changes in humans subjected to severe, selective calorie restriction for two years in Biosphere 2: health, aging, and toxicological perspectives. Toxicol Sci 1999;52:61–5.

91. Walford RL, Mock D, Verdery R, et al. Calorie restriction in biosphere 2: alterations in physiologic, hematologic, hormonal, and biochemical parameters in humans restricted for a 2-year period. J Gerontol A Biol Sci Med Sci 2002;57: B211–24.

92. Fontana L, Meyer TE, Klein S, et al. Long-term calorie restriction is highly effective in reducing the risk for atherosclerosis in humans. Proc Natl Acad Sci U S A 2004;101:6659–63.

93. Racette SB, Weiss EP, Villareal DT, et al. One year of caloric restriction in humans: feasibility and effects on body composition and abdominal adipose tissue. J Gerontol A Biol Sci Med Sci 2006;61:943–50.

94. Redman LM, Heilbronn LK, Martin CK, et al. Effect of calorie restriction with or without exercise on body composition and fat distribution. J Clin Endocrinol Metab 2007;92:865–72.

95. Fontana L, Villareal DT, Weiss EP, et al. Calorie restriction or exercise: effects on coronary heart disease risk factors. A randomized, controlled trial. Am J Physiol Endocrinol Metab 2007;293:E197–202.

96. Heilbronn LK, de Jonge L, Frisard MI, et al. Effect of 6-month calorie restriction on biomarkers of longevity, metabolic adaptation, and oxidative stress in overweight individuals: a randomized controlled trial. JAMA 2006;295:1539–48.

97. Larson-Meyer DE, Heilbronn LK, Redman LM, et al. Effect of calorie restriction with or without exercise on insulin sensitivity, beta-cell function, fat cell size, and ectopic lipid in overweight subjects. Diabetes Care 2006;29:1337–44.

98. Lefevre M, Redman LM, Heilbronn LK, et al. Caloric restriction alone and with exercise improves CVD risk in healthy nonobese individuals. Atherosclerosis 2009;203:206–13.

99. Lane MA, Ingram DK, Cutler RG, et al. Dietary restriction in nonhuman primates: progress report on the NIA study. Ann N Y Acad Sci 1992;673:36–45.

100. Lane MA, Ingram DK, Roth GS. Calorie restriction in nonhuman primates: effects on diabetes and cardiovascular disease risk. Toxicol Sci 1999;52:41–8.

101. Colman RJ, Roecker EB, Ramsey JJ, et al. The effect of dietary restriction on body composition in adult male and female rhesus macaques. Aging (Milano) 1998;10:83–92.

102. Verdery RB, Walford RL. Changes in plasma lipids and lipoproteins in humans during a 2-year period of dietary restriction in Biosphere 2. Arch Intern Med 1998;158:900–6.

103. Rezzi S, Martin FP, Shanmuganayagam D, et al. Metabolic shifts due to long-term caloric restriction revealed in nonhuman primates. Exp Gerontol 2009;44: 356–62.

Primary and Secondary Prevention of Cardiovascular Disease in Older Adults: A Status Report

Peter Kriekard, MD[a], S. Michael Gharacholou, MD[b,c],
Eric D. Peterson, MD, MPH[d,e,*]

KEYWORDS

- Prevention • Cardiovascular disease • Older adults
- Status • Risk factors

Cardiovascular disease (CVD), comprising heart disease, peripheral arterial disease, and stroke, remains the number one killer in the United States, accounting for 35% of all deaths in 2005. The population of older adults is disproportionately affected due to higher CVD prevalence. It is estimated that 80% of deaths from CVD occur in individuals older than 65 years and that 60% of all myocardial infarction (MI)-related deaths occur in individuals older than 75 years.[1] The large burden of CVD in older adults will be further magnified by the rapid growth of this segment of the population in the next several decades. Particularly striking will be the demographic of adults over the age of 85 years, which will represent 25% of the population aged 65 years and older by 2050 (**Fig. 1**).[2]

Although CVD remains the dominant mortal disease in developed societies, its ravages are not inevitable. Men and women who reach age 50 years without cardiac risk factors (including high blood pressure, hypercholesterolemia, smoking, and diabetes) have only a 5% and 8% lifetime risk, respectively, of ever developing CVD.[3]

---

[a] Department of Internal Medicine, Duke University Medical Center, Box 31181, Durham, NC 27710, USA
[b] Department of Internal Medicine, Division of Cardiology, Duke University Medical Center, Box 31262, Durham, NC, 27710, USA
[c] Department of Internal Medicine, Division of Geriatrics, Duke University Medical Center, Box 31262, Durham, NC, 27710, USA
[d] Department of Internal Medicine, Division of Cardiology, Durham, NC 27710, USA
[e] Duke Clinical Research Institute, 2400 Pratt Street, Durham, NC 27705, USA
* Corresponding author. Duke Clinical Research Institute, 2400 Pratt Street, Durham, NC 27705, USA.
E-mail address: peter016@mc.duke.edu (E.D. Peterson).

Clin Geriatr Med 25 (2009) 745–755
doi:10.1016/j.cger.2009.07.008
0749-0690/09/$ – see front matter © 2009 Elsevier Inc. All rights reserved.

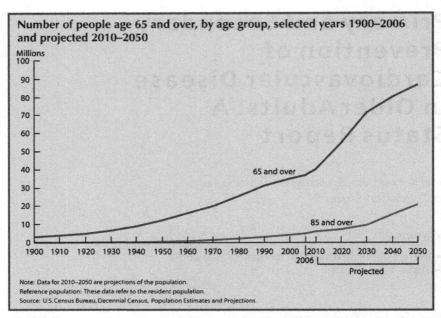

Fig. 1. Number of people aged 65 years and older and projected numbers up to 2050. *Data from* U.S. Census Bureau. US population projections. Available at: http://www.census.gov/population/www/projections/summarytables.html. Accessed April 8, 2009.

Greater emphasis on early recognition, patient awareness, and effective treatment of cardiovascular risk factors represents the critical prevention strategy that must take place among middle-aged and older adults to improve health outcomes in later life.

The multidimensional health status of older adults presents challenges and missed opportunities to further explore functional status, existing health conditions, and patient-centered care discussions, factors that may be impacting the evidence gap for prevention strategies. These issues may contribute to the therapeutic inertia that exists in implementing CVD prevention strategies in older adults. Current guidelines focus on preventing CVD through risk reduction for hypertension,[4] cholesterol management,[5] healthy lifestyle modification, and strong recommendations for extending preventative strategies to older adults. However, older adults remain an under-recognized and under-treated high-risk population. Therefore, the public health importance of translating guidelines into clinical practice among older patients must get moving; the inertia is costing too many lives!

This article reviews the practicality of implementing prevention strategies in older patients by highlighting results from recent clinical studies related to primary and secondary prevention of CVD in older adults. Many of these studies have demonstrated that greater absolute reductions in important cardiovascular events are achieved when implemented among older, higher-risk populations. Guideline recommendations for CVD risk factor modification are also reviewed with emphasis on issues pertaining to the older adult population.

RISK REDUCTION FOR PREVENTION IN OLDER ADULTS

Among older US adults participating in the National Health and Nutrition Examination Survey (NHANES) III (1988–1994 and 1999–2004), there was a 10% increase in the prevalence of hypertension among those aged 60 years and older, among both sexes, and among participants with CVD and diabetes mellitus.[6] The higher prevalence was accompanied by improvements in hypertension awareness, medication treatment, and control (systolic blood pressure <140 mm Hg and diastolic blood pressure <90 mm Hg) in participants 60 years of age or older between the 2 periods of the survey. However, although control was significantly better between study periods in those 60 to 69 years old, control was not significantly improved in those 70 years of age or older (n = 5503).[6] More recently, NHANES 2005 to 2006 revealed a similar disappointing trend in patients older than 60 years with hypertension, demonstrating that although 77% were receiving medical therapy for hypertension, only 58% were controlled (less than 140/90 mm Hg). The percentage at goal was lower in women (53%) than in men (64%).[6] Thus, more than one-third of patients older than 60 years on therapy for hypertension are being suboptimally treated. Furthermore, of all patients over the age of 60 years with hypertension, only 45% are at goal.[7] These observations suggest that, despite improved awareness and treatment of hypertension, optimizing therapy to recommended targets, particularly among older adults, will be essential to close the existing gap in primary and secondary prevention.

Hypertension

High blood pressure, or hypertension, is a known risk factor for CVD including stroke, coronary artery disease (CAD), heart failure (HF), peripheral artery disease (PAD), and renal failure. In addition to increasing prevalence, the pattern of blood pressure elevation changes with advancing age. Before the age of 50 years, most patients with hypertension have elevated diastolic blood pressure. However, after the age of 50 years systolic blood pressure rises and diastolic blood pressure falls, making isolated systolic hypertension (ISH) the predominate form in the elderly. In most cases ISH is caused by atherosclerosis and reduced compliance of the arterial system that progresses with age.[8] This is concerning as systolic hypertension is more important as a cardiovascular risk factor than elevated diastolic pressure in patients older than 50 years, and it is also more difficult to control.[9]

The cardiovascular benefits of treating hypertension, particularly systolic hypertension, among older adults have been well established. In the Systolic Hypertension in the Elderly Program (SHEP) trial, 4376 patients with a mean age of 72 years and mean systolic blood pressure of 170 mm Hg at baseline were randomized to antihypertensive treatment or placebo and assessed for cardiovascular events during an average follow-up period of 4.5 years. The study demonstrated a 36% reduction in stroke, a 27% reduction in coronary heart disease, and a 55% reduction in HF in the treatment group.[10] A 14-year follow-up from the SHEP trial was recently published and demonstrated a 14% relative risk reduction (adjusted RR = 0.86; 95% CI, 0.76–0.98; P = .026) of cardiovascular mortality in the chlorthalidone-based antihypertensive treatment arm, as well as a nonsignificant decrease in all-cause mortality and stroke mortality.[11]

Although treatment of blood pressure among older adults is beneficial, the value of treating hypertension in patients older than 80 years has been less certain. A retrospective cohort study of patients older than 80 years reported lower survival for those with systolic blood pressure less than 140 mm Hg.[12] In an attempt to further elucidate the risk of treating hypertension in the elderly, a subgroup meta-analysis of clinical trial participants older than 80 years treated with antihypertensive drugs was published in 1999. The Individual Data Analysis of Antihypertensive Drug Intervention Trials (INDI-ANA) group concluded that drug treatment was associated with a 36% reduction in stroke and a 22% reduction in cardiovascular events, but there was a trend toward a 6% increase in all-cause mortality (95% CI, −5% to +18%).[13]

The Hypertension in the Very Elderly Trial (HYVET) was a randomized, double-blind, placebo-controlled trial performed in 3845 patients aged 80 years or older with systolic blood pressure greater than 160 mm Hg. Patients were randomized to receive either indapamide, with or without the angiotensin-converting enzyme (ACE) inhibitor perindopril, or placebo. The target systolic blood pressure was less than 150/80 mm Hg. The trial was stopped early at approximately 2 years at the recommendation of the data safety and monitoring board as a result of benefit in all-cause mortality in the active drug arm. The study demonstrated that treatment with antihypertensive therapy resulted in a 30% relative reduction in the risk of stroke, a 64% relative reduction in the risk of HF, and a 21% relative reduction in the risk of death from any cause (95% CI, 4–35; P = .02).[14] This timely and pivotal clinical trial demonstrated that modest reduction in blood pressure among the elderly translated into improved clinical outcomes.

Even as the benefits of treating hypertension in the elderly are becoming more evident, the preferred class of drugs for this age group remains controversial. Three trials, Antihypertensive and Lipid-Lowering Treatment to Prevent Heart Attack Trial (ALLHAT), Losartan Intervention for Endpoint Reduction (LIFE) trial, and Avoiding Cardiovascular Events through Combination Therapy in Patients Living with Systolic Hypertension (ACCOMPLISH), compared different classes of antihypertensive medication, but did not specifically look at the elderly population. For example, ALLHAT, published in 2002, enrolled more than 33,000 patients over the age of 55 years, with a median age of 67 years.[15] The study concluded that a thiazide diuretic (chlorthalidone) was superior to a calcium-channel blocker (amlodipine), an a-blocker (doxazosin), and an ACE inhibitor (lisinopril) in preventing some cardiovascular outcomes, such as HF. A subgroup analysis of patients older than 65 years showed similar results with chlorthalidone being noninferior to amlodipine (RR = 0.95; 95% CI, 0.89–1.01), and superior to lisinopril (RR = 0.88; 95% CI, 0.83–0.94) with respect to combined cardiovascular outcomes.[15]

The LIFE study, also published in 2002, enrolled more than 9000 patients aged 55 to 80 years. This study found that losartan, an angiotensin-II receptor antagonist, prevented more cardiovascular events and deaths than the β blocker atenolol (HR = 0.87; 95% CI, 0.77–0.98).[16] These results argue against the use of β blockers as first-line treatment of primary hypertension in older adults; however, the average age of study participants was only 67 years.

More recently, the ACCOMPLISH trial found that the combination of an ACE inhibitor plus a dihydropyridine calcium-channel blocker (benazepril-amlodipine) was superior to the combination of an ACE inhibitor plus a thiazide diuretic (benazepril-hydrochlorothiazide). The trial enrolled more than 11,500 patients aged 65 years or older with a mean age of 68 years. Although blood pressure reduction was similar in the 2 groups, the composite end point of death from cardiovascular causes and incident cardiovascular events was lower in the benazepril-amlodipine group (HR = 0.80; 95% CI, 0.72–0.90).[17]

The optimal classes of antihypertensive medications in the elderly population remain unclear, as efforts to find safe and effective therapies, including those which have demonstrable benefits on health outcomes, remain an active area of ongoing research. The Blood Pressure Lowering Treatment Trialist Collaboration (BPLTTC) sought to answer the question of class effect on blood pressure lowering and prevention of cardiovascular events through a meta-analysis of randomized controlled trials. The investigators found that the benefits of different antihypertensive drug classes were similar across age groups, including those older than 65 years, but effects in persons older than 80 years were not evaluated. Nonetheless, all major randomized trials with large numbers of elderly patients included either a diuretic or calcium-channel blocker as first-line therapy.[18] This is in agreement with the most recent Joint National Committee on Prevention, Detection, Evaluation, and Treatment of High Blood Pressure (JNC-7) guidelines. Current recommendations are to initiate drug therapy with a thiazide diuretic in most patients with hypertension, in the absence of certain comorbid conditions. For patients with blood pressures greater than 20/10 mm Hg above goal, initial therapy should include 2 medications, 1 of which should be a thiazide diuretic. Older persons are at greater risk for postural symptoms and adverse drug reactions; therefore, low doses should be used initially with gradual titration before adding a second agent.[4]

Hyperlipidemia

Hyperlipidemia, especially elevated low-density lipoprotein (LDL), is a major risk factor for CVD. In 2006, almost 100 million adults in the United States had hyperlipidemia (total cholesterol >200 mg/dL), representing almost 45% of the population. In addition, 16% of adults had serum total cholesterol levels of 240 mg/dL or greater.[19]

The association between LDL reduction (specifically, the use of HMG CoA reductase inhibitors [statins] to achieve this reduction) and lower cardiovascular event rates has been studied extensively. However, early primary prevention trials excluded the very elderly. For example, the West of Scotland Coronary Prevention Study (WOSCOPS) and the Anglo-Scandinavian Cardiac Outcomes Trial – Lipid Lowering Arm (ASCOT-LLA) either excluded patients older than 65 years (WOSCOPS) or excluded patients older than 80 years (ASCOT-LLA).[20,21] Therefore, although there is ample evidence for treating younger adults with lipid-lowering drugs, the evidence for treating the very old is sparse.[22]

The Scandinavian Simvastatin Survival Study (4S) was the first large secondary prevention trial to demonstrate beneficial effects of lipid-lowering therapy among patients 65 to 70 years of age. In this study, simvastatin reduced the risk of all-cause mortality and major coronary events by more than 30% in older adults. Moreover, compared with patients less than 65 years of age, older patients had greater absolute risk reductions in adverse outcomes.[23,24] The Prospective Study of Pravastatin in the Elderly at Risk (PROSPER) trial enrolled 5804 patients aged 70 to 82 years with a history of vascular disease (secondary prevention) or cardiovascular risk factors (primary prevention). Patients were randomized to receive pravastatin 40 mg daily versus placebo. The treatment group showed a 15% relative risk reduction and a 2.1% absolute risk reduction in the primary end point (coronary heart disease death, nonfatal MI, or stroke) during the treatment duration of 3 years (number needed to treat [NNT] to prevent 1 event = 48). There was a 25% reduction of transient ischemic attacks in the treatment group that did not reach significance. There was, however, no difference in all-cause mortality between treatment assignments. In the primary prevention group (ie, without previous vascular disease), which had 3239 patients (56% of study population), there was no significant reduction in the composite end point (HR = 0.94; 95% CI, 0.77–1.15).[25]

More recently, the Justification for the Use of Statins in Prevention: an Intervention Trial Evaluating Rosuvastatin (JUPITER) study examined statin use in patients with LDL-cholesterol levels less than 130 mg/dL but with high-sensitivity C-reactive protein (CRP) levels greater than or equal to 2.0 mg/L. More than 17,000 men aged 50 years or older and women aged 60 years or older were randomized to rosuvastatin 20 mg daily or placebo. At 1.9 years follow-up, the rosuvastatin group showed a 44% decrease in the combined primary end point (MI, stroke, arterial revascularization, hospitalization for unstable angina [UA] or death from cardiovascular causes; HR = 0.56; 95% CI, 0.46–0.69).[26] Extrapolating these data to the US population, an additional 3.9 million men over the age of 50 years and 2.6 million women over the age of 60 years could potentially be candidates for statin therapy.[27]

In the Heart Protection Study, more than 20,000 patients up to 80 years old with known coronary disease, vascular disease, or diabetes were enrolled. Patients were randomized to receive simvastatin 40 mg daily or placebo. The treatment group showed a 27% reduction in coronary events and a 13% reduction in all-cause mortality. In the subgroup of patients older than 75 years, simvastatin was associated with a 28% relative risk reduction and 9% absolute risk reduction in major vascular events (23.1% versus 32.3%; NNT to prevent 1 event = 9; P = .0002). The magnitude of benefit in the older subgroup was similar to that seen in younger patients.[28] Among the 2565 patients in the secondary prevention cohort of PROSPER, treatment with pravastatin 40 mg daily was associated with a 22% relative risk reduction and 4.3% absolute risk reduction in cardiovascular events (NNT to prevent 1 event = 23).[25]

In a post-hoc analysis from the Pravastatin or Atorvastatin Evaluation and Infection Therapy Thrombolysis in Myocardial Infarction (PROVE IT-TIMI 22) trial, the benefits of statins were evaluated in 634 patients aged 70 years or older who achieved an LDL-C level of less than 70 mg/dL. Compared with older patients who did not achieve an LDL-C level of less than 70 mg/dL, those who did experienced a 40% relative risk reduction and an 8% absolute risk reduction in the composite end point of death, MI, or hospitalization for UA (13.5% versus 21.5%; P = .008).[29] Compared with patients less than 70 years of age who achieved an LDL-cholesterol level of less than 70 mg/dL, the net benefit was greater among the elderly, as reflected in the NNT to prevent 1 event, which was 12.5 in older patients versus 43.5 in younger patients.

Current guidelines developed by the National Cholesterol Education Program (NCEP) Adult Treatment Panel (ATP-III) for the treatment of hyperlipidemia provide similar recommendations for younger and older adults. Lifestyle changes including diet, weight loss, and exercise are the preferred initial management. Lipid-lowering drugs, particularly statins, may be considered in older patients who are at high risk and whose LDL-cholesterol levels remain higher than recommended targets despite therapeutic lifestyle changes. In patients with known CAD or risk equivalents, the guidelines advocate LDL lowering to less than 100 mg/dL regardless of age, with the option of treating to less than 70 mg/dL in high-risk patients, such as those with CAD and diabetes.[5] The numbers of preventable events at 2 years resulting from achieving the NCEP optional goal of 70 mg/dL with statins by age group are shown in **Table 1**.[29]

OTHER SECONDARY PREVENTION STRATEGIES
Antiplatelet Therapy

Antiplatelet therapy has repeatedly been shown to benefit patients with CVD, including the elderly. The Antiplatelet Trialists' Collaboration, published in 1994, examined 145 randomized trials of antiplatelet therapy, predominantly aspirin. More than 14,000 patients with CAD aged 65 years or older were included in the analysis. The benefits of aspirin in reducing death, recurrent MI, and stroke were unequivocal (P<.00001). The absolute benefit of aspirin use was greater in patients older than 65 years due to the higher baseline risk in this age group.[30]

More recently, 3 major trials have evaluated clopidogrel in patients with CAD. The Clopidogrel versus Aspirin in Patients at Risk of Ischemic Events (CAPRIE) trial found that compared with aspirin, clopidogrel was associated with a modest 0.5% annual risk reduction for stroke, MI, and cardiovascular death. The CAPRIE trial did not exclude patients based on age, but the mean age was 62 years and subgroup analysis

Table 1
Expected number of preventable[a] cardiovascular events at 2 years in patients achieving LDL-C less than 70 mg/dL at 30 days for every 1000 patients treated by age

	Age Group	
Cardiovascular Events	<70 years old	≥70 years old
Death	5	43
MI	12	58
UA requiring hospitalization	9	14
Coronary revascularization after 30 days	15	43
Stroke	5	1
Death, MI, or UA requiring rehospitalization	23	80
Death, MI, UA requiring rehospitalization, or stroke	29	75

The analysis considers only patients alive at day 30 who reach the LDL-C goal, and assesses subsequent events after day 30.
[a] First event only.
Data from Ray KK, Bach RG, Cannon CP, et al. Benefits of achieving the NCEP optional LDL-C goal among elderly patients with ACS. Eur Heart J 2006; 27:2310–6.

by age was not reported.[31] The Clopidogrel in Unstable Angina to Prevent Recurrent Events (CURE) trial found that patients with recent UA/non–ST-elevation MI treated with clopidogrel plus aspirin had a 2.1% absolute risk reduction in death, MI, or stroke (RR = 0.80; 95% CI, 0.72–0.90) compared with aspirin alone.[32,33] The absolute risk reduction was similar in patients older than 65 years (2.0%) relative to younger patients (2.2%). There was a higher risk of bleeding with high-dose aspirin (160–325 mg) versus low-dose aspirin (75–100 mg) when combined with clopidogrel in the trial.[33]

The Clopidogrel for High Atherothrombotic Risk and Ischemic Stabilization, Management, and Avoidance (CHARISMA) trial examined the addition of clopidogrel to aspirin in patients with stable CAD. The investigators concluded that clopidogrel added to aspirin was not significantly more effective than aspirin alone in reducing MI, stroke, or death from CVD in patients with stable CAD. The CHARISMA trial did not exclude older individuals and enrolled patients up to 95 years of age, with a mean age of 64 years.[34] These studies indicate that the benefits of antiplatelet therapy, including treatment with clopidogrel, extend to the elderly population, but at a cost of an increased risk of bleeding. Daily low-dose aspirin is recommended for all elderly patients with chronic CAD in the absence of contraindications. The addition of clopidogrel to aspirin is indicated in patients with acute coronary syndromes, regardless of whether they are treated medically or with revascularization, but more research is needed to clarify the optimal duration of dual antiplatelet treatment, especially among older adults.

Other Medications in Secondary Prevention

ACE inhibitors and β blockers are recommended for patients with HF or CAD, including the elderly. In the Heart Outcomes Prevention Evaluation (HOPE) trial, patients older than 55 years with vascular disease (80% with CAD) or diabetes plus an additional risk factor were randomized to receive ramipril 10 mg daily or placebo. Treatment with an ACE inhibitor in this high-risk group resulted in a 3.8% absolute risk reduction for the composite outcome of MI, stroke, or cardiovascular death (RR = 0.78; 95% CI, 0.70–0.86).[35]

Therapy with β blockers in the elderly has increased risk due to more prevalent conduction system disease. Nonetheless, current data support their use in several situations. Following acute MI, elderly patients derive similar or greater survival benefit from β blockers compared with younger patients. Elderly patients with HF and CAD also benefit from β blocker therapy added to an ACE inhibitor. Three trials, the Metoprolol CR/XL Randomized Intervention Trial in CHF (MERIT-HF), Carvedilol Prospective Randomized Cumulative Survival Study (COPERNICUS), and Carvedilol Post-Infarct Survival Control in LV Dysfunction (CAPRICORN) study all showed that β blockers reduced mortality.[36–38] Based on these results, elderly patients with HF and reduced left ventricular systolic function should be treated with an ACE inhibitor and β blocker for secondary prevention. Careful monitoring of renal function, potassium, and orthostasis is necessary to reduce the risk of adverse events.

Smoking Cessation

The association of smoking with CVD, including the relationship between smoking and adverse vascular events and death, is well established. From a prevention standpoint, abstinence remains the best method to avoid the adverse cardiovascular effects of smoking. Quitting smoking has an early impact on mortality risk, reducing mortality by as much as 50% in those with prior MI, with most of this mortality benefit occurring in the first year.[39] In patients over the age of 70 years with CAD participating in the Coronary Artery Surgery Study (CASS) registry, morbidity and mortality rates were reduced among those who stopped smoking, with risk reductions similar to those seen among younger patients.[40] Intervention programs that use behavioral approaches, physician counseling, close clinical follow-up, and pharmacologic therapy are recommended to help older adults who are tobacco dependent.[41]

SUMMARY

Although older adults have often been excluded from clinical trials, either explicitly or implicitly, results from primary and secondary prevention studies have demonstrated that older patients derive similar or greater benefits from preventive therapies compared with younger patients. These studies support guideline recommendations to include older patients in most risk reduction and prevention strategies. Unfortunately, there is evidence of a "disconnect" between what is known about the benefits of prevention and the application of preventive measures in real-world practice, particularly in elderly patients. This therapeutic inertia is exemplified by, for example, blood pressure control rates remaining well below the target for Healthy People 2010.[42]

Some of the treatment gap in the elderly may be attributed to heightened vulnerability to adverse drug reactions, increased comorbidity, reduced access to health care, socioeconomic issues, cognitive status, and hearing or visual impairment. These are important patient variables that present challenges to health care providers when implementing prevention strategies in older adults. As a result, many high-risk elderly patients are managed more conservatively than younger individuals. Addressing these issues may require greater integration of key components within health care (nursing, social services, telemedicine, rehabilitation, and pharmacists), as well as support from policy makers to revamp the current approach to prevention so that equitable and effective therapies are provided to our increasingly aging society. The solution to therapeutic inertia will require substantial interdisciplinary efforts to move prevention to the forefront of health care as a critical element for improving public health for people of all ages.

REFERENCES

1. American Heart Association. Heart disease and stroke statistics–2009 update. Dallas (TX): American Heart Association; 2009.
2. U.S. Census Bureau. US population projections. Available at: http://www.census.gov/population/www/projections/summarytables.html. Accessed April 8, 2009.
3. Lloyd-Jones DM, Leip EP, Larson MG, et al. Prediction of lifetime risk for cardiovascular disease by risk factor burden at 50 years of age. Circulation 2006;113: 791–8.
4. Chobanian AV, Bakris GL, Black HR, et al. The seventh report of the Joint National Committee on Prevention, Detection, Evaluation, and Treatment of High Blood Pressure: the JNC 7 report. JAMA 2003;289:2560–72.
5. Executive summary of the third report of the National Cholesterol Education Program (NCEP) expert panel on detection, evaluation, and treatment of high blood cholesterol in adults (ATP III). JAMA 2001;285:2486–97.
6. Ostchega Y, Dillon CF, Hughes JP, et al. Trends in hypertension prevalence, awareness, treatment, and control in older U.S. adults: data from the National Health and Nutrition Examination Survey 1988 to 2004. J Am Geriatr Soc 2007; 55:1056–65.
7. Ostchega Y, Toon SS, Hughes J, et al. Hypertension awareness, treatment, and control – continued disparities in adults: United States, 2005–2006. NCHS data brief no. Hyattsville (MD): National Center for Health Statistics; 2008.
8. Chobanian AV. Isolated systolic hypertension in the elderly. N Engl J Med 2007; 357:789–96.
9. Izzo JL Jr, Levy D, Black HR. Clinical advisory statement. Importance of systolic blood pressure in older Americans. Hypertension 2000;35:1021–4.
10. Prevention of stroke by antihypertensive drug treatment in older persons with isolated systolic hypertension: final results of the Systolic Hypertension in the Elderly Program (SHEP). SHEP Cooperative Research Group. JAMA 1991; 265:3255–64.
11. Patel AP, Kostis JB, Wilson AC, et al. Long-term fatal outcomes in subjects with stroke or transient ischemic attack: fourteen-year follow-up of the Systolic Hypertension in the Elderly Program (SHEP). Stroke 2008;39:1084–9.
12. Oates DJ, Berlowitz DR, Glickman ME, et al. Blood pressure and survival in the oldest old. J Am Geriatr Soc 2007;55:383–8.
13. Gueyffier F, Bulpitt C, Boissel JP, et al. Antihypertensive drugs in very old people: a subgroup meta-analysis of randomized controlled trials (INDIANA). Lancet 1999;353:793–6.
14. Beckett NS, Peters R, Fletcher AE, et al. Treatment of hypertension in patients 80 years of age or older (HYVET). N Engl J Med 2008;358:1887–98.
15. Major outcomes in high-risk hypertensive patients randomized to angiotensin-converting enzyme inhibitor or calcium channel blocker vs diuretic: the Antihypertensive and Lipid-Lowering Treatment to Prevent Heart Attack Trial (ALLHAT). ALLHAT Officers and Coordinators for the ALLHAT Collaborative Research Group. JAMA 2002;288:2981–97.
16. Dahlof B, Devereux RB, Kjeldsen SE, et al. Cardiovascular morbidity and mortality in the Losartan Intervention For Endpoint reduction in hypertension study (LIFE): a randomised trial against atenolol. Lancet 2002;359:995–1003.
17. Jamerson K, Weber MA, Bakris GL, et al. Benazepril plus amlodipine or hydrocholorthiazide for hypertension in high-risk patients. N Engl J Med 2008;359: 2417–28.

18. Blood Pressure Lowering Treatment Trialists' Collaboration. Effects of different regimens to lower blood pressure on major cardiovascular events in older and younger adults: meta-analysis of randomized trials. BMJ 2008;336:1121–3.

19. Schober SE, Carroll MD, Lacher DA, et al. High serum total cholesterol – an indicator of monitoring cholesterol lowering efforts; U.S. adults, 2005–2006. NCHS data brief no 2. Hyattsville (MD): National Center for Health Statistics; 2007.

20. Shepherd J, Cobbe S, Ford I, et al. Prevention of coronary heart disease with pravastatin in men with hypercholesterolemia. West of Scotland Coronary Prevention Study Group (WOSCOPS). N Engl J Med 1995;333:1301–7.

21. Sever PS, Dahlof B, Poulter NR, et al. Prevention of coronary and stroke events with atorvastatin in hypertensive patients who have average or lower-than-average cholesterol concentrations, in the Anglo-Scandinavian Cardiac Outcomes Trial–Lipid Lowering Arm (ASCOT-LLA): a multicentre randomised controlled trial. Lancet 2003;361:1149–58.

22. Weverling-Rijnsburger AW, Blauw GJ, Lagaay AM, et al. Total cholesterol and risk of mortality in the oldest old. Lancet 1997;350:1119–23.

23. Scandinavian Simvastatin Survival Study Group. Randomised trial of cholesterol lowering in 4444 patients with coronary heart disease: the Scandinavian Simvastatin Survival Study (4S). Lancet 1994;344:1383–9.

24. Miettinen TA, Pyorala K, Olsson AG, et al. Cholesterol-lowering therapy in women and elderly patients with myocardial infarction or angina pectoris: findings from the Scandinavian Simvastatin Survival Study (4S). Circulation 1997;96:4211–8.

25. Shepherd J, Blauw GJ, Murphy MB, et al. PROSPER Study Group. Pravastatin in elderly individuals at risk of vascular disease (PROSPER): a randomized trial. Lancet 2002;360:1623–30.

26. Ridker PM, Danielson M, Fonseca F, et al. JUPITER Study Group. Rosuvastatin to prevent vascular events in men and women with elevated C-reactive protein. N Engl J Med 2008;359:2195–207.

27. Michos ED, Blumenthal RS. Prevalence of low low-density lipoprotein cholesterol with elevated high sensitivity C-reactive protein in the US. J Am Coll Cardiol 2009; 53:931–5.

28. Heart Protection Study (HPS) Collaborative Group. MRC/BHF Heart Protection Study of cholesterol lowering with simvastatin in 20,536 high-risk individuals: a randomized placebo-controlled trial. Lancet 2002;360:7–22.

29. Ray KK, Bach RG, Cannon CP, et al. Benefits of achieving the NCEP optional LDL-C goal among elderly patients with ACS. Eur Heart J 2006;27:2310–6.

30. Antiplatelet Trialists' Collaboration. Collaborative overview of randomised trials of antiplatelet therapy–I: Prevention of death, myocardial infarction, and stroke by prolonged antiplatelet therapy in various categories of patients. BMJ 1994;308: 81–106.

31. A randomised, blinded, trial of clopidogrel versus aspirin in patients at risk of ischaemic events. CAPRIE Steering Committee. Lancet 1996;348:1329–39.

32. Peters RJ, Mehta SR, Fox KAA, et al. Effects of aspirin dose when used alone or in combination with clopidogrel in patients with acute coronary syndromes: observations from the Clopidogrel in Unstable Angina to Prevent Recurrent Events (CURE) study. Circulation 2003;108:1682–7.

33. Yusuf S, Zhao F, Mehta SR, et al. Effects of clopidogrel in addition to aspirin in patients with acute coronary syndromes without ST-segment elevation. N Engl J Med 2001;345(7):494–502.

34. Bhatt DL, Fox KAA, Hacke W, et al. Clopidogrel and aspirin versus aspirin alone for the prevention of atherothrombotic events. N Engl J Med 2006;354:1706–17.

35. Yusuf S, Sleight P, Pogue J, et al. Effects of an angiotensin-converting-enzyme inhibitor, ramipril, on cardiovascular events in high risk patients. The Heart Outcomes Prevention Evaluation (HOPE) Study Investigators. N Engl J Med 2000;342:145–53.

36. Hjalmarson A, Goldstein S, Fagerberg B, et al. Effects of controlled-release metoprolol on total mortality, hospitalizations, and well-being in patients with heart failure. The Metoprolol CR/XL Randomized Intervention Trial in congestive heart failure (MERIT-HF). JAMA 2000;283:1295–302.

37. Packer M, Fowler MB, Roecker EL, et al. Effect of carvedilol on the morbidity of patients with severe chronic heart failure: results of the Carvedilol Prospective Randomized Cumulative Survival (COPERNICUS) study. Circulation 2002;106: 2194–9.

38. Effect of carvedilol on outcome after myocardial infarction in patients with left-ventricular dysfunction: the CAPRICORN randomised trial. The CAPRICORN Investigators. Lancet 2001;357:1385–90.

39. Sparrow D, Dawber T, Colton T. The influence of cigarette smoking on prognosis after first myocardial infarction. J Chronic Dis 1978;31:415–32.

40. Hermanson B, Omenn GS, Kronmal RA, et al. Beneficial six-year outcome of smoking cessation in older men and women with coronary artery disease: results from the CASS registry. N Engl J Med 1988;319:1365–9.

41. Williams MA, Flegg JL, Ades PA, et al. Secondary prevention of coronary heart disease in the elderly (with emphasis on patients ≥ 75 years of age). Circulation 2002;105:1735–43.

42. U.S. Department of Health and Human Services. Health People 2010: Understanding and Improving Health. 2nd edition. Washington, DC: US Government Printing Office. November 2000.

Index

Note: Page numbers of article titles are in **boldface** type.

A

ACCOMPLISH trial, 748
ACCORD trial, 613
ACE inhibitors, in vascular diseases, 751–752
ADVANCE trial, 613
Aging, cardiovascular physiology of, 678
    heart disease and, 733–734
    noncardiovascular physiology of, 678–680
    physiology of, 678
Air Force/Texas Coronary Atherosclerosis Prevention Study, 597
ALLHAT trial, 748
Antihypertensice therapy, effect on cardiovascular events, 581–582
Antihypertensive drug therapy, adverse effects of, 582–584
    in elderly, 581–582
    in persons with associated medical conditions, 584–585
Antiplatelat therapy, in cardiovascular disease, 750–751
Antiplatelet agents, in type 2 diabetes, 630, 631–632
Aortic stenosis, 571
Aortic valve sclerosis, 570–571
Aortic valve thickening and calcification, 570–571
Apoptosis, in age-related heart remodeling, 720
Arrhythmias, in cardiovascular disease, 571–572
ASCOT-LLA trial, 617
Atrial fibrillation, incidence of, 572
    prevalence of, 572
Autophagy, importance for cardiomyocyte health and survival, 721

B

Balance and stability, physical activity and, 685
Beta blockers, in vascular diseases, 751, 752
    precautions in use of, 583
Bile acid sequestrants, in hyperlipidemia, 602
Blood pressure, physical activity and, 682–683
Blood pressure control, in type 2 diabetes, 624–627, 635
Blood Pressure Lowering Treatment Tialist Collaboration (BPLTTC), 748–749
Body composition, effect of resistance training on, 706–707
Body fat, increases with age, 679
    physical activity and, 681
Body mass index, abdominal fat, and intentional weight loss, outcomes of, 653

United States Postal Service

Statement of Ownership, Management, and Circulation
(All Periodicals Publications Except Requester Publications)

1. Publication Title
Clinics in Geriatric Medicine

2. Publication Number
0 0 0 - 7 0 4

3. Filing Date
9/15/09

4. Issue Frequency
Feb, May, Aug, Nov

5. Number of Issues Published Annually
4

6. Annual Subscription Price
$208.00

7. Complete Mailing Address of Known Office of Publication (Not printer) (Street, city, county, state, and ZIP+4®)
Elsevier Inc.
360 Park Avenue South
New York, NY 10010-1710

Contact Person
Stephen Bushing

Telephone (Include area code)
215-239-3688

8. Complete Mailing Address of Headquarters or General Business Office of Publisher (Not printer)
Elsevier Inc., 360 Park Avenue South, New York, NY 10010-1710

9. Full Names and Complete Mailing Addresses of Publisher, Editor, and Managing Editor (Do not leave blank)

Publisher (Name and complete mailing address)
John Schrefer, Elsevier, Inc., 1600 John F. Kennedy Blvd. Suite 1800, Philadelphia, PA 19103-2899

Editor (Name and complete mailing address)
Yonah Korngold, Elsevier, Inc., 1600 John F. Kennedy Blvd. Suite 1800, Philadelphia, PA 19103-2899

Managing Editor (Name and complete mailing address)
Catherine Bewick, Elsevier, Inc., 1600 John F. Kennedy Blvd. Suite 1800, Philadelphia, PA 19103-2899

10. Owner (Do not leave blank. If the publication is owned by a corporation, give the name and address of the corporation immediately followed by the names and addresses of all stockholders owning or holding 1 percent or more of the total amount of stock. If not owned by a corporation, give the names and addresses of the individual owners. If owned by a partnership or other unincorporated firm, give its name and address as well as those of each individual owner. If the publication is published by a nonprofit organization, give its name and address.)

Full Name	Complete Mailing Address
Wholly owned subsidiary of	4520 East-West Highway
Reed/Elsevier, US holdings	Bethesda, MD 20814

11. Known Bondholders, Mortgagees, and Other Security Holders Owning or Holding 1 Percent or More of Total Amount of Bonds, Mortgages, or Other Securities. If none, check box ☐ None

Full Name	Complete Mailing Address
N/A	

12. Tax Status (For completion by nonprofit organizations authorized to mail at nonprofit rates) (Check one)
The purpose, function, and nonprofit status of this organization and the exempt status for federal income tax purposes:
☐ Has Not Changed During Preceding 12 Months
☐ Has Changed During Preceding 12 Months (Publisher must submit explanation of change with this statement)

PS Form 3526, September 2007 (Page 1 of 3 (Instructions Page 3)) PSN 7530-01-000-9931 PRIVACY NOTICE: See our Privacy policy in www.usps.com

---

13. Publication Title
Clinics in Geriatric Medicine

14. Issue Date for Circulation Data Below
May 2009

15. Extent and Nature of Circulation		Average No. Copies Each Issue During Preceding 12 Months	No. Copies of Single Issue Published Nearest to Filing Date
a. Total Number of Copies (Net press run)		1520	1381
b. Paid Circulation (By Mail and Outside the Mail)	(1) Mailed Outside-County Paid Subscriptions Stated on PS Form 3541 (Include paid distribution above nominal rate, advertiser's proof copies, and exchange copies)	683	605
	(2) Mailed In-County Paid Subscriptions Stated on PS Form 3541 (Include paid distribution above nominal rate, advertiser's proof copies, and exchange copies)		
	(3) Paid Distribution Outside the Mails Including Sales Through Dealers and Carriers, Street Vendors, Counter Sales, and Other Paid Distribution Outside USPS®	271	235
	(4) Paid Distribution by Other Classes Mailed Through the USPS (e.g. First-Class Mail®)		
c. Total Paid Distribution (Sum of 15b (1), (2), (3), and (4)) ►		954	840
d. Free or Nominal Rate Distribution (By Mail and Outside the Mail)	(1) Free or Nominal Rate Outside-County Copies Included on PS Form 3541	52	70
	(2) Free or Nominal Rate In-County Copies Included on PS Form 3541		
	(3) Free or Nominal Rate Copies Mailed at Other Classes Through the USPS (e.g. First-Class Mail)		
	(4) Free or Nominal Rate Distribution Outside the Mail (Carriers or other means)		
e. Total Free or Nominal Rate Distribution (Sum of 15d (1), (2), (3) and (4)) ►		52	70
f. Total Distribution (Sum of 15c and 15e) ►		1006	910
g. Copies not Distributed (See instructions to publishers #4 (page #3)) ►		514	471
h. Total (Sum of 15f and g) ►		1520	1381
i. Percent Paid (15c divided by 15f times 100) ►		94.83%	92.31%

16. Publication of Statement of Ownership
☐ If the publication is a general publication, publication of this statement is required. Will be printed in the **November 2009** issue of this publication. ☐ Publication not required

17. Signature and Title of Editor, Publisher, Business Manager, or Owner

Stephen R Bushing
Stephen R Bushing – Subscription Services Coordinator

Date
September 15, 2009

I certify that all information furnished on this form is true and complete. I understand that anyone who furnishes false or misleading information on this form or who omits material or information requested on the form may be subject to criminal sanctions (including fines and imprisonment) and/or civil sanctions (including civil penalties).

PS Form 3526, September 2007 (Page 2 of 3)

Moving?

Make sure your subscription moves with you!

To notify us of your new address, find your **Clinics Account Number** (located on your mailing label above your name), and contact customer service at:

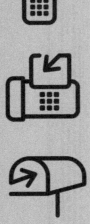

Email: journalscustomerservice-usa@elsevier.com

800-654-2452 (subscribers in the U.S. & Canada)
314-447-8871 (subscribers outside of the U.S. & Canada)

Fax number: 314-447-8029

Elsevier Health Sciences Division
Subscription Customer Service
3251 Riverport Lane
Maryland Heights, MO 63043

Printed in the United States
By Bookmasters